IAP Clinical Examination in
PEDIATRICS

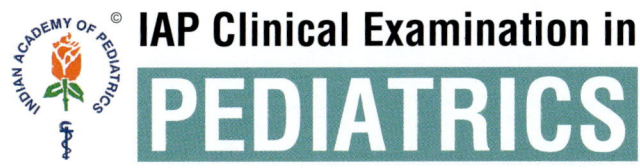

IAP Clinical Examination in PEDIATRICS

Editor

Baldev Prajapati
MD DPed FIAP MNAMS
Professor and Head
Department of Pediatrics
GCS Medical College, Hospital and
Research Center, Ahmedabad
Aakanksha Children Hospital and
Postgraduate Institute
Ahmedabad, Gujarat, India

Forewords

Digant D Shastri
Santosh T Soans
Bakul Jayant Parekh

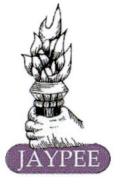

JAYPEE BROTHERS MEDICAL PUBLISHERS
The Health Sciences Publisher
New Delhi | London

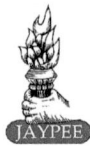 **Jaypee Brothers Medical Publishers (P) Ltd.**

Headquarters
Jaypee Brothers Medical Publishers (P) Ltd
EMCA House, 23/23-B
Ansari Road, Daryaganj
New Delhi 110 002, India
Landline: +91-11-23272143, +91-11-23272703
+91-11-23282021, +91-11-23245672
Email: jaypee@jaypeebrothers.com

Corporate Office
Jaypee Brothers Medical Publishers (P) Ltd
4838/24, Ansari Road, Daryaganj
New Delhi 110 002, India
Phone: +91-11-43574357
Fax: +91-11-43574314
Email: jaypee@jaypeebrothers.com

Overseas Office
J.P. Medical Ltd
83 Victoria Street, London
SW1H 0HW (UK)
Phone: +44 20 3170 8910
Fax: +44 (0)20 3008 6180
Email: info@jpmedpub.com

Website: www.jaypeebrothers.com
Website: www.jaypeedigital.com

© 2021, Indian Academy of Pediatrics

The views and opinions expressed in this book are solely those of the original contributor(s)/author(s) and do not necessarily represent those of editor(s) of the book.

All rights reserved. No part of this publication may be reproduced, stored or transmitted in any form or by any means, electronic, mechanical, photocopying, recording or otherwise, without the prior permission in writing of the publishers.

All brand names and product names used in this book are trade names, service marks, trademarks or registered trademarks of their respective owners. The publisher is not associated with any product or vendor mentioned in this book.

Medical knowledge and practice change constantly. This book is designed to provide accurate, authoritative information about the subject matter in question. However, readers are advised to check the most current information available on procedures included and check information from the manufacturer of each product to be administered, to verify the recommended dose, formula, method and duration of administration, adverse effects and contraindications. It is the responsibility of the practitioner to take all appropriate safety precautions. Neither the publisher nor the author(s)/editor(s) assume any liability for any injury and/or damage to persons or property arising from or related to use of material in this book.

This book is sold on the understanding that the publisher is not engaged in providing professional medical services. If such advice or services are required, the services of a competent medical professional should be sought.

Every effort has been made where necessary to contact holders of copyright to obtain permission to reproduce copyright material. If any have been inadvertently overlooked, the publisher will be pleased to make the necessary arrangements at the first opportunity. The **CD/DVD-ROM** (if any) provided in the sealed envelope with this book is complimentary and free of cost. **Not meant for sale.**

Inquiries for bulk sales may be solicited at: jaypee@jaypeebrothers.com

IAP Clinical Examination in Pediatrics

First Edition: 2021
Reprint: **2023**
ISBN: 978-93-89776-37-9

Printed at: Samrat Offset Pvt. Ltd.

Contributors

Aloka Santosh Hedau
DNB FICO FPOS
Pediatric Ophthalmologist and
Squint Specialist
Dr Aloka's Eye Care
Hyderabad, Telangana, India

Anand Rao
MD Fellowship Pediatric Rheumatology
Director
Pediatric Rheumatology Clinic
Manipal Hospital, Bengaluru
Indira Gandhi Institute of
Child Health
Bengaluru, Karnataka, India

Archana Kadam MD (Ped) DNB
Developmental Pediatrician
KEM Hospital and
Jehangir Hospital
Pune, Maharashtra, India

Bakulesh Chauhan MD PGDAP
Professor
Department of Pediatrics
KG Patel Children Hospital
Vadodara, Gujarat, India

Baldev Prajapati
MD DPed FIAP MNAMS
Professor and Head
Department of Pediatrics
GCS Medical College, Hospital and
Research Center, Ahmedabad
Aakanksha Children Hospital and
Postgraduate Institute
Ahmedabad, Gujarat, India

Chandrika S Bhat
MBBS MD RCPCH Fellowship Pediatric Rheumatology
Consultant Pediatric and
Rheumatologist
Department of Rheumatology
Rainbow Children's Hospital
Bengaluru, Karnataka, India

MMA Faridi MD DCH MAMS FIAP FNNF
Principal, Dean and Professor
Department of Pediatrics
Era's Medical College
Lucknow, Uttar Pradesh, India

Mukund Vaghela
MBBS MS (Otolaryngology)
Consultant ENT Surgeon
Kundan ENT Hospital
Ahmedabad, Gujarat, India

R Madhu MD (Dermatologist) DCH
Associate Professor
Department of Dermatology
Madras Medical College
Chennai, Tamil Nadu, India

Rajal Prajapati MD DPed
Former Professor
Department of Pediatrics
AMC MET Medical College
VS General Hospital
Ahmedabad, Gujarat, India

Rhishikesh Thakre
DM (Neo) MD DNB DCH FCPS FIAP
Director
Neo Clinic and Hospital
Aurangabad, Maharashtra, India

Satish Tiwari MD (Pediatrics) LLB FIAP
Professor
Department of Pediatrics
Dr PDM Medical College
Amravati, Maharashtra, India

Sudhir Mishra MD (Pediatrics)
Chief Consultant and Head
Tata Main Hospital and
Manipal Tata Medical College
Jamshedpur, Jharkhand, India

Suktara Sharma
MBBS MS (Otolaryngology)
Assistant Professor
Department of ENT
GCS Medical College, Hospital
and Research Center
Ahmedabad, Gujarat, India

Vijay Bhaskar MBBS MD (DERM) DCH
Associate Professor
Department of Dermatology
Madras Medical College
Chennai, Tamil Nadu, India

Vikram Bhaskar MD (Pediatrics)
Assistant Professor
Department of Pediatrics
University College of
Medical Sciences and
Guru Teg Bahadur Hospital
New Delhi, India

Foreword

Indeed, it is a proud privilege for me to write "foreword" for *IAP Clinical Examination in Pediatrics*.

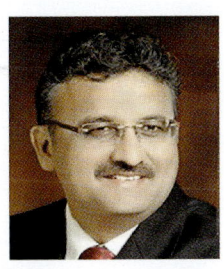

Even though the medical science has expanded by leaps and bounds and there are many diagnostic modalities available, still clinical examination is the key to early and appropriate diagnosis without submitting the patient for a battery of investigations. A detailed history taking and thorough clinical examination can definitely contribute to the accurate early diagnosis and save on time and money both. In an era of consumerism, Google-learned patients, and cut throat competition, it is imperative to have strong clinical knowledge and skill. A strong foundation of the same can be created while the person is in medical training (during undergraduate and postgraduate studies).

With an aim to strengthen the clinical skills of students and young practitioners the Indian Academy of Pediatrics (IAP) envisaged to come out with a book on *IAP Clinical Examination in Pediatrics* under action plan 2018-19. We feel blessed to have Dr Baldev Prajapati and team as editorial board members who have taken pains and have carefully drafted this book.

Apart from chapters on History Taking and Clinical Examination the book has sections on some of the overlooked skills—Anthropometry and Assessment of Growth and Assessment of Diet and Feeding Practices. It has also included some non-medical sections like: Communication with Child and Parents and Ethical and Legal Issues in Pediatric Practice.

I am sure reading this comprehensive book on clinical skills will be a big boon as they do not need to refer several books and it will contribute to capacity/skill building for the PG students.

My heartiest congratulations to editorial team as well as contributors for coming out with this compact but comprehensive book on clinical skills. I am sure it will be popular amongst readers.

Digant D Shastri
President, 2019
Indian Academy of Pediatrics

Foreword

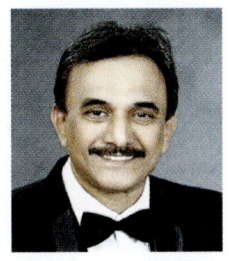

In the field of modern as well as ancient medicine, clinical examination has played a pivotal role and has been taught the students to be good clinicians. Though there are many books available on this subject, we have never had a comprehensive book from Indian Academy of Pediatrics. This made us to initiate this project.

As we thread into the early part of the 21st century with newer technologies changing the way of diagnosis, sometimes we wonder whether the period of clinical examination with inspection-palpation-percussion is over. But I am sure a proper history and clinical examination will give you a diagnosis in almost 80% of the cases. As teachers it is our duty to make sure that our future students are trained well in clinical examination.

The *IAP Clinical Examination in Pediatrics* will be an excellent trestle for students of pediatrics, be it undergraduate, postgraduate, or fellowship student with depth and clarity.

First and foremost I wish to congratulate Dr Baldev Prajapati who took on this project almost single-handedly. He has been able to bring out the book within the time limit, which is highly appreciable. I also thank other team members for taking up the onerous task of compiling this book and enthusiastically pursuing this project to fruition. They have envisioned a comprehensive coverage of clinical examination in this book with Indian focus and perspective in mind. I am also glad to see that a large number of experts in this field have contributed chapters and made this into a genuine team effort.

IAP is a professional organization whose mission statement is improvement of child health and it is committed to the mental and physical wellbeing of all children with various academic and social activities. IAP fulfills this mission by updating the knowledge, attitude, and skills of her members by various academic events and publications. Over the last many years, IAP publications, being very popular, are well read, accepted, and appreciated.

Any organization can thrive only when it is focused on its core purpose. IAP has a long-standing track record of outstanding academic activity. It can be reinvigorated only when we continue to produce an academic output of excellent quality. This book is a step forward in that direction. I wish to convey the academy's gratitude to all those who have been involved in this effort, chiefly the editors and contributors for giving life to the IAP's vision for emerging as a professional organization of repute.

Santosh T Soans
President, 2018
Indian Academy of Pediatrics

Foreword

In this modern era of sophisticated technology for laboratory and radio imaging diagnosis and their easy availability, the art of clinical diagnosis is gradually vanishing. With reference to it, several members of IAP including office bearers and executive board members felt a need of a book on clinical examination, helping the students to understand the importance of 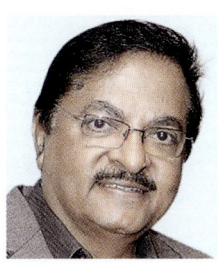 bedside clinical examination and diagnosis. To impart thorough clinical knowledge and skill to the students, the book should be small in volume, in simple language, and easy to understand. With this thought, IAP decided to bring out this publication, *IAP Clinical Examination in Pediatrics*.

It is our great pleasure and privilege to have Dr Baldev Prajapati, Professor and Head, Department of Pediatrics, GCS Medical College, Hospital and Research Center and Aakanksha Children Hospital and Postgraduate Institute, Ahmedabad, Gujarat, India as the Editor and other eminent teachers as contributors. Baldev Prajapati is very well-known as an eminent teacher across the country. He is known for his bedside teaching, clinical acumen, and analytic approach based on detail history and thorough clinical examination to any given case.

This book contains unique chapters on communication skill, ethical and legal issues in practice, and diagnosis of death which are hardly found in other books. The special aspects of child health like Developmental assessment, Diet in young children, Anthropometry, and Growth assessment are covered very nicely. Besides all the systems, it also includes Newborn, Eye, ENT, Skin, and Musculoskeletal system examination. A chapter on Common procedures is relevant to daily practice. The book has been made self-explanatory by many original clinical pictures and tables.

This book would become a most practical and useful tool to the students in their training in clinical medicine. I hope this book will find its place on shelf of each library.

Bakul Jayant Parekh
President, 2020
Indian Academy of Pediatrics

Preface

Over the last few decades, the science of medicine has progressed very rapidly not only in the field of therapeutics, but also in the field of diagnostic technology. But, it is a sad reality that there is a gradual rusting of clinical medicine and lack of interest for bedside diagnosis among us. Detail history, thorough physical examination, and good communication skill are major pillars of clinical medicine. Medicine is not only science, but it is also an art. It is learnt only by methodological and well-organized clinical examination which requires continuous practice and special efforts. During bedside teaching in my daily round and conducting undergraduate as well as postgraduate examinations, I felt the need of a handbook on clinical examination in pediatrics which is simple, easy to understand, and can be practiced daily. Meanwhile, I received a request from the office of our central Indian Academy of Pediatrics to prepare a book, *IAP Clinical Examination in Pediatrics* under my Editorship with the help of eminent teachers, I accepted it immediately with a great pleasure.

The book has been written to provide a simplified clinical approach to children with various medical disorders. The focus is mainly on clinical methods to elicit physical symptoms and signs. The book is phased into 18 chapters, beginning with a chapter on communication with child and parents. It has been observed that communication skill is lacking with many of us as it was not taught to us during our training period. It provides knowledge, skills, and philosophy to handle the children and their parents with concern and compassion. Breastfeeding and feeding practices in young children, anthropometry and assessment of growth, and developmental assessment have unique place in pediatrics. Breastfeeding and related practical issues, diet in young children, interpretation of anthropometric parameters and assessment of growth, body index mass (BMI), use of growth charts, and importance of developmental screening and assessment have been covered in view of its importance in health and disease of children. Besides all the major systems, it also includes examination of newborn, eye, ENT, skin, and its appendages and musculoskeletal system. There are plenty of tables and our own original clinical photographs for good visual impression and easy retrieval of information. With availability of most advanced life-supporting systems for the management of critically ill patients, many a times it is a dilemma for a treating physician to diagnose death with reference to modern medicine and law. For this reason, a separate chapter on Diagnosis of Death is devoted. In this modern era, it is essential for every clinician to be well versed regarding ethical and legal issues in our daily practice. The expert in the field has made it simple for us. A chapter on Common Procedure in Pediatrics is relevant to this book.

Baldev Prajapati

Acknowledgments

I would like to thank Dr Bakul Jayant Parekh, President IAP–2020, Dr Digant D Shastri, President IAP–2019, Dr Santosh T Soans, President IAP–2018, Dr Remesh Kumar R, Honorable Secretary, IAP 2018–19 and all the members of the executive board, IAP for giving me the opportunity to prepare this book. I remain grateful to all the authors for their contributions, without whose help it would not have been possible. I am thankful to all my colleagues from Department of Pediatrics, GCS Medical College, Hospital and Research Center, Ahmedabad, Gujarat, India; Aakanksha Children Hospital and Postgraduate Institute, Ahmedabad, Gujarat, India for their help in preparing this book. No amount of words can express my gratitude to my wife, Dr Rajal Prajapati, my daughters, Dr Aakanksha and Dr Aalapi, and my son-in-law, Dr Mukund, who allowed me ample time for completing this book.

I thank the faculties Drs Ami Patel, Hetal Jiyani, Bhanu Desai, Pinakin Trivedi, Harsh Mod, Prarthana Kharod-Patel, Rutvik Parikh, and Sheena Sivanandan and all the Resident Doctors, Department of Pediatrics, GCS Medical College, Hospital and Research Centre, Ahmedabad for their contribution for clinical photographs and other helps.

I like to thank Nisarg Shah for type setting and composing.

I also like to thank Shri Jitendar P Vij (Group Chairman), Mr Ankit Vij (Managing Director), Mr MS Mani (Group President), Ms Chetna Malhotra Vohra (Associate Director—Content Strategy), Ms Pooja Bhandari (Production Head), Ms Prerna Bajaj (Development Editor), and the staff of M/S Jaypee Brothers Medical Publishers (P) Ltd, New Delhi, India, for giving a go-ahead at the very beginning and helping us in every way possible to bring out this book.

I welcome comments for omissions and errors as well as suggestions for future editions.

Contents

1. **Communication and Counseling in Pediatric Practice** 1
   MMA Faridi

2. **History Taking** 12
   Baldev Prajapati

3. **General Physical Examination** 31
   Baldev Prajapati

4. **Infant and Young Child Feeding** 90
   Bakulesh Chauhan, Baldev Prajapati

5. **Anthropometry and Assessment of Growth** 111
   Vikram Bhaskar

6. **Developmental Assessment** 129
   Rhishikesh Thakre, Archana Kadam

7. **The Alimentary System and Abdomen** 157
   Baldev Prajapati

8. **The Respiratory System** 194
   Baldev Prajapati, Rajal Prajapati

9. **The Cardiovascular System** 221
   Baldev Prajapati

10. **The Nervous System** 265
    Baldev Prajapati

11. **Examination of the Newborn** 336
    Rhishikesh Thakre

12. **The Musculoskeletal System** 362
    Chandrika S Bhat, Anand Rao

13. **Examination of Skin and Its Appendages** 373
    Vijay Bhaskar, R Madhu

14. **Examination of Eye** 395
    Aloka Santosh Hedau

15. **Examination of Ear, Nose, and Throat** 417
    Suktara Sharma, Mukund Vaghela

16. **Ethical and Legal Issues in Pediatric Practice** 437
    Satish Tiwari

17. **The Diagnosis of Death** 443
    Sudhir Mishra, Satish Tiwari

18. **Common Procedures in Pediatrics** 450
    Baldev Prajapati

Index 501

Communication and Counseling in Pediatric Practice

CHAPTER 1

MMA Faridi

INTRODUCTION

A famous saying is that sword and words have the same letters; strangely they also have the same effect if not handled properly.

Disease is an entity comprising of some physiological disturbances frequently coupled with anatomical changes and histopathological derangement that manifests in the form of symptoms and signs. Patient on the other hand is an individual who feels pain, and agony; needs help and support for self and personal care, and requires careful evidence-based measures to diagnose the disease and institution of rational therapy for cure or palliation. Patient is not alone in this hour of disease and discomfort but there are family and friends, and healthcare providers around. It is easy to prescribe medicines and surgical interventions to the patient; changes in lifestyle and diet can also be very easily advised. However, acceptance of the reality, gravity and long-term prognosis of the ailment by the patient and the family, and coming to terms with the social impact of the disease and quality of life may differ from person to person and family to family. This may add many dimensions to the disease management. Treating a patient and treating a disease is, therefore, not same. It is easy to treat disease but extremely difficult to treat a patient.

An infant or child patient throws some more peculiar challenges. If their capacity to react to disease insult is limited, then more often it is stereotypic to many serious illnesses. Initially parents may not consider signs and symptoms serious as they continue to "play" and behave "normally" till the disease is well entrenched with complications; it is late. Often parents feel guilt and are inconsolable seeing their child in serious and grave situation.

Once a child patient is admitted in the health facility, the mother remains the main caregiver except in the neonatal intensive care unit (NICU) and pediatric intensive care unit (PICU). The routine of the entire family gets disturbed, parents do not get enough rest, and absence of facilities for basic comfort and unfamiliar and not-so-friendly hospital rules and regulations make the parents and other relatives jittery and frustrated. This sets the milieu for patient/family dissatisfaction and aggressive behavior and results into accusations and complaints landing in the consumer court.

Active communication with the patient and family may mitigate some of the concerns and anxiety of the parents including ethical dilemma and social issues. Counseling is the way of working with the people. Counseling truly reflects empathy towards the patient and the family and empowers them to understand the disease, its treatment and prognosis and to take most appropriate decision best suited to their situation. Spending some time with the patient and family gives big dividends to the treating physician and nurses. This helps building trust between the patient/family and the healthcare providers and gives confidence to them to follow treatment plan and advice. A good rapport and communication also enhance early recovery and well-being of the patient and ensures timely follow-up.

However, it is important that doctors should have detached empathy with the patient and are not involved sentimentally. Otherwise, it may lead to "burn out" and "sympathetic" actions which are perceived irrational. This may also lead to insinuations and doubts by the patient, family and friends later on. The attributes of active communication are described in **Box 1**. Counseling is to give professional help and recommendation to someone. There are three components of counseling **(Flowchart 1)**.

Box 1: Attributes of active communication.
- Explaining nature of the disease and its consequences in simple language and nonthreatening manner
- Understanding patient/family concerns and difficulties
- Giving relevant information enabling them for making informed decision/s
- Exploring and evaluating with the patient and family all possible treatment options
- Giving few suggestions not commands
- Skill building and mentoring to ensure patient and family understand the treatment plan and enable them to take care at home

Flowchart 1: Components of counseling.

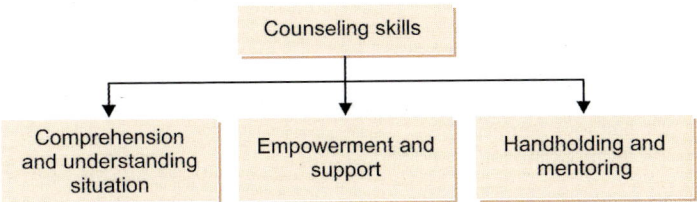

> **Box 2:** Steps of facilitate comprehension and understanding situation.
> - Making appropriate ambience and presentation
> - Asking open or factual questions
> - Showing interest by responses and gestures during communication
> - Paraphrasing or reflecting back what the patient/family says and thinks
> - Empathizing with the patient/family what he/she feels and experiences
> - Avoiding judging words during conversation

COMPREHENSION AND UNDERSTANDING SITUATION

It is extremely important to first find out sociocultural background, economic status, education level, religious beliefs, community practices, and past experience of the patient/family before offering any help and support regarding the present disease and its sequelae. The learning of the above aspects may be facilitated by a set of steps, described in **Box 2**.

MAKING APPROPRIATE AMBIENCE AND PRESENTATION

Active communication and counseling should be done at a quiet and reasonably comfortable place. All family members—parents, grandparents, friends, and distant relatives—present at the time of counseling should be invited, greeted, and seated in the chair. Pediatrician/senior resident/junior resident should also sit in the chair without any table between the doctor and the attendees to remove any barrier. Doctor should introduce himself and then ask all the person their name and relationship with the patient.

Maintain social distance while talking to the patient/family; neither too close nor too far. Always look towards the person you are talking. It is a common mistake that while talking to the patient or her relative, the doctor is busy with the papers/case sheet or calling

> **Box 3:** Kinesics (Nonverbal communication skills).
> - Posture—head level
> - Distance—social distance
> - Eye contact
> - Have time
> - Remove barrier
> - Appropriate touch and handshake

other staff for some work or attending phone. Never look towards the watch while in conversation. This indicates that you are in a hurry and do not have enough time for them. Always show to the patient and the family that you have plenty of time for them and that you enjoy talking to them. When patient talks or family shares some facts then show response by nodding, smiling or saying "achha", "un hoon" or exclaiming "oh my dear" or "is that so", etc. Touch and patting are a great gesture and shows respect, friendship, and bonding. Doctor can appropriately touch and pat the patient and relatives else you can touch the child. But be careful of the societal values. In our culture, male doctor touching a woman is generally not appreciated but with time once you command faith then you can gently pat the mother/father on the shoulder assuring her/him of your availability for any clarification or consultation any time. The above measures are also referred as nonverbal communication or body language. The nonverbal communication skills are summarized in **Box 3**.

Adequate measures should be taken for privacy and confidentiality. For eliciting history of HIV and some hereditary disease, it is better to talk one to one or in front of a person whom patient or family is comfortable with. Do not show anger and make such gestures which amount to disapproval or inappropriateness. Always end the conversation with saying thank you and reassurance of your availability and support anytime.

ASKING OPEN OR FACTUAL QUESTIONS

Questions are of two types, open question and closed question. An open question is one which elicits a response from the patient/family. It is very useful in taking history and learning situation of the patient/family in shorter time and without speaking much.

Communication and Counseling in Pediatric Practice

Table 1: Examples of closed and open questions.	
Closed questions	Open questions
• Do you wash hands before taking meals? • Can you donate blood? • Can you look after this baby at home?	• How do you ensure hygiene before taking meals? • How will you arrange blood? • Who will look after this baby at home?

It allows more time to the patient/family to speak and encourage them to share more information. The open question starts with when, how, why, where, etc. The closed question elicits answer as yes or no. Patient does not feel like telling details and is frequently leading type and ends up with judging words. For example, is your child well? It is a closed question because answer to the question will be either yes or no. Here "well" is a judging word that may make mother confused as to what exactly you mean by "well". If you ask an open question, then judging word will disappear. How is your baby?

If you want to know whether mother is breastfeeding? You may ask the mother "are you breastfeeding?" The answer may be, yes, I am breastfeeding, or I am not. It does not tell anything more. But if you ask the mother how are you feeding your child? The answer may be, I am breastfeeding but sometimes my child cries more in the evening, so I give powder milk by a bottle. I do it two to three times in a week. So, mother gives more information about feeding the child. Factual question is a type of closed question, but it is asked when factual information is required, e.g. what is your age? how many children do you have? are you pregnant? etc. Example of closed and open questions are in **Table 1**.

PARAPHRASING OR REFLECTING BACK WHAT THE PATIENT/FAMILY SAYS AND THINKS

Listen to the patient/family patiently. In order to know more about a point or narration, patient is making or expressing his/her opinion. It is advisable to repeat the same or paraphrase the sentence said by him/her. Reflecting back encourages the parents and patient to tell more about their concerns and apprehensions and reassures them that doctor is listening to them and that healthcare provider is responsive and interested.

Example, mother says "I do not have enough breast milk that is why I give cow's milk twice a day, in the morning and night, as my son is 4 months old now".

Doctor can say "you think you do not have sufficient breast milk" or "how did you get this idea?" or simply "you think so".

Mother will now give reasons and tell more about why she thinks her milk is not enough for the child. She may inform you that she has to join job next month and she wants that child is able to feed on the animal milk while she is away in the office. She further informs that her sister says it is better to start bottle feeding at least a month before joining duties as child can learn to take top feed. Thus, reflecting back on the patient or parents helps you understand the situation. It will now be easy for the doctor to give information on the signs of insufficiency of breast milk and offer suggestions as to how a woman can breastfeed when she is away from her child.

You will appreciate that disagreeing with the mother or questioning her on her decision of top feeding or telling her about the dangers of top feeding in the beginning will vitiate the atmosphere and make mother/father unwilling to follow your advice and suggestions. However, one should be careful that while you are reflecting back you do not sound sarcastic or judgmental or insensitive.

EMPATHIZING WITH THE PATIENT/FAMILY WHAT HE/SHE FEELS AND EXPERIENCES

Empathy is an essential component of counseling and active communication. It means expressing to the patient/parents that you understand their concerns and agony and respect their feelings. Try to find out occasions, while talking to the patient/parents, where you can show empathy. Using empathy is a great skill which makes the person comfortable from inside that doctor understands his/her worries and concerns. If you empathize then parents may share several things and enrich patient's history by telling things without being asked. If a child patient with

> **Box 4:** Steps for building confidence with parents.
> - Accept what parents think, believe or feel
> - Identify what parents/patient are doing right and praise for that
> - Give little practical help to make them comfortable
> - Give relevant information
> - Use simple language
> - Make few suggestions not commands

respiratory distress comes to casualty and you show empathy to the parents by saying "I can understand you are quite worried about the child". Father may tell you in chocked voice that "he lost elder child with similar complaints 2 years ago". You can imagine the kind of feelings and apprehension this family has which you do not know when patient walks in the emergency room. You can identify with the pain and anguish of the family by saying "loosing child is always very painful to parents". This is empathy. If you say "it was so bad, God willed that way". This is sympathy and this does not sooth the traumatized feelings of the parents. So do not show sympathy and sentiments.

The next important step in counseling is building confidence and checking understanding of the patient/parents. It is very important that you must assess what patient/family has understood about the disease and its treatment at the end of conversation. The steps as mentioned in **Box 4** can help in building the confidence with parents.

ACCEPT WHAT PARENTS THINK, BELIEVE OR FEEL

It has been seen that disagreement during conversation with a person on a mistaken idea makes him/her annoyed, resistant and possessive of his/her ideas and opinion. In turn he/she often loses confidence and does not accept suggestions. Agreement with a mistaken idea is vulnerable because then one cannot offer suggestions for correction later on. Therefore, one should neither agree nor disagree with the parents or patient if they harbor a wrong and unscientific idea; instead a neutral response should be given. The neutral statement could be in the form of reflecting back or empathy.

A mother says "my 1-month-old daughter cries in the night and wants breastfeed too often. She perhaps remains hungry as my milk is not enough for her". Doctor can say that mother's milk is never in short supply. Child feeds two hourly in early infancy throughout the day including night and circadian rhythm of the infant is such that he/she gets up in the night and more playful; your baby is alright. These statements are scientifically correct but smell of disagreement. Mother may not be satisfied with this response. Rather she may lose confidence as she may feel she does not know physiology of her child. However, if doctor says to the mother that "you are obviously worried about your child", "both of you then are not able to sleep", "I understand you are worried about breast milk supply" he is seen polite and gives feelings of being sensitive towards the mother. These statements are showing empathy and giving neutral response to the mistaken idea expressed by the mother. Another example, a mother comes with her daughter to the Well Baby Clinic. The nurse advises immunization to the child, but she refuses citing that it will cause pain and fever. What will you say?

- No, you should not refuse immunization. It will prevent many diseases.
- There will be some pain and fever, but benefits outweigh these.

You are concerned with the discomfort the immunization will cause? Is that so? Accept what the person thinks and feels in a neutral fashion.

IDENTIFY WHAT PARENTS/PATIENT ARE DOING RIGHT AND PRAISE FOR THAT

Praising is liked by every individual. This boosts the morale of the person, enhances confidence, makes him to do same thing again and again if appreciated for that and encourages him/her to accept suggestions given by the person who praises him/her. Doctors have to learn praising as a communication skill. They have to find out something being done right by the parents or the patient himself/herself and praise them for even in worst scenario.

A mother brings 1-year-old child to the OPD with the complaints of loose motions and fever. Child is feeding on diluted cow's milk by bottle from the age of 3 months and is malnourished. Mother is carrying old patient record including discharge ticket given at birth. A doctor generally becomes judgmental in this situation and accuses the mother for being responsible for this sorry state of her child. Remember mother will never harm her child. So how can a doctor praise the mother in this situation? See mother is carrying old patient record and a discharge ticket indicating birth weight and other information. Doctor can praise the mother that old patient record will be very helpful in understanding the situation and managing the patient. It will boost her morale and she will feel happy.

GIVE RELEVANT INFORMATION

Doctors are busy persons. They should use communication skills that encourage parents/patient to tell history correctly and convey the message that doctor is sensitive and empathic. It is very important that doctor gives relevant information about the disease and treatment in one sitting. One or more sittings may be arranged depending on the course of the disease and situation. A mother comes to Well Baby Clinic for immunization of her 6 weeks old infant. Mother may be given information about the three doses of pentavalent vaccine, oral poliovirus vaccines (OPV) and *Rota virus* vaccine which will be administered at 6, 10, and 14 weeks of age. Pneumococcal and fractionated inactivated polio vaccine will be administered at 6 and 14 weeks of age. Child may have some fever for which medicine (paracetamol) will be given. Breastfeeding should continue. There is no need to tell about Measles-Rubella (MR) vaccine at 9 months and then booster doses of diphtheria-pertussis-tetanus (DPT), etc. at this time. This is relevant information.

The relevant information should be in positive manner. Negative information is perceived as threatening and may down the confidence of the parents/patient if they are doing that. For example, information on excessive viewing of the mobile by the child can be given by two ways:
- Spending less time on mobile chatting enhances school performance. Exclusive breastfeeding till 6 months of age makes the baby grow strong and healthy. This are relevant information in a positive manner.

- If you spend more time on mobile chatting, you will fail in the examination. Mixed feeding or top feeding will cause diarrhea and pneumonia. These are relevant information albeit in negative frame.

The information should be provided as a scientific fact in general terms and not specifically addressing the patient or the parents. The language should be simple and comprehensible by the nonmedical person. Remember, even well-literate people do not understand medical terminology.

MAKE FEW SUGGESTIONS NOT COMMANDS

Doctors are trained to give orders. Even the prescription paper begins with R. This tells "I order in the name of God" the following medicines. Command or order is not liked by any person. Commands are not generally adhered to. Alternatively, suggestions do make a difference. Suggestion gives a person choice and authority to carry it out or not. How one will feel if somebody says, please close the door or will you please close the door? Former is an order to close the door; there is no choice. But later statement gives a choice to the person to say no if he does not want to close the door. Former is a command and later is a suggestion. After giving primary immunization to a 6 weeks child, the nurse tells the mother to come after a month for second dose without looking at her and busy in writing records in the register. Obviously, immunization coverage is not satisfactory. If nurse says to the mother that three doses of pentavalent vaccine will prevent diphtheria, pertussis, tetanus, hepatitis B and *Haemophilus influenzae* meningitis (use local language for the diseases) in the child. You are a good and responsible mother that you were on time for first vaccination. The next immunization will be after a month say on January 29. Can you come for immunization? Now mother will think for a moment and can say yes. It is possible she may say "no, I have parent child meeting (PTM) in my elder son's school or there is family function. I cannot come on January 29". Now nurse may give mother other suggestions like immunization can be done after 4 weeks. So, nurse can suggest that she can come on January 28, for immunization. It is important to give suggestions and not commands for carrying out treatment and taking informed consent. This is a very useful communication skill which is immensely appreciated by the parents and the patient.

CHECKING UNDERSTANDING OF THE PATIENT/PARENTS

It is not enough to give relevant information and suggestions. The parents/patient has to understand the disease, its implications, treatment modalities and long-term effects including adverse effects of the drugs and nutritional rehabilitation. Doctor should always determine that parents have learnt and internalized the whole conversation about the disease. It should be done in a manner that it does not sound like appearing in an examination. Doctor can start by saying, well we have discussed many things today. Can we revise or recollect what we have discussed? Now information may be elicited and supported and completed by the doctor. He may finish the session by assuring the parents that at any time, something is not clear they can approach him.

CHAPTER 2

History Taking

Baldev Prajapati

INTRODUCTION

When the parents contact the pediatrician for any health issue of their child, the pediatrician has to derive the diagnosis before he suggests any remedy. There are three tools in clinical medicine to reach the diagnosis and they are detailed history, thorough clinical examination and relevant, and necessary investigations. Before he suggests investigations, he should have clinical diagnosis. History and clinical examination are important components to derive clinical diagnosis.

History taking is the most important among them, because not only history taking will guide examination and investigations, but in many cases, history is the only indicator of the disease. Many a times, physical examination and investigations have a complementary role. It also provides an opportunity to build rapport with the child and the parents, which helps in planning the management of the child.

The broad principles and the format of history taking in children are the same as in adults, the important differences are noteworthy as follows:

- Pediatric history is generally derived from parents or relatives and not directly from the child and it may be influenced by their own concerns, beliefs and emotions toward the child. The interpretations may be biased by the parents, which may be away from reality.
- Childhood is a dynamic phase like newborn, infant, toddler, older child, and adolescent in life and history taking in children must be modified according to their age with different areas of emphasis for different age groups.
- Perinatal history, developmental, dietary, and immunization histories are additional components in pediatric history taking.

Although tight compartment-wise format of history taking cannot be recommended, this chapter outlines broad principles and guidelines within traditional structured format.

PREREQUISITES FOR GOOD HISTORY TAKING

History taking is not merely a collection of data concerning health and disease, but also the process of getting important information. The interview should be a pleasant experience and should help in establishing a good relationship.

A good history taking needs a reliable informant, development of a good rapport with the child and the parents, appropriate questioning, correct interpretation of responses, and meticulous documentation of information for future use and record. Some essential points for obtaining good history are discussed.

Setting

History must be recorded in a quiet and comfortable place with consideration of their privacy, especially in case of adolescents. Adolescent girls must be interviewed only in the presence of mother or a female nurse. There should be sitting arrangement for the patient and his parents.

Rapport Building

Development of a good rapport with the child and his parents is essential for collection of reliable information. Following points are important to establish a rapport:
- Medical person should wear descent clothes with an apron
- Greeting the child and the parents
- Introducing yourself
- Addressing the child with his name
- Establish a good eye contact
- Conversing in an empathetic manner
- Patient hearing is one of the good qualities of the clinician. Patient listening that patient wants to tell is not the waste of time, but may offer a clue to diagnosis. Information provided by the patient is never vague

- Avoid distractions, e.g. phone calls during history taking
- Assure them regarding confidentiality of information
- Try to collect the information in shortest time
- Avoid recording unnecessary, lengthy narration.

Informant

A mother is the most reliable informant. The father may not be knowing all details. The grandparents may exaggerate the illness. Sometimes, relatives and caregivers may be helpful. If necessary, history may be crosschecked with other parent or relatives. Children above the age of 7 years often provide good information themselves, they should be made the primary informant or contributors. They may provide details of present illness, but development history and immunization details should be obtained from parents.

Collecting Information

Collecting information should be in a form of conversation rather than in an interrogation.

- Begin with open-ended questions, e.g. what is wrong... and let the informant narrate the story of illness in his words without interruptions. Open-ended questions also allow parents to reveal their perception about illness of the child.
- Subsequently, identify the issue that needs further clarifications and use close-ended questions to get the desired answer, e.g. "Is it the first time ...?"
- Ask about each complaint separately to ensure accurate response. Let the older child participate in providing detailed information.
- Choice of language should be one which is understood by the patient and parents.
- Follow the broad sequence of format of history taking so that important information is not missed.
- In case of chronic or recurrent illnesses, the parents may be knowing details of diagnosis and management, e.g. bronchial asthma, nephrotic syndrome, drug allergy, etc.
- In summary, the history should be accurate, brief, and clear.

Assessment of Response

Response from the informant to questions asked in the history is often influenced by their intellectual level, profession, awareness of the problem, emotional reactions, and net or Google information.

Listen carefully to the narration by the informants. Also observe their behavior, body language, hesitancy or avoidance of a certain question, change in tone or attitude, lack of concern, etc. Avoid argument and embarrassment. Never laugh at their answers and reactions.

Documentation

It is essential to maintain record for future reference and for legal implications. Consider the following points:
- History should be recorded in a prestructured format, once the interview is over. Do not interrupt the process of narration for the sake of recording the history.
- History should be narrated in the words of parents or patient, regardless of your interpretations.
- Avoid abbreviations and medical jargon as much as possible.
- Use diagrams to depict pictorial information, e.g. distribution of skin rash, areas of body involved in burus with their severity in percentage.
- Mention date and time of history recording. Name and signature of the interviewer should be there on record.
- During interview, it is important to show your concern with the illness of the child and anxiety of parents. The parents should be allowed to talk freely and express their concerns. During the process of interview, interviewer should look at the child and informant intermittently and not only at writing instruments.

An empathetic interviewer who addresses the parent and child by name frequently obtains more accurate information than a person who is in hurry and nonconcerned. Careful observation during the interview many a times uncovers their stress, anxiety, and concerns.

Closure

At the end of interview, ask for any other concern or questions that the parents have, may not be related to medical problem.

Appreciate them for their cooperation toward giving a detailed history and their initiative to seek medical advice. Offer your services and availability at any time if they need.

COMPONENTS OF HISTORY TAKING

The following major components should be included in history taking as a general, may vary in an individual case according to clinical situation:

- General information (demographic data)
- Presenting complaints (chief complaints)
- History of present illness (origin, duration, and progress)
- Past history
- Antenatal, natal, and postnatal history
- Developmental history
- Dietary history
- Family history
- Immunization history
- Personal history
- Socio economic history
- Environmental history.

It is very essential to look toward the child before starting history taking. A mere look at the patient from distance may offer an important clue (first impression) to the condition and is a certainly important parameter which guides for urgent intervention. A child with altered sensorium, respiratory distress, petechial or purpuric spots on the skin, very sick looking (toxic look) child, etc. are important observations which require urgent attention and prompt action before detailed history taking. Infants and young children should be offered a soft toy or rattle. School going children feel at ease when they are directly called by their name, details about school, hobbies, and health problems. Avoid staring toward the child. This will help in establishing rapport with the child and parents and thereby assisting in a good history taking.

General Information (Demographic Data)

This is essential not only for identity of the patient but also helping in analysis the clinical problem and follow-up. A record of

> **Box 1:** General information.
> - Name (full name)
> - Age (date of birth)
> - Sex
> - Complete address
> - Telephone number (S)
> - Religion
> - Caste
> - Date and time of history taking

demographic data is also essential for medico legal and insurance purposes. The important components of general information are name, age, sex, complete address, telephone number, religion, caste, date, time of history taking **(Box 1)**.

- *Name:* It must be recorded correctly with the spelling, which is there on his school record or birth certificate. It should be full name (child's name, father's name, and surname). Addressing the child with his name helps to develop good rapport with him and parents.
- *Age:* Record the birth date. Age should be calculated accordingly, in hours for initial 3–5 days, in days for a neonate, in months for infants and in years thereafter. If the parents do not recall the birth date of the child, information may be obtained in reference to important events like festivals or family functions.

  Besides identity of the child, age also helps in differential diagnosis as certain diseases are more common in specific age groups. Congenital anomalies and genetic disorders usually manifest in neonatal period or early infancy. Infections and injuries are more common in toddlers. Connective tissue diseases like systemic lupus erythematosus (SLE) are uncommon before adolescence. The common age-wise distribution of few childhood diseases is shown in **Table 1**.
- *Gender (sex):* It must be recorded carefully, especially in newborns. In case of ambiguous genitalia, sex should be assigned only after thorough investigations.

  Gender is also important in considering or excluding certain conditions as certain diseases in children have a distinct

Table 1: Common age for certain childhood diseases.

Disease	Age
Febrile seizures	6 months–5 years
Bronchiolitis	Infants
Infantile tremor syndrome (ITS)	6 months–2 years
Kawasaki disease	Less than 5 years
Rheumatic fever	5–15 years
Minimal change nephrotic syndrome (MCNS)	3–8 years
Wilson disease	More than 5 years
Slipped upper femoral epiphyses	Adolescents
Systemic lupus erythematosus (SLE)	Adolescents

gender bias. X-linked recessive disorders like Duchenne muscular dystrophy and glucose 6 phosphate dehydrogenase (G6PD) deficiency almost always manifest only in males and females asymptomatic carriers. Other X-linked recessive diseases in males are hemophilia A and B, Fragile X syndrome, Hunter syndrome, etc. SLE is more common in females.

- *Religion and caste:* Certain diseases are common in specific religion and caste which information helps in diagnosis like sickle cell disease in tribals and thalassemia in Kutchi, Lohana, Thakkar, Jain, etc.
- *Residence (origin and ethnic background of the family):* It should be recorded in details. The complete postal address and phone numbers will be helpful for follow-up of the case. In migrants, both present and permanent addresses to be recorded. Certain diseases are known for their geographical distribution like kala azar in Bihar and eastern part of our country, Japanese encephalitis in Uttar Pradesh, West Bengal, Karnataka, etc. Rickettsial diseases in West Bengal, Karnataka, South Maharashtra, etc. help to consider those possibilities when the patient is from specific area. Correct address also helps to public health authorities for taking necessary preventive measures during outbreaks.

Presenting Complaints (Chief Complaints)

The chief complaints form the basis for clinical history and convey the main reason for seeking medical advice. Important aspects of writing the chief complaints are as follows:
- All presenting complaints must be recorded in the chronological order of appearance along with the duration of complaints.
- All the complaints must be recorded in form of a list along with brief description and duration.
- Try to define the prominent chief complaint which may be attention seeking and responsible for the whole illness. Other complaints may be associated with it or secondary to main complaint.
- Record chief complaints in a chronological order according to sequence of events. It may indicate progress of the disease and may suggest clinical diagnosis. For example:
  - 1-year male
  - High-grade fever 5 days
  - Irritability, excessive crying, and vomiting 3 days
  - Convulsions and unconsciousness today.

  An infant presents with high grade fever of 5 days duration, likely some infection, followed by irritability, excessive crying and vomiting (raised intracranial pressure) indicates localization of infection at central nervous system (CNS), convulsions and unconsciousness (acute febrile encephalitic syndrome), favors possibility of acute bacterial meningitis.
- Complaints should be recorded in the exact words of the parents or patient. Do not translate it in medical terminology. Do not mention your interpretations, e.g. write yellow eyes and yellow urine, not the jaundice, bluish discoloration of lips and nails, not cyanosis, etc.
- In cases of chronic illnesses like cerebral palsy, bronchial asthma, nephrotic syndrome, etc. chief complaints may be structured to include the whole duration of illness. In a chronic disease, it is possible that with every episode, chief complaints may be almost same or may overlap. An effort should be made to make it concise and condense.

- A known diagnosis from the past should be included before listing the complaints to assist in the process of analysis. For example, begin with "a known case of nephrotic syndrome, presenting with complaints of..." However, before stating that a known case of..., one should verify that it was confirmed diagnosis in the past. It should be made clear, when it was first diagnosed, diagnosis was confirmed, number of episodes in the past, management of every episode, development of any complication, response to various drugs, etc. and chief complaints at present...

History of Present Illness (Origin, Duration, and Progress)

This includes detailed description of current health problem as listed in chief complaints. It also includes important positive points favoring possibilities of conditions considered in differential diagnosis and negative points favoring exclusion of conditions in list of differential diagnosis. These positive points and negative points included in the history should be relevant to the present illness, not just to complete the list.

- The history of present illness should be written in a concise manner in a story like format. There should be continuous flow of the information. Elaborate on each complaint in details with reference to mode of onset, duration, and progress. It should also include localization of illness, its severity, aggravating or relieving factors, medicines taken their effect, etc. as shown in **Table 2**.
- Details of note of each consultant, consulted before approaching you, investigations performed and their interpretations, treatment received and its effect on illness, etc. should be recorded. In a case of chronic illness with multiple consultations and several investigations, information should be recorded in tabulation form for information at a glance.

Past History

It should include all significant health-related events prior to onset of present illness with special emphasis on major infections, hospitalization, blood component transfusion,

Table 2: Points to be recorded in relation to complaints in history of present illness.

Points	Defining variable
Symptoms	Fever, cough, vomiting, diarrhea, pain in abdomen, headache, seizures, and breathlessness
Onset of illness	Sudden (hyperacute), acute, subacute, and chronic
Duration	Hours/days/weeks/months… years
Severity	Mild, moderate, and severe
Course of illness	Static, progressive, recurrent, episodic, waxing, and waning
Aggravating/relieving factors	Effect of posture, food, cough, etc. During sleep—whether the symptoms persist or disappear
Interventions	Investigation, hospitalization, medications, etc.

Box 2: Important points to be included in past history.

- History of hospitalization
- History of measles, whooping cough
- History of chronic suppurative otitis media
- History of pica
- History of worms infestations
- History of convulsions
- History of adverse reaction following medication or vaccination
- History of blood component or immunoglobulin therapy
- History of surgical intervention

immunoglobulin therapy, medications, surgical interventions, adverse reactions following medication or vaccination, etc. **(Box 2)**.

Many of childhood morbidities have an important correlation with the past history. For example:
- A child presenting with convulsions may have past history of febrile convulsions, hypoglycemia, meningitis, head injury, etc.
- A child presenting with hearing impairment may have past history of bacterial meningitis, chronic ear infection, or ototoxic drug therapy like aminoglycosides, quinine, etc.
- A child presenting with history of recurrent chest infections may have history of foreign body aspiration.
- A child presenting with gastroesophageal reflux disease (GERD) may have past history of surgery for tracheoesophageal fistula.

Antenatal, Natal, and Postnatal History

The aim is to correlate the present illness with antenatal, perinatal, or early postnatal events. It is more relevant in cases of infants and young children with congenital malformation, developmental delay or unexplained chronic diseases like cerebral palsy, recurrent convulsions, etc.

Antenatal History

The following information is important:
- *Maternal age:*
  - Advanced maternal age during pregnancy is risk factor for Down syndrome
  - Pregnancy in a young girl carries more problems and complications.
- *Maternal nutrition and pregnancy:* Poor maternal nutrition, severe iron deficiency anemia, and other nutritional factors deficiency adversely affect the growth of the fetus.
- *Maternal illness during pregnancy:*
  - Infants of diabetic mothers are vulnerable to develop malformations, metabolic disorders, maturity related problems, and other complications.
  - Various infections to mother in first trimester are known for congenital infections and malformations to baby.
  - Malaria during pregnancy can lead to various problems like abortion, intrauterine growth restriction (IUGR), etc.
  - Hepatitis B and tuberculosis to mother during pregnancy can affect the fetus in various ways.
- Bad obstetric history with previous abortions, still births, or neonatal deaths.
- *Antenatal care received:* Antenatal visits, tests done during pregnancy like hemoglobin (Hb) level, blood group of mother ABO Rh type, status of other tests like hepatitis B surface antigen (HbsAg), hepatitis C virus (HCV), human immunodeficiency virus (HIV), etc. Other specific tests, if performed. Ultrasonography (USG) scanning, etc. Ideally, USG study is recommended four times during pregnancy. The scan at 18–20 weeks of pregnancy is important to study congenital malformation, if any.

- Potential exposure to infections, drugs, toxins, and radiation during pregnancy.
- Antenatal complications like pregnancy-induced hypertension, eclampsia, bleeding per vagina, etc.

Birth History

- *Place of delivery:* Hospital or home. In a case of home delivery details, who conducted, how umbilical cord was cut, aseptic, and antiseptic precautious, if any taken
- *Mode of delivery:* Vaginal, instrumental, vacuum, and operative
- Obstetric complications like meconium stained liquor and prolonged labor
- Apgar score, neonatal resuscitation—need, mode, etc. neonatal intensive care unit (NICU) admission
- Gestational age and birth weight of baby.

Early Neonatal History

- Prelacteal feed
- When breastfeeding started
- Any top feeding—details which milk, how was it given, etc.
- *Postnatal complications:* Icterus, sepsis, seizures, and hypoglycemia
- Neonatal intensive care unit admission
- Injection vitamin K given or not
- *Vaccines given:* Bacillus Calmette-Guérin (BCG), oral polio vaccine (OPV), and hepatitis B.

The following examples are a few of the possible association between the antenatal, natal, and postnatal history and their implications:

- Periconceptional folic acid supplementation for prevention of neural tube defects
- *Delayed passage of meconium*: Cystic fibrosis and Hirschsprung's disease
- *Delayed cry (perinatal birth asphyxia):* Cerebral palsy and delayed development
- *Infant of diabetic mother:* Large for date baby, hypoglycemia, perinatal complications, congenital malformations, hematological problems, etc.

- *Maternal SLE:* Neonatal complete heart block
- *Intracranial hemorrhage/neonatal meningitis:* Hydrocephalus in infancy
- *History of delayed fall of umbilical cord (>3 weeks):* Leukocyte adhesion defect and factor XIII deficiency.

Family History

Family history provides information regarding several important aspects like genetic factors playing the role for illness, environmental risk factors influencing health of child, tuberculous contact in the family, etc. For getting a reliable family history, one should have established good rapport with the family and should be reassured about the confidentiality. Main aspects to be included in family history are as follows:

- Consanguinity is defined as one between blood relatives who have at least one common ancestor, no more remote than a great great grandparent. Consanguinity of the parents should be inquired as it is common in some communities and poses an increased risk of transmission of genetic diseases, especially autosomal recessive diseases.

    The degree of consanguinity is defined as shown in **Table 3**.
- Prepare a family pedigree chart **(Fig. 1)** including three generations—siblings, parents, and grandparents to assess the possibility of genetic basis and mode of inheritance.
- Pedigree chart is defined as a diagram of family history indicating the normal and the affected individuals and their relationships with the proband as well as their status with respect to a particular genetic disorder.

Table 3: Degree of consanguinity.

Degree	Relationship	% of sharing the genes
First degree	• Sibling and sibling • Parent and child	50
Second degree	• Uncle and niece • Aunt and nephew • Stepbrother and stepsister • Grandparents and grant children	25
Third degree	First cousins	12.5

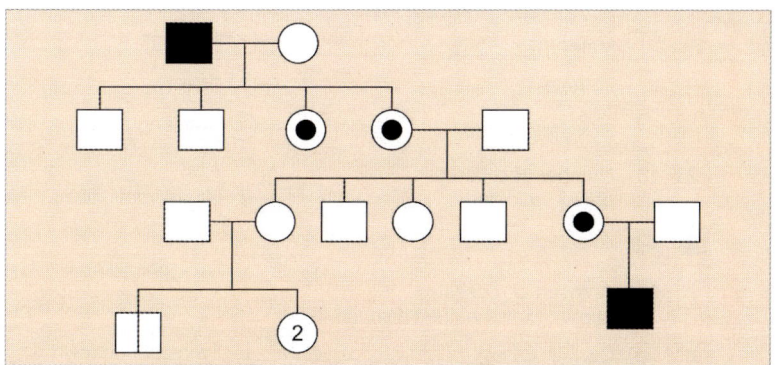

Fig. 1: Typical pedigree chart—X-linked recessive.

- All the members of the same generation, living or dead, should be placed in the same line and each generation should be denoted by Roman numerals on the left (I, II, and III). Conventionally, the male members are placed on the left side of the chart.
- The commonly used symbols in the pedigree chart are shown in **Figure 2**
- Record the history of similar illness in family members, may be indicating common genetic or environmental factors like infections or toxic exposure.
- Search for contact with infectious diseases not only in the family but also in other household members, relatives, and neighbors in the present or past, especially tuberculosis.
- History of contact with tuberculosis is an important component of family history in pediatrics. It is considered to be positive if the child is in contact with a person who is open case [discharging acid fast bacillus (AFB), sputum positive for AFB] on antituberculous treatment or has completed the treatment within the past 2 years.
- Assess the psychosocial environment of the family especially marital conflicts, psychiatric illnesses, substance abuse, child rearing practices, etc.

Developmental History

Developmental history is a special feature of pediatric history and is very important. Development is age dependent and is

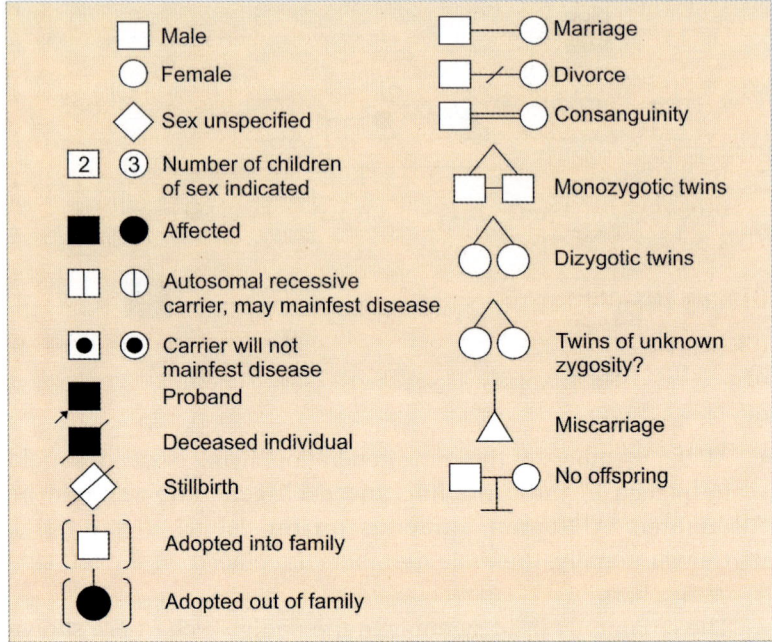

Fig. 2: Commonly used symbols in pedigree charts.

more relevant in cases where history suggests a neurological, developmental, or behavioral problem. The important aspects of developmental history are as follows:
- Developmental history is recorded under four headings, gross motor, fine motor, personal and social, and language development. The details have been described in chapter on development.
- Age of achievement of these milestones should be compared with normal standards to identify any deviation from normal. The marginal delay should not be given undue importance. It can be compared with the sibling.
- In a case of delayed development, try to assess whether all milestones are uniformly delayed in more than two fields (global delayed development) or isolated delay in one or two fields with normal development in other fields. It may be due to other reasons like delayed language may be due to hearing impairment and only gross motor involvement in a case of severe malnutrition or chronic illness.

- In a case of abnormal development, try to find out whether some milestones were never achieved (delayed development) or they have lost after the initial achievement (regression of milestones). The regression of milestones is an important clue to neurodegenerative disorders.
- In school going children, academic performance and social interactions with other students are also useful indicators for assessment of development.

Dietary History

It is age dependent and aims to assess any role of diet in causation of present illness, e.g. malnutrition, obesity, etc. It also helps to differentiate between malnutrition and organic cause for failure to thrive. Dietary history should include feeding in early infancy (first 6 months of age), complementary feeding and present diet with calculation of consumption of total calories and protein. Salient features of dietary history are as follows:

- *In infants younger than 6 months of age:*
  - When breastfeeding was started after delivery? [Within half an hour in a case of normal delivery and 4 hours in a case of lower segment cesarean section (LSCS)].
  - Any prelacteal feed given?
  - Was it exclusive breastfeeding for first 6 months of age?
  - Any top feeding—milk, powder milk.
  - By spoon and katori or bottle.
- *In children 6 months–2 years of age:*
  - Complementary feeds—when and which food?
  - Whether along with breastfeeding or not
  - Calculation of consumption of calories and protein.
- *In children more than 2 years of age:*
  - Calculate dietary intake for 24 hours, before the onset of illness
  - Calculation consumption of calories and proteins in 24 hours
  - See whether it is adequate or not as shown in **Table 4**.

Immunization History

Immunization history is a special feature of pediatric history taking, which hardly gets attention in other specialties. It helps to

Table 4: Energy and protein requirements in children.

Body weight (kg)	Requirements
Energy	
<10	100 cal/kg/day
10–20	1000 + 50 cal for every additional kilogram of body weight above 10 kg
>20	1500 cal + 20 cal/kg/day above 20 kg
Proteins	
<10	2.9/kg/day
>10	1.5 g/kg/day (minimum 20 g/day)

assess the possibility of vaccine preventable diseases and adverse reactions to vaccines in causation of present illness. It is best recorded by reviewing immunization record often available with the parents. If the record is not available, some points on interrogation can also be helpful as follows:

- Presence of BCG scar on left deltoid can be checked.
- MR vaccine is usually given on right shoulder.
- Timing and doses of vaccines can be helpful, e.g. three doses of vaccine given at 6, 10, and 14 weeks, are likely pentavalent (DPT + HBV + HIB).
- Oral vaccines may be OPV or rotavirus vaccines.
- Vaccines given at age of 18 months and 5 years are likely boosters.
- Information regarding national campaign vaccines like pulse polio and MR vaccines received or not should also be documented.

Information should also be obtained about adverse event following any vaccine.

It should also be asked whether child received any product for passive immunization like immunoglobulins, fresh frozen plasma, etc. It helps to know what was the indication for such therapy and possibility of any relation with present illness.

Personal History

Personal history may provide an important clue for certain conditions. The important information include eating habits, bladder and bowel control, sleeping patterns, temperament and behavioral problems, interactions with siblings, friends and parents, any drug abuse, total screen time (television, mobile, videogames, laptop, etc.). Menstrual history is very important for girls.

Social History

Social history helps in several ways like any risk factor for causation of disease and the most suitable diagnostic, therapeutic and rehabilitative interventions that are most appropriate for the parents. Three important components of social history include such as parental education status, parental occupation and family income. Kuppuswamy scale is most popular for assessment of socioeconomic status as per prevalent consumer price index of 2017 **(Table 5)**.

Table 5: Modified Kuppuswamy scale.

Variables	Score
Educational status	
• Profession or honors • Graduate or postgraduate • Intermediate or post-high school • High school • Middle school • Primary school • Illiterate	• 7 • 6 • 5 • 4 • 3 • 2 • 1
Occupational status	
• Professional • Semiprofessional • Clerical, shop owner, farmer • Skilled worker • Semiskilled worker • Unskilled worker • Unemployed	• 10 • 06 • 05 • 04 • 03 • 02 • 01
Monthly family income (Rupees)	
• >41,430 • 20,175–41,429 • 15,536–20,714 • 10,357–15,535 • 6,214–10,356 • 2,092–6,213 • <2,091	• 12 • 10 • 06 • 04 • 03 • 02 • 01

Contd…

Contd...

Variables	Score
Socioeconomic classification	
• Upper (I) • Upper middle (II) • Lower middle (III) • Upper lower (IV) • Lower (V)	• 26–29 • 16–25 • 11–15 • 5–10 • <5

> **Box 3:** Making presentation of history.
> - Greet the patient, teacher, or examiner
> - Inform regarding your presentation to the patient and teacher
> - You should be loud enough to listen
> - Language should be simple and grammatically correct with clear pronunciations
> - Presentation should be impressive, continuous flow, and sequential
> - The presentation should be story like, clear narration, and precise. Do not mention unnecessary negative points in the history. The point should be relevant to the present illness, either strengthening your possibility or excluding the condition
> - Unnecessary, lengthy, boring presentation should be avoided
> - Analyze and keep a track of time available for presentation
> - Conclude with brief summary

Environmental History

It indicates any environmental indoor or outdoor risk factor for health of the child. Like,

- Overcrowding
- Air quality assessed by ventilation, pollution of cooking fuel, passive smoke, construction activity, chemical or toxic fumes, etc.
- Water quality from its source, storage, and purification method of drinking water
- Sanitation—hygiene awareness and practices especially during food preparation, consumption and excreta disposal.

Some practical tips for presenting the history are as shown in Box 3.

General Physical Examination

CHAPTER 3

Baldev Prajapati

INTRODUCTION

After the detailed history, thorough general clinical examination is essential to derive the clinical diagnosis. General physical examination in children is the combination of art and science. This chapter deals with essential prerequisites for physical examination, an approach, interpretation of examination findings, and to derive logical conclusion. To become well-verse, regarding normal and abnormal findings on general physical examination, the students should examine several neonates, infants, and children.

- The examination of the child should be performed in proper setting, warm, well-illuminated, and comfortable room with all tools needed for examination. One should never do cursory examination at home, in the corridor or social gathering because in this type of set up, there are very high chances of missing important findings and diagnosis. The setting for examination is often unfamiliar for child causing undue anxiety. It is, therefore, important to make the environment pleasant and the atmosphere friendly. The yellow- or blue-colored curtains in the room should be avoided as they may interfere with the assessment of jaundice and cyanosis in the child. Daylight available in the examination room is very crucial.

  The tools required for clinical examination should include stethoscope, torch light, a measure tape made up from nonstretchable material like fiberglass, weighing machine, tongue spatula, blood pressure instrument, clinical digital thermometer, and some tools for assessment of development **(Fig. 1)**.

- The child should be in proper position so that he allows maximum access for examination.

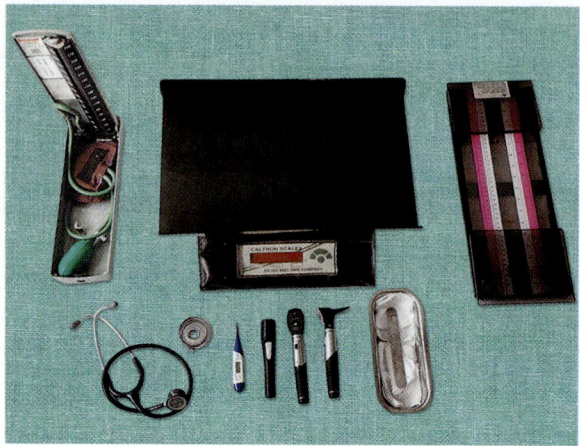

Fig. 1: Common tools required for clinical examination: Stethoscope, torch, a measure tape, weighing machine, infantometer, tongue spatula, BP instrument, digital thermometer, otoscope, ophthalmoscope, etc.

- Children between 3 months and 1 year are more comfortable in mother's lap.
- Between the age of 1 year and 3 years, child may be examined in sitting or standing position or in mother's lap.
- Children more than 3 years can be examined on examination table. Older children are usually cooperative and allow examination in different positions. If good rapport is established prior to examination with an adolescent, his cooperation is easily available.
- The adolescents must always be examined in the presence of the parents or paramedical staff.
- If the child is sleeping, try to examine him without disturbing much. An unpleasant examination should be performed at the end of examination, for example, throat examination by spatula, otoscopic examination, per rectal examination, etc. If the child cries during examination, wait for some time, if required, ask the mother to feed the child. Use of age-appropriate toys such as rattles, soft balls, blocks to keep the child engaged, distract his attention, etc., is quite rewarding.
- Proper exposure of an area to be examined is quite essential. If the child is to be undressed in order to examine, request

the mother or an attendant to do so and older child can be requested to do himself. Cover the patient as soon as possible once the task is over.
- Frequent eye contact with the child is necessary for smooth and successful examination.

Somebody rightly said, "Eyes, ears, nose, and palpating fingers are the real gems of physician and intact analytic brain is the necklace." They contribute in a following way:
- Sharp and keen observation
- Hearing (listen, percussion, and auscultation)
- Smell (ketosis, uremia, poisons, pus, fetor hepaticus, etc.)
- Touch (gentleness, sensitive, and dedicated hands)
- Analytic mind

THE FIRST IMPRESSION

Though a systemic approach and methodological examination are imperative, an initial impression (general appearance) of the child can often clinch the diagnosis. The important points to be noted on observation are listed in **Box 1**.
- *Severity of illness:* Appearance of a well-nourished, active, and alert child usually rules out a serious disease. There are certain red flag signs which should be noted and their presence indicates need of immediate attention and prompt action. These signs are listed in **Box 2**.
- *Nutrition and growth:* Is the child suffering from failure to thrive (FTT)? Is the child wasted, stunted? Is the child obese? Any obvious reason for obesity—syndrome, endocrinal or overeating? Signs of marasmus **(Fig. 2)** and kwashiorkor are obvious.

Box 1: Important points on observation.
- Look of face
- Dysmorphic facial features
- Posture and attitude
- Nutrition
- Breathing
- Nature of cry
- Mental status
- Abnormal movements

> **Box 2:** Red flag signs on general appearance.
> - Ill look/sick look
> - Altered sensorium (drowsiness, irritable)
> - Lethargic/generalized weakness (poor perfusion)
> - Abnormal posture (dyskinesia, dystonia, opisthotonic posture)
> - Respiratory distress
> - Petechial/purpuric spots on skin (sepsis/meningococcemia/dengue fever)
> - Faucial membrane (diphtheria)

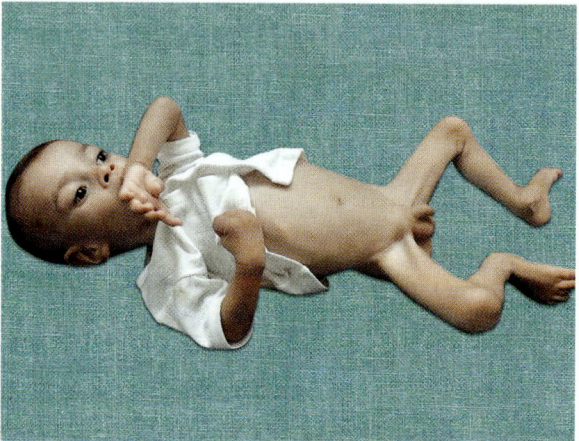

Fig. 2: Marasmus. Note the loss of fat from thighs, buttocks, groin and trunk. But the look is bright.

- *Facial dysmorphism:* Does the child have facial dysmorphism (abnormal physical features)? The phenotypic features of the child may suggest some of the syndromes like Down syndrome **(Fig. 3)**, Turner syndrome, Noonan syndrome **(Figs. 4A and B)**, Marfan syndrome, etc.
- *Pallor/cyanosis/jaundice:* One should check for pallor, cyanosis or jaundice. Severity of pallor, cyanosis, and jaundice should be assessed.
- *Hydration:* Assessment of hydration is very vital. Check for signs of dehydration and its severity.
- *Skin and its appendages:* Skin color, texture and signs of vitamins, and trace elements deficiency should be checked. Look for color of hair and check nails for clubbing or koilonychia.

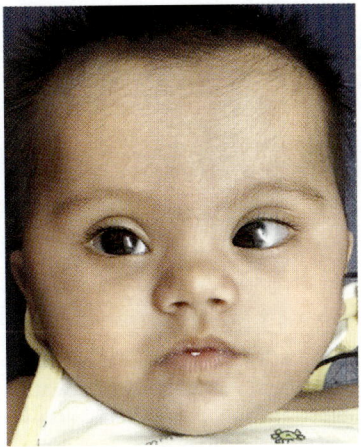

Fig. 3: Down syndrome. Note the slanting of eyes, depressed nasal bridge and hypertelorism.

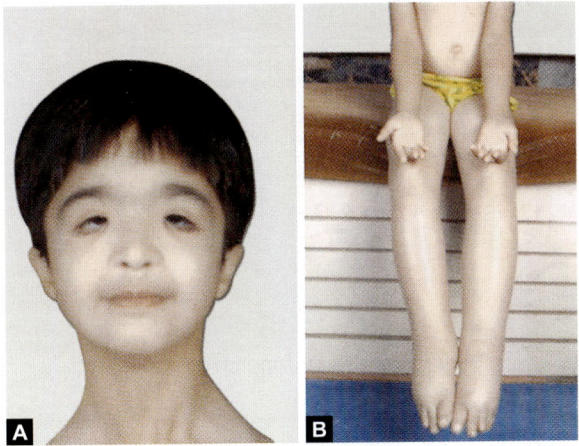

Figs. 4A and B: Noonan syndrome with nonpitting edema.

- *Behavior and responsiveness:* Is the child alert and active? Behavior should be observed, whether it is normal or abnormal. Is the child ill looking, sick looking or normal looking? Is the child lethargic, drowsy or unconscious? This information will help you to decide the gravity of the problem and necessity of prompt action.

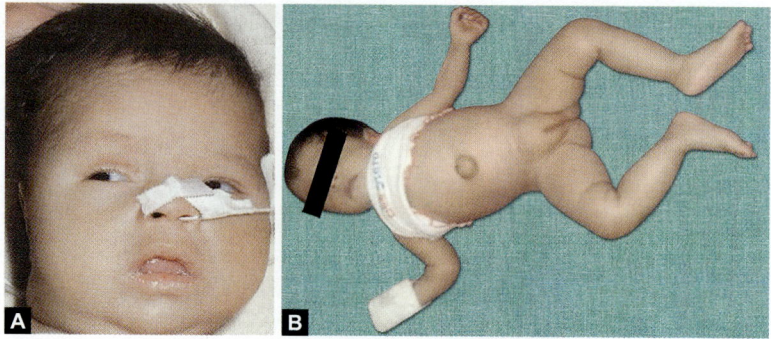

Figs. 5A and B: Hypothyroidism. (A) Coarse facial features in hypothyroidism; (B) Hypothyroidism in a neonate as floppy infant with coarse facial features, persistent neonatal jaundice and umbilical hernia.

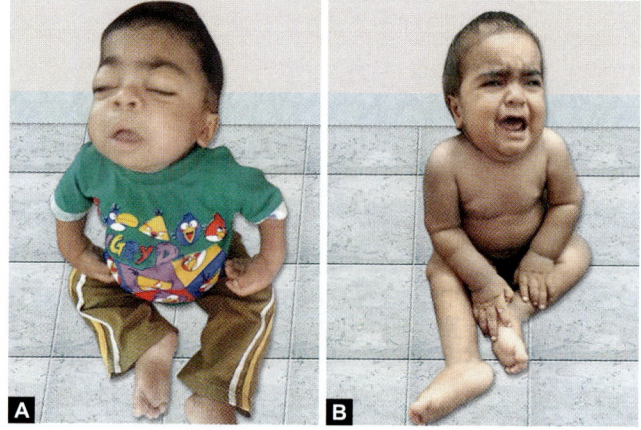

Figs. 6A and B: Mucopolysaccharidosis.

Other Abnormalities

Look for skin rash, edema, posture, and limb anomalies. Coarse facial features suggest hypothyroidism **(Figs. 5A and B)**, mucopolysaccharidosis **(Figs. 6A and B)**, etc.

VITAL PARAMETERS

The vital parameters include temperature, pulse (heart) rate, respiratory rate, blood pressure, capillary refill time (CRT), hydration, and oxygen saturation by pulse oximetry **(Box 3)**.

> **Box 3:** Vital parameters.
> - Temperature
> - Pulse (heart) rate
> - Respiratory rate
> - Blood pressure
> - Capillary refill time (CRT)
> - Hydration
> - Oxygen saturation

Temperature

The normal body temperature is 98.4°F (37°C). Body temperature fluctuates in the defined normal range 97.9–100.2°F (36.6–37.9°C), rectally. It is high in evening and low in the morning. Fever is defined as rectal temperature ≥100.4°F (38°C). The mild degrees of fever are more likely to be recognized in the evenings, so called as evening rise of temperature. Fever should always be measured by thermometer and documented. Palpation of skin to assess body temperature is widely used by the parents; it is less accurate and falsely labels children as having fever. Therefore, correct assessment of fever by using a proper and accurate temperature-measuring device is essential.

Measurement of Body Temperature

The measurement of body temperature should reflect the core temperature. The thermometer should be easy, comfortable to use, and give rapid results. It should not cause cross infection. It should not be influenced by room temperature, should be safe and cost-effective. There are several devices available at present to measure the body temperature, but no ideal method has been found yet. The various available thermometers are as shown in **Figures 7A to C**. The different methods of measuring body temperature are as follows:

- *Axillary temperature:* For accurate measurement of temperature, care must be taken that axilla is dry. The thermometer is kept in axilla with the bulb of the thermometer toward apex of axilla, the elbow is flexed, and the arm is held close to the chest wall. If mercury thermometer is used, it should be kept

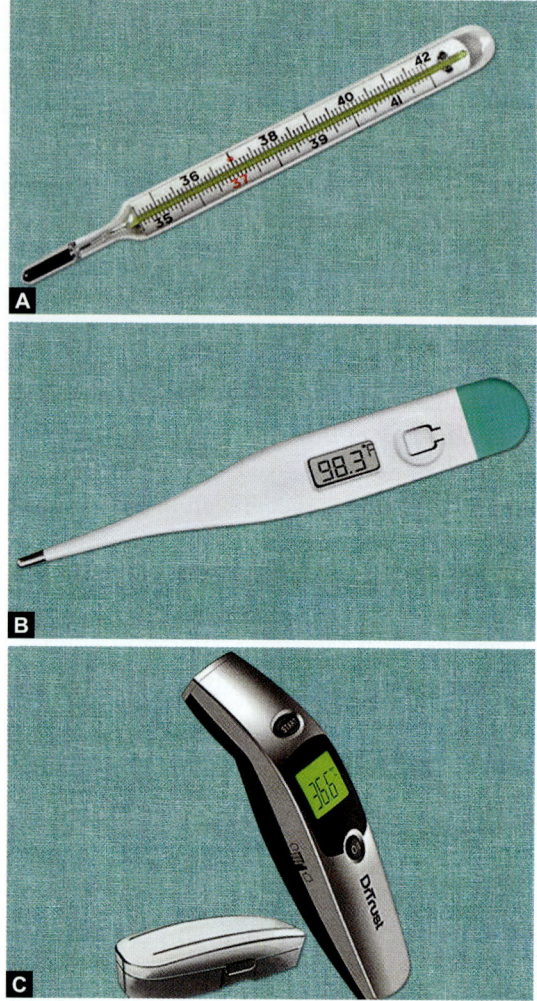

Figs. 7A to C: Different thermometers. (A) Mercury clinical thermometer; (B) Digital thermometer; (C) Infrared thermometer.

in place for 3 minutes. While using a digital thermometer, switch on the thermometer, and keep the bulb at the apex of dry axilla till its final beep. The thermometer should be cleaned with 70% isopropyl alcohol after each use, dried, and kept in its container. The axillary temperature is 1°C less than rectal temperature.

- *Sublingual (oral) temperature:* It reflects the temperature of lingual arteries. This method can be used in children older than 5 years. The mercury thermometer should not be used in this method to prevent accidental exposure and poisoning of mercury in case child bites the thermometer and breaks it. The mouth should remain sealed, with the tongue depressed for 3–4 minutes. The oral temperature is 0.5–1°C higher than axillary temperature.
- *Rectal temperature:* Rectal temperature is considered as most reliable temperature in children and is recommended for newborns and infants. The rectal thermometer is different from clinical thermometer, having rounded bulbous tip and low reading (30–40°C). The rectal thermometer should be cleaned with soap and water, wiped dry, and then used. Water-based jelly or lubricant is applied on the tip. Put the baby on his back on a firm surface. Hold the baby's ankles and lift both the legs. Gently, introduce the thermometer in the rectum, directing its tip posteriorly toward the back up to a depth of 2.5 cm. Hold the thermometer till it beeps. Remove the thermometer and read the temperature on the digital display. Clean it properly and keep in proper container. Due to accidental perforation of rectum, it is not routinely recommended.
- *Tympanic thermometer:* The degree of temperature of blood supplying to tympanic membrane and that of to the hypothalamus are very close to each other. Therefore, it is the ideal location for core temperature estimation. They measure the thermal radiation emitted from the tympanic membrane and the ear canal and are called infrared radiation emission detectors (IRED). The amount of thermal radiation emitted in proportion to the membrane's temperature, IRED accurately estimates tympanic membrane temperature. Crying, otitis media or earwax have not been shown to change tympanic readings significantly.
- *Temporal artery thermometer:* It reads the infrared heat released by the temporal artery, which runs across the forehead just below the skin. It can be used in 3 months and older children. Before the age of 3 months, it is used as a screening device. The temperature should be taken on the side of forehead.

Examination of Pulse

- *Definition of pulse:* Pulse is defined as expansion of the vessel wall due to propagation of wave produced by movement of blood column ejected from the heart during each systolic contraction which is felt by a palpating finger.
- *Presence of peripheral pulsations:* The radial pulse is examined using index, middle, and ring fingers with the arm in semipronation and the wrist slightly flexed. If the radial pulse is feeble or absent, check the pulsations of bigger arteries like brachial, femoral, carotid, etc. The radial pulsations may be feeble or absent when the patient is in shock. The femoral pulsations may be diminished while other pulsations may be good in coarctation of the aorta. The upper limb pulsations may be weak or absent in Takayasu arteritis.

  In an obese child, radial artery located behind radius bone or an aberrant pathway of vessel, it may be difficult to palpate radial pulsations or may not be palpable.
- *Pulse rate:* Pulse rate should be counted when the child is relaxed and comfortable. In an irritable or crying child, pulse rate may be high which should not be mistaken for tachycardia. The pulse should be counted for a complete minute. In an emergency situation, count the pulse for 6 seconds and multiply it by 10 to get the pulse rate per minute.

  In conditions like irritable, excessive crying child, fever, and thyrotoxicosis, there may be tachycardia. The pulse rate increases by 10 for each degree of rise in body temperature. If it is not proportionate, it is called as relative bradycardia. The relative bradycardia is seen in enteric fever and brucellosis. Relative bradycardia in enteric fever is not common in young children; it may be seen in older children and adults. The sleeping tachycardia is considered as pathognomic sign of rheumatic fever. Tachycardia may be the early sign of poor perfusion or shock.
- *Rhythm:* Assess the rhythm of the pulse. The pulse may vary with respiration (sinus tachycardia—heart rate increases with inspiration, sinus bradycardia—heart rate decreases with expiration), which is called as physiological arrhythmia.

If the pulse is irregular, try to define its pattern, atrial fibrillation, atrial flutter, extrasystoles or missed beats.
- *Volume:* The uplifting of middle finger (thrust) measures the pulse volume. Low volume pulse is observed in shock, aortic stenosis, cardiomyopathy, and vasculitis. High volume pulse is present in conditions with hyperdynamic circulation like anemia, thyrotoxicosis, high-grade fever, etc. It is also found in aortic regurgitation (AR), mitral regurgitation, patent ductus arteriosus (PDA), hypertension, arteriovenous fistula, etc.
- *Force:* The pressure required to feel the arterial pulsation is called force. It indicates systolic blood pressure.
- *Tension:* The pressure required to obliterate the pulsations is called tension. It indicates diastolic blood pressure.
  The proximal finger is pressed to obliterate radial pulsations felt by middle finger. The distal finger is pressed to prevent the pulsations from ulnar artery being conducted into the radial artery through palmar arch.
- *Radiofemoral delay:* Feel the radial and femoral pulsations simultaneously, they are felt together. If femoral pulsations are delayed to radial pulsations, it is called as radiofemoral delay and it indicates coarctation of aorta.
- *Radioradial delay:* Feel both radial arteries at the same time; if there is delay in left radial arterial pulsations, it indicates preductal coarctation of aorta.
- *Pulse apex deficit:* Presence of a disparity of 10 or more between auscultated heart rate and the palpated radial arterial pulse rate, both estimated at the same time for a full 1 minute, is called as pulse apex deficit. In atrial fibrillation, ventricular premature beats-like conditions manifest with pulse apex deficit.
- Vessel wall is normal in children. It is thickened in old age people due to atherosclerosis.
- *Bounding (hyperkinetic) pulse:*
  - Bounding pulse is characterized by high amplitude, large volume pulse with rapidly rising ascending wave.
  - Present in conditions with high cardiac output with decreased peripheral arterial resistance and wide pulse pressure, e.g. anxiety, exercise, fever, anemia, thyrotoxicosis, beriberi, arteriovenous fistula, AR, ventricular septal defect (VSD), PDA, etc.

- *Water hammer (collapsing) pulse:* A large volume pulse with abrupt and rapid upstroke followed by equal downstroke due to the rapid and reverse diastolic run off into the left ventricle in AR, PDA, etc. and rapid run off to the peripheral vessels due to decreased systemic peripheral vascular resistance in hyperkinetic states like anemia, fever, pregnancy, thyrotoxicosis, etc.
- *Hypokinetic pulse:* It is characterized by weak, small volume pulse felt with difficulty. It is found in conditions with low cardiac output, shock, severe cardiac failure, myocarditis, coarctation of aorta, cardiac tamponade, etc.

Pulsus Paradoxus

The term pulsus paradoxus is a misnomer as it represents an exaggeration of a normal phenomenon. There is marginal physiologic decrease in systolic BP during inspiration, from 5 mm Hg to 10 mm Hg. Pulsus paradoxus is defined as difference of BP more than 10 mm Hg taken during expiration and inspiration. Often, this difference is more than 20 mm Hg.

Respiration

While assessing the respiration, note the respiratory rate, its depth, regularity, and any specific type, if it is there.
- *Respiration rate:* The respiratory rate should be counted for complete 60 seconds when the child is quiet (not crying) or sleeping. The normal respiratory rates vary with age of the child. Age-specific normal respiratory rates are shown in **Table 1**.

Table 1: Age-specific normal respiratory rates.	
Age	*Respiratory rate (breaths/min)*
Premature	40–60
Term newborn	30–50
1 month to 1 year	20–40
1–5 years	20–30
5–10 years	15–25
Above 10 years	15–20

Table 2: Cut-off for tachypnea at different age groups.

Age	Respiratory rate
0 to 2 months	≥60/min
2 months to 1 year	≥50/min
1 year to 5 years	≥40/min
>5 years	≥30/min

The cut-off rates for tachypnea at different ages are shown in **Table 2**. Bradypnea refers to decreased respiratory rate and is seen in hypothyroidism, increased intracranial pressure, and alkalosis.

- *Type of respiration:* The respiration is usually abdominal or abdominothoracic in infants and thoracic in older children. In normal inspiration, the thorax and abdomen move out and converse occurs in expiration. Paradoxical respiration occurs in diaphragmatic paralysis when the movement of abdomen is inward in inspiration. In unilateral diaphragmatic paralysis, there is decreased movement of diaphragm on the affected side.
- *Rhythm:*
  - Periodic breathing occurs normally in neonates. In periodic breathing, there are alternate periods of rapid respiration and apnea. The rapid respiration is followed by apnea which is not longer than 20 seconds and is not associated with bradycardia or cyanosis.
  - Cheyne–Stokes breathing is similar to periodic breathing (period of apnea), but occurs in older children with cardiac failure or cerebral edema.
  - Biot's breathing is characterized by apnea followed by four to five normal breaths. It is seen in conditions with raised intracranial pressure.
- *Work of breathing:* The increased work of breathing is characterized by tachypnea, use of accessory muscles of respiration, and different sounds **(Box 4)**. The presence of common respiratory sounds denotes their site of origin **(Table 3)** which helps to decide the site of pathology and likely etiology.

Box 4: Signs of increased work of breathing.
- Tachypnea
- Flaring of alae nasi
- Retractions (subcostal/intercostal/suprasternal)
- Use of accessory muscles of respiration (sternocleidomastoid)
- Tracheal tug (inward movement of trachea during inspiration)
- Head bobbing
- Various sounds (stridor/wheezing/grunting)
- Cyanosis

Table 3: Common respiratory sounds and their site of origin.

Sound	Site of origin	Phase of respiration when heard
Snuffle	Nasal passage	Inspiration/expiration
Snore	Oropharyngeal airway	Inspiration/expiration
Stridor	Extrathoracic airway	Inspiration
Wheeze	Intrathoracic airway	Expiration
Grunt	Lung parenchyma	Expiration

- *Depth of respiration:* The normal sequence of respiration is inspiration–expiration–pause. The respiration may be shallow in narcotic poisoning and cervical cord compression. It may be rapid and deep in metabolic acidosis (diabetic ketoacidosis, severe dehydration, acute renal failure, inborn error of metabolism, salicylate poisoning, etc.). Kussmaul breathing is characterized by deep breathing (increased tidal volume), seen in children with metabolic acidosis. Rapid and shallow breathing is seen in pleurisy.
- *Adventitious sounds:* Presence of audible adventitious sounds without use of stethoscope is of great clinical importance **(Table 3)**.

Blood Pressure

Blood pressure is defined as the lateral pressure exerted on the vessel wall by the blood, while flowing through it. The systolic blood pressure is chiefly determined by the force of contraction of the left ventricle. The diastolic blood pressure is regulated by the arteriolar resistance. Blood pressure should be measured routinely as a part of the physical examination of children. Every child over the age of 3 years should have his blood pressure measured once a year and during every visit to the doctor during adolescence. The blood pressure should be measured in all the four limbs.

Measurement of Blood Pressure

There are four methods by which blood pressure can be measured:
1. Sphygmomanometer method
2. Flush method (mainly for newborns)
3. Oscillometer method
4. Doppler method

Sphygmomanometer method:
- *Prerequisites:* It is a conventional method. In routine daily practice, the blood pressure is measured in the upper arm (brachial artery). The child should be lying comfortably in bed or sitting with arm kept at the level of heart. The appropriate size of cuff which covers two-thirds of upper arm (or width of the cuff should be 40% of the circumference of the arm) should be used. The recommended cuff size in infants below age of 1 year is 2.5 cm, 1–4 years is 5 cm, 5–9 years is 9 cm, and over 10 years is 13 cm. The use of a narrow blood pressure cuff is associated with high systolic blood pressure reading and vice versa. The cuff is applied snugly over the upper arm by keeping its lower edge at least 2 cm above the cubital fossa. The manometer should be kept at the level of heart and should be conveniently placed for the observer to see it easily.
- *Method of measuring blood pressure:*
  - *Palpatory method:* Inflate the pressure cuff while palpating the brachial pulse. The reading at which brachial pulse disappears is suggesting systolic blood pressure.
  - *Auscultatory method:* Inflate the cuff 20–30 mm Hg above the reading of palpatory method and then listen through the diaphragm of stethoscope placed over the brachial artery. Deflate the cuff slowly by decrements of 2–3 mm Hg and the point when Korotkoff sounds are first heard is indicating systolic blood pressure. When the cuff is further deflated,

the Korotkoff sounds become muffled and finally disappear which indicates diastolic blood pressure. Sometimes, the Korotkoff sound does not disappear and in that case muffling of sounds is taken as criterion for diastolic blood pressure.

For recording lower limb blood pressure, the child is asked to lie in prone position. The cuff is applied over the thigh and stethoscope is placed over the popliteal artery in the popliteal fossa. Normally, the lower limb systolic blood pressure is more by 10–30 mm Hg while the diastolic blood pressure is identical in upper and lower limbs. The pulse pressure is the difference between the systolic and diastolic blood pressure and is indicative of pulse volume. Ideally, blood pressure should be measured in all the four limbs, especially when coarctation of aorta or Takayasu disease is suspected.

Flush method: The limb should be raised and squeezed till the hand or foot becomes pale. The cuff should be rapidly inflated so that blanching is noted. The pressure should be gradually and slowly released by 5 mm holding for about 5 seconds at each step. The point at which the flushing of the hand or foot is seen represents the systolic pressure which is about 5 mm Hg less than that obtained by the auscultatory method. The diastolic pressure cannot be recorded by this technique. Flush pressure is not affected by the cuff size to any great degree. Flush method is mainly used in newborns.

Oscillometer method: When the pressure in the cuff is released, the point at which the oscillometer needle begins to flick regularly is the systolic BP and the point where the oscillations are maximal denotes the diastolic pressure.

Doppler method: This is the most reliable method. The baby is made to lie in supine position and an approximate-sized cuff is fitted around the arm. The probe of the ultrasonic Doppler is placed over the radial artery at an angle of 15°. The exact position of the radial artery is located by listening to the hissing sound through the headphone attached to the Doppler cuff which is inflated quickly till the hissing sound ceases. Then the pressure is gradually released and the point at which the hissing sound reappears corresponds to the systolic pressure. Diastolic pressure cannot be recorded by this method.

Normally, standing pressure is higher than supine pressure. The difference between the leg and arm BP is normally 10–15 mm Hg. In children, both diastolic and systolic BP increase with emotional tension. Most children have high BP in the late afternoon or evening than in the morning.

Blood pressure varies with the age of the child and is closely related to height and weight. Significant increases occur during adolescence. Serial measurements should always be obtained in the evaluation of the patient with hypertension.

Capillary Refill Time

Capillary refill time is a very useful bedside test to assess the peripheral perfusion of tissues. It is also called as capillary filling time (CFT). It is performed by pressing a thumb against bony prominence (sternum or forehead) for 5 seconds and allows the skin to be blanched. Note the time taken for the skin to regain its normal color. In a normal child with good perfusion, skin regains the normal pink color within 3 seconds. CRT is said to be delayed if it is ≥3 seconds and it indicates poor perfusion and shock. It can also be tested by blanching the finger pulp or nail beds, provided that hands are warm.

Assessment of Hydration

Assessment of hydration is an integral part of general physical examination of any child and especially in a child presenting with diarrhea. The following signs are used to assess the hydration:
- Assess the sensorium and general condition of the child. See whether the child is alert, lethargic, restless/irritable or drowsy. Offer the water to the child to drink and note whether he accepts readily (thirsty) or refuses to drink.
- Sunken eye balls are a sign of dehydration. It may not be a reliable sign in a marasmic child.
- *Look for skin turgor (skin elasticity):* Pinch the skin over abdomen, midway between the umbilicus and flank, release it.

Table 4: Assessment of severity of dehydration.

Criteria	Some dehydration	Severe dehydration
Sensorium*	Restless and irritable	Lethargic or unconscious
Eyes*	Sunken	Very sunken
Skin pinch*	Skin goes back slowly	Skin goes back very slowly (>2 seconds)
Oral mucosa	Dry	Very dry
Thirst	Drinks eagerly	Unable to drink
Urine output	Decreased	Very decreased or absent

Note: As per Integrated Management of Neonatal and Childhood Illness (IMNCI) any of the two signs marked as "*" should be present in a child to label as some or severe dehydration.

The skin goes back immediately in a normal child with good hydration. If it goes back very slowly (more than 2 seconds) or slowly (skin stays up even for a brief instant), it indicates presence of dehydration. In a marasmic child, the skin may go back slowly even if the child is not dehydrated. The reverse may occur in an obese child or a child with abdominal wall edema. Therefore, this sign is not reliable to assess the hydration in children with marasmus, obesity or abdominal wall edema like nephrotic syndrome.

- The severity of dehydration is assessed as shown in **Table 4**. The child with no dehydration is alert, with moist oral mucosa, the skin pinch goes back immediately, the child is not thirsty, and has normal urine output.

Oxygen Saturation

Oxygen saturation is an important parameter and this can be assessed at bedside by noninvasive modality of pulse oximetry. It measures the percentage saturation of hemoglobin bound with oxygen in the blood.

- *Method:* An oxygen saturation probe is attached to a pulse oximeter applied across a capillary rich area like pulp of finger or toe or ear lobule. The right middle finger is desirable site for it. The infrared rich light source allows light to pass through tissues and depending upon the concentration of

oxygenated hemoglobin, some of the light is absorbed and what comes out at the receiving end of the probe is analyzed by a microprocessor. The values are expressed as percentage of oxygen saturation of hemoglobin. Saturation less than 90% indicates hypoxemia.
- *Advantage and disadvantages:* The main advantages of pulse oximetry are that it is noninvasive, reproducible, requires minimal training, and very useful for bedside use. However, it has some limitations like its accuracy is less when oxygen saturation is <70%, hemoglobinopathies, hypotension, hypothermia or carbon monoxide poisoning.

Anthropometry

Anthropometric data are useful to assess the nutrition and growth of the child. It is quite essential to measure the parameters like weight, length/height, head circumference, mid-arm circumference, and upper segment and lower segment ratio as a part of general examination of every child. One should also calculate body mass index (BMI) of every child. These parameters should be plotted on appropriate growth charts and assess the nutrition and growth of the child. Anthropometry has been discussed in detail separately.

HEAD-TO-TOE EXAMINATION
Examination of Head

- *Size and shape of head:*
  - Head circumference should be measured and compared with normal values for the age and sex of the child.
  - Microcephaly is defined as head circumference <3 SD below normal. It can be primary or secondary. Slanting forehead is very often associated with microcephaly. Primary microcephaly is when the brain is inherently small since birth with or without its potential for growth. It may be familial and child is asymptomatic with normal development. It may be associated with genetic disorders. The secondary microcephaly occurs due to primary insult to growing brain. It is often associated with global developmental delay. The common causes of primary and secondary microcephaly are shown in **Table 5**.

Table 5: Causes of primary and secondary microcephaly.

Primary microcephaly	Secondary microcephaly

Familial	• Intrauterine infections:
	  – Cytomegalovirus
	  – Rubella
	  – Toxoplasmosis

• Chromosomal:
  – Down syndrome
  – Edward syndrome
  – Rubinstein–Taybi syndrome
	• Intrauterine toxins:
	  – Fetal alcohol syndrome
	  – Fetal hydantoin syndrome

	• Perinatal and postnatal insults:
	  – Birth asphyxia
	  – Meningitis
	  – Encephalitis

- *Macrocephaly:* It is defined as head circumference >2 SD above normal. Common causes of macrocephaly are listed in **Box 5**.
- *Shape of head:* Look for shape of head whether it is normal or abnormal. The abnormal shapes of the skull are described in **Box 6**.
- *Sutures:* All the sutures should be palpated and see whether they are normal, prematurely closed or widely separated. Early closure may indicate craniosynostosis and widely separated sutures may be due to hydrocephalus **(Fig. 8)**, rickets, raised intracranial pressure, congenital hypothyroidism or skeletal dysplasia like achondroplasia or osteogenesis imperfecta.
- *Fontanels:* Palpate all the fontanels. A neonate has normally six fontanels, anterior, posterior, two mastoid, and two sphenoid. Examine the fontanels in details whether they are open/closed, large/small, bulging/sunken, pulsatile/nonpulsatile, etc.
  - The rhomboid-shaped anterior fontanel (AF), located at the junction of the two parietal and two frontal bones, is the most prominent and important in clinical examination. The AF measures 2.5 × 2.5 cm at birth in a term baby. The posterior fontanel (PF) at birth usually is the size of tip of the little finger (0.5 cm).
  - Usually, AF closes between 9 months and 18 months of age while the PF closes by 6 weeks of age.

General Physical Examination

Box 5: Common causes of macrocephaly.

- Familial
- Hydrocephalus (congenital/acquired)
- Mucopolysaccharidosis
- White matter degenerative disorders like Canavan and Alexander diseases
- Neurocutaneous disorders like neurofibromatosis, tuberous sclerosis, etc.
- Cerebral gigantism (Sotos syndrome)

Box 6: Abnormal shapes of the skull.

- *Brachycephaly:* It is due to premature closure of coronal sutures. The head cannot grow in the anteroposterior (AP) diameter and grows only in transverse diameter, resulting in square and short skull, e.g., Down syndrome
- *Scaphocephaly (dolichocephaly):* It is due to premature closure of sagittal sutures. The head grows only in AP diameter, resulting in anteroposteriorly elongated skull. The parietal eminences are usually absent. May be seen in Hurler syndrome
- *Trigonocephaly:* It is due to early closure of metopic sutures. It is pointed skull, prominent mid forehead ridging
- *Oxycephaly (acrocephaly/turricephaly):* There is early closure of multiple sutures. This leads to compensatory upward growth of skull, resulting in elongation of skull like a tower. It is seen in Apert and Carpenter syndrome
- *Plagiocephaly:* It is due to unilateral premature closure of coronal or lambdoid sutures. It results in skewing of skull. It may be a flattened occiput. Viewed from above, it looks like a parallelogram. This is usually a postural deformity in early infancy that often gets corrected as the child grows

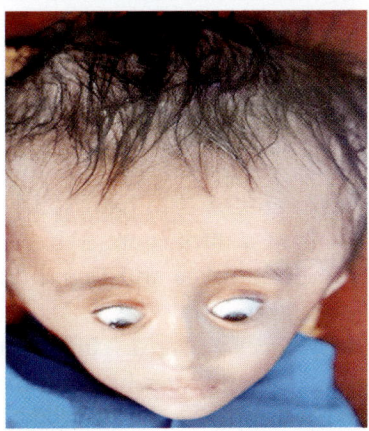

Fig. 8: Hydrocephalus. Note Sun-setting sign.

- The AF should be palpated when the infant is quiet and sitting or held upright with the head lifted up. A bulging AF in a crying child does not necessarily mean increased intracranial pressure.
- The tension in AF is important in deciding whether there is an increased intracranial pressure (bulging and non-pulsatile) or dehydration (depressed/sunken).
- A bulging AF in cases of raised intracranial pressure is seen in meningitis, hydrocephalus, intracranial hemorrhage, benign intracranial hypertension, etc.
- If a bulging and tense AF is accompanied by a large head and separated sutures, then the raised intracranial pressure is the most likely cause.
- Delayed closure of AF can occur in rickets, congenital hypothyroidism, hydrocephalus **(Fig. 8)**, Down syndrome, skeletal dysplasia like achondroplasia, osteogenesis imperfecta, etc.
- Small AF or early close of AF may be due to craniosynostosis.
- Prominent scalp veins may be seen in hydrocephalus.

- *Craniotabes:* Craniotabes refers to a reduction in rigidity of the cranial bones. Its presence indicates softening of skull bones which may get indented like a ping pong ball when pressed away from the lines. Craniotabes is a characteristic of rickets. It is also normally seen in skull of premature babies.
- *Frontal bossing of skull:* It is present in rickets, Hurler syndrome, and thalassemia.
- *Transillumination:* Transillumination should be performed, if subdural effusion, hydrocephalus **(Fig. 8)**, porencephaly or hydranencephaly is suspected. Illuminate with a torch light with a rubber foam cuff or cold light source over the frontal and occipital areas in a dark room. When transillumination exceeds 2.5 cm in frontal area and 1 cm in the occipital area, it is considered as abnormal.
- *Cracked pot sign (Macewen sign):* This should be performed only in children whose fontanels have been closed. A positive sign indicates raised intracranial pressure. The head of the child should be raised. Tap lightly on one side of the parietal

eminence and listen to the reverberating sound on the opposite parietal eminence. The stethoscope can also be used to listen the quality of sound. A characteristic sound as if coming from a cracked pot suggests raised intracranial pressure.
- *Cranial bruits:* It should be auscultated for over vertex, occipital, and temporal regions. Its presence suggests vascular malformation like vein of Galen.

Face

Looking at face may provide important clues for clinical diagnosis, especially in a child with dysmorphic features. Observe symmetry of the face, record any malformation of the eyes, ears, nose, mouth, teeth, hairline, forehead, etc., if present. Some characteristic facies are shown in **Figures 9A to D**.

Eyes

Examination of eyes may provide important information which may be useful for clinical diagnosis. Observe for any anatomical, congenital, and acquired defect, test the functions of extraocular muscles, acuity of vision, color vision, light reflex, etc. Examine the pupil in details for its size, reaction to light, unequal or equal on both sides, etc. Lastly, carry out the fundus examination.
- *Size of eyeballs:* Eye balls may be prominent (exophthalmos), deep (enophthalmos), small (microphthalmos) or enlarged (buphthalmos). Exophthalmos may be seen in hyperthyroidism, Crouzon syndrome, neuroblastoma, retinoblastoma, etc. Enophthalmos is seen in Horner syndrome or post-traumatic, microphthalmia may be seen in congenital infections like, CMV, rubella, etc.
- *Placement:* The distance between the two eyes may be measured in terms of inner canthal distance, midpupillary distance, and outer canthal distance. The distance between the inner corners of both eyes is called intercanthal distance. Normally, the intercanthal distance is equal to the distance between the inner corner and outer corner of each eye equaling the width of the eye. If the intercanthal distance is more than width of the eye, it may be telecanthus or hypertelorism.

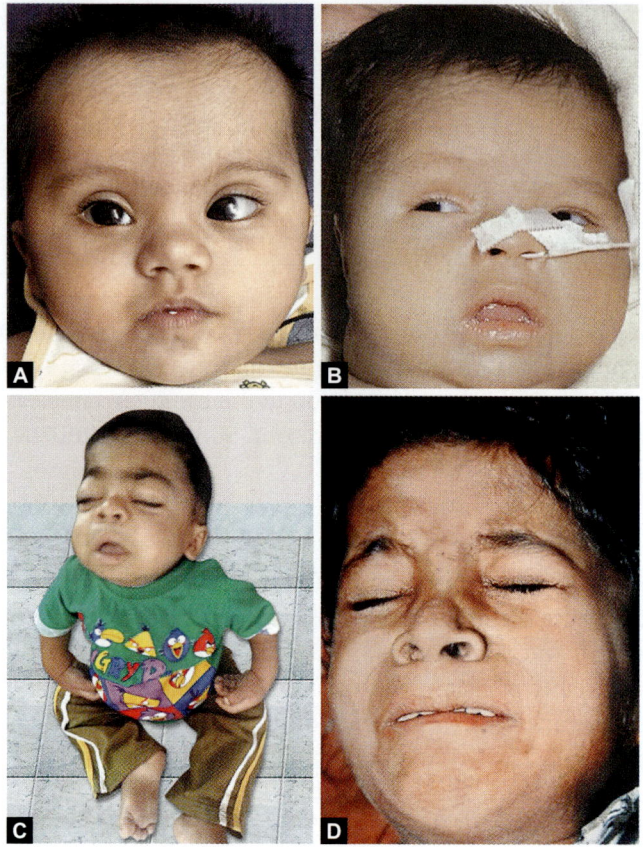

Figs. 9A to D: Characteristic facies. (A) Down syndrome. Note slanting of eyes, depressed nasal bridge, hypertelorism; (B) Hypothyroidism with coarse facial features; (C) Mucopolysaccharidosis; (D) Risus sardonicus in a case of tetanus.

If the intercanthal distance is increased, but interpupillary distance is normal, it indicates telecanthus, but if both are increased, it indicates hypertelorism. Hypertelorism may be seen in Down syndrome **(Fig. 3)**, Turner syndrome, Noonan syndrome **(Figs. 4A and B)**, cretinism, thalassemia, etc. Hypotelorism may be seen in trisomy 13 (Patau syndrome).
- *Slanting of eyes:* A palpebral slant wherein the outer canthus is higher than the inner canthus is called mongoloid or

upward slant. It is seen in Down syndrome **(Fig. 3)**, Prader–Willi syndrome, ectodermal dysplasia, etc.

If the inner canthus is higher than the outer canthus, it is called downward slant (antimongoloid slant). It is seen in Treacher Collins syndrome, Turner syndrome, Apert syndrome, Noonan syndrome, Cri-du-chat syndrome, etc.

- *Epicanthic folds:* Epicanthic folds are folds of skin which project from the upper lid over the medial epicanthus. Epicanthic folds are seen in Down syndrome **(Fig. 3)**, Turner syndrome, Noonan syndrome, Cornelia de Lange syndrome, etc.
- *Eyelids:* Look for developmental defects like coloboma. Eyelid edema is very common. It can be seen in renal causes like acute nephritis, renal failure, pertussis, conjunctivitis, infectious mononucleosis, etc. Ptosis (drooping of eye lids) can be congenital or acquired, unilateral or bilateral. Ptosis is seen in Horner syndrome, oculomotor nerve palsy, myasthenia gravis **(Fig. 10)**, botulism, etc.
- *Eyebrows and eyelashes:*
  - Eyebrows are sparse in premature babies and hypothyroidism. Eyebrows meeting in midline (synophrys) are seen in Cornelia de Lange syndrome **(Fig. 11)** and Waardenburg syndrome.

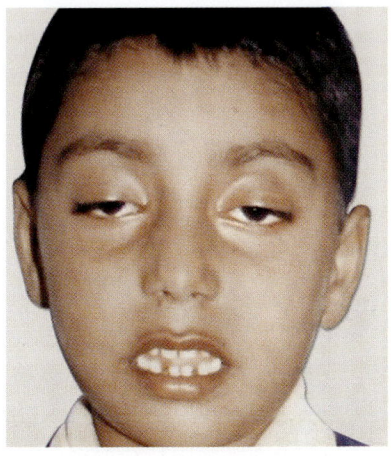

Fig. 10: Ptosis in a case of myasthenia gravis.

- Scanty or absent eyelashes are seen in ectodermal dysplasia **(Fig. 12)** cartilage hair hypoplasia, Treacher Collins syndrome, etc.
- Long and curly eyelashes are seen in Cornelia de Lang, syndrome **(Fig. 11)**.
- Hypopigmentation of eyebrows and eyelashes occurs in children with albinism.

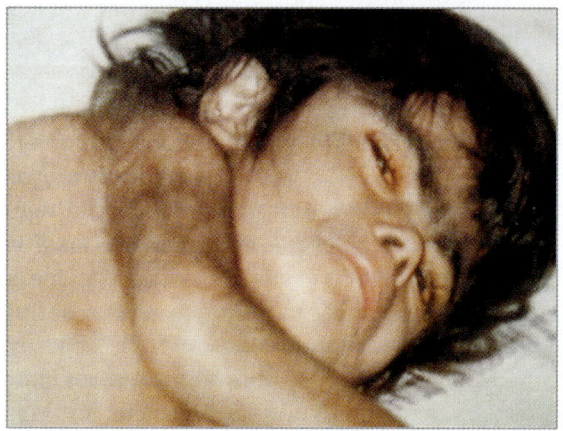

Fig. 11: Cornelia de Lange syndrome. Note the long philtrum, up turned nostrils, excessive eyebrows, long eye lashes and hypertrichosis.

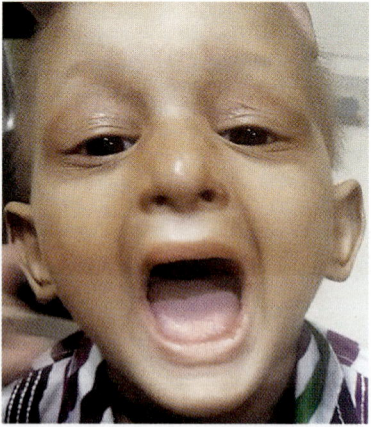

Fig. 12: Ectodermal dysplasia. Note absence of eyebrows, eyelashes and teeth.

- *Conjunctiva:* Examine conjunctiva for dryness (vitamin A deficiency), scarring (trachoma), hemorrhages **(Fig. 13)** (whooping cough, scurvy), and vascularization (riboflavin deficiency)
  - Look for pterygium.
  - Look for any infection (conjunctivitis).
  - Look for conjunctival injection (Bilateral nonpurulent in Kawasaki disease).
  - Pallor of conjunctiva indicates anemia.
- *Cornea:*
  - Dryness and ulceration (keratomalacia) is seen in vitamin A deficiency.
  - Look for microcornea (<10 mm) and megalocornea (>13 mm).
  - Kayser–Fleischer (KF) ring is a brownish ring around the cornea and is characteristic of Wilson disease **(Fig. 14)**. If it is not seen by naked eye, it should be examined by slit-lamp examination. It can also be seen in chronic liver disease.
  - Clouding of cornea is common in Hurler syndrome, Morquio syndrome, Scheie syndrome, tyrosinosis, etc.
  - Interstitial keratitis is seen in syphilis.
- *Sclera:*
  - Sclera is made up of yellow elastic fibers, a type of connective tissues.
  - *Look for yellow sclera (jaundice):* As bile salts and bile pigments have affinity for yellow elastic fibers, in a case of jaundice, they are getting deposited in sclera.
  - With thinning or stretching of sclera, the presence of venous plexus behind the sclera makes it bluish. Blue sclera **(Fig. 15)**

Fig. 13: Subconjunctival hemorrhage.

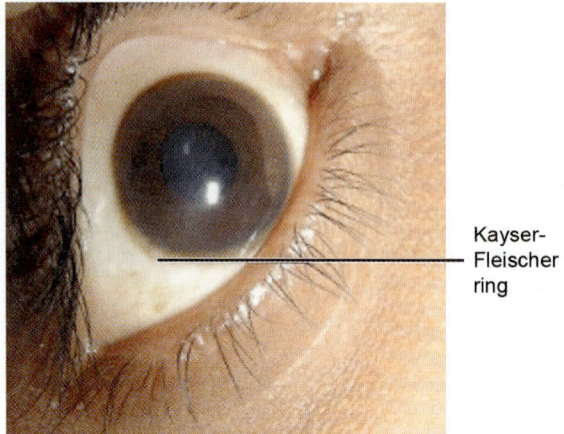

Fig. 14: Kayser–Fleischer ring in a case of Wilson disease.

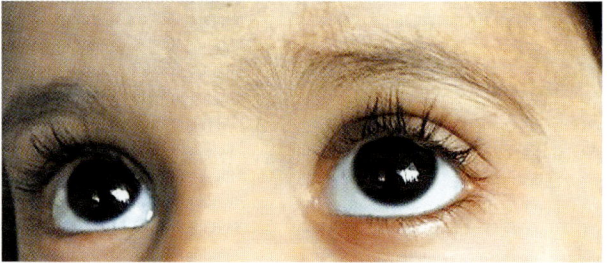

Fig. 15: Blue sclera.

can be normal in preterm babies. It can also be seen in normal children. Blue sclera is seen in osteogenesis imperfect, Ehlers–Danlos syndrome, Marfan syndrome, etc.
- *Pupils:* Look for pupil size, symmetry, and reaction to the light.
- *Iris:* Look for absent iris (aniridia) seen in Wilms tumor and brushfield spots (seen in Down syndrome). Lisch nodules may be seen in neurofibromatosis.
- *Lens:*
    - Cataract (lenticular opacity) may be congenital in TORCH infection—especially rubella, Marfan syndrome, homocystinuria, Down syndrome, etc. It can be acquired due to radiation therapy, steroid therapy for long time, trauma, etc.

- Lens may be dislocated or subluxated in case of Marfan syndrome, homocystinuria, etc.
- White reflex in the eye is the characteristic of retinoblastoma.

- *Lacrimal glands:* Look for dacryocystitis which is seen commonly in neonates due to congenital nasolacrimal duct obstruction.
- *Tears:* Congenital absence of tears occurs in familial dysautonomia syndrome. Decreased tear production may be seen in Sjögren's syndrome, vitamin A deficiency, and some drug therapies like antihistaminics, decongestants, etc.

  Watering eye (epiphora) means overflow of tears onto the face, occurs due to blocked tear ducts or excessive production of tears. Excessive production of tears may be due to some chemicals, fumes, onions, allergic conjunctivitis, infective conjunctivitis, ectropion, Bell's palsy, etc.
- *Vision:* Acuity of vision should be tested by Snellen chart in older children. Color vision can be tested by Ishihara chart.
- *Fundoscopy:* An ophthalmoscopic examination for fundus is essential and every pediatrician should know it.
  - Look for optic disk margins and depth of the optic disk.
  - Papilledema is seen in conditions with raised intracranial pressure.
  - Look for any retinal hemorrhage, optic therapy, chorioretinitis, etc.
  - Cherry red spot **(Fig. 16)** may be seen in Tay–Sachs disease and gangliosidosis.

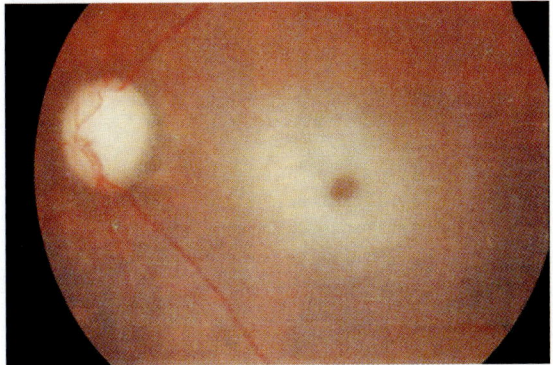

Fig. 16: Cherry red spot in Tay-Sachs disease and gangliosidosis.

- Choroid tubercles are seen in a case of military tuberculosis.
- Roth spot is seen in a case of bacterial endocarditis.

Examination of Ears

The ear examination should include its anatomical position (placement), any external ear anomaly, infection, otoscopic examination, and hearing.

- *Anatomical position—low set or normal?:* A horizontal line drawn joining both the medial canthi and extended outward, the helix usually lies above this line. If the helix lies below this line, the ears are said to be "low set". Low-set ears are seen in Down syndrome, Turner syndrome, Noonan Syndrome, DiGeorge syndrome, and other congenital anomalies.
- *External ear anomalies:*
  - External ear may be small and dysplastic (microtia) or absent (anotia).
  - Preauricular tags **(Fig. 17)** or pits are often seen due to maldevelopment of the first bronchial arch. Renal anomalies may be associated with these anomalies, it should be ruled out.
  - Large ears—bat-like ears are seen in fragile X syndrome.

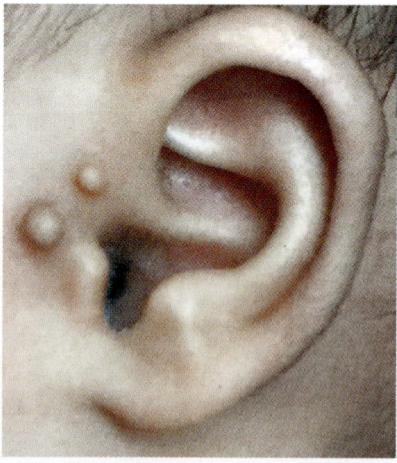

Fig. 17: Preauricular skin tags.

- *Otoscopic examination:* Every pediatrician should know the otoscopic examination in children and it should be integral part of clinical examination. It will be useful to diagnose otitis media, foreign body, and wax.
    - The pinna of ear is pulled horizontally in infants and upward and backward in older children while holding the handle of the otoscope between the thumb and the index finger.
    - The cone of light which extends from the tip of the handle of malleus downward and forward may be obliterated in ear infections, while the handle of the malleus may become more prominent in retraction of the tympanic membrane.
    - Observe the tympanic membrane for color (dusky), tension (bulging, retracted) or perforation.

Examination of Nose

Examination of nose is very crucial especially for dysmorphism and congenital anomalies.

- *Size and shape:* The nasal length from the root of the nose to the highest concavity at the tip of the nose in a vertical axis ranges from 20 mm to 32 mm at birth in term neonates. The nasal width approximates the distance between the medial margins of the nostrils.

  The nose may be small (Down syndrome, Edward syndrome, Apert syndrome) or large (Seckel dwarf). Beaking of the nose is seen in Apert syndrome, progeria, etc. Rudimentary nose is seen in holoprosencephaly. The depressed nasal bridge is seen in syphilis, Down syndrome, Hurler syndrome, hemolytic anemia, etc. The hypoplastic alae nasi may be seen in infants of diabetic mothers.

- *Nares:* Exclude choanal atresia by passing a nasogastric tube through each nostril one by one. In bilateral choanal atresia, the baby breathes through mouth and becomes bluish on taking breastfeeding, immediately baby cries and becomes pink. Absence of one of the nostrils may be seen rarely.

- *Nasal cavity:* Look for any foreign body, purulent nasal discharge, nasal crusts, or polyps using a nasal speculum. The deviated nasal sputum is very common on examination.

Nasal snuffle since birth may be a sign of congenital syphilis. Occasionally a CSF leak may be responsible for recurrent meningitis in a case of crack in cribriform plate.

Examination of Oral Cavity

Examination of oral cavity includes examination of lips, angle of mouth, philtrum, buccal mucosa, gum, palate, tongue, teeth, tonsils, and oropharynx. It should be performed at the end of clinical examination as it is unpleasant for the child and you may lose his cooperation for rest of examination.

- *Mouth:* Look for the symmetry of the mouth when the child is crying or laughing. The asymmetric face may be due to unilateral facial nerve palsy or hypoplasia of the depressor anguli oris muscle. Parotid gland swelling may be there, unilateral or bilateral in a case of mumps. Recurrent parotid swelling may be due to parotid duct obstruction or HIV.
- *Lips:*
  - Cleft lip **(Fig. 18)** may be found in neonates or infants, unilaterally or bilaterally with or without cleft palate.
  - The lips may show edema (angioneurotic edema) **(Fig. 19)**, pallor, cyanosis, infection (herpes simplex) or signs of vitamin deficiency.

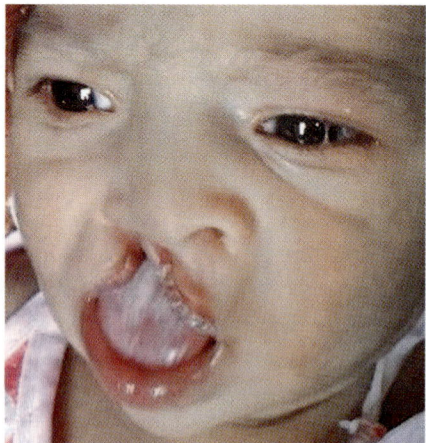

Fig. 18: Cleft lip.

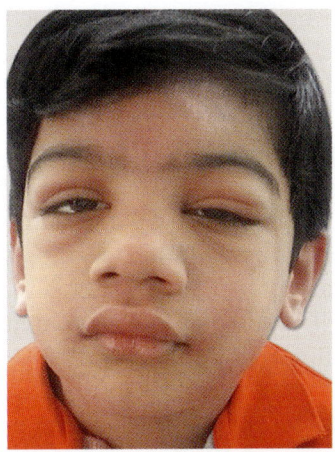

Fig. 19: Angioneurotic edema. Note the swelling of eyelids and lips.

- Dryness, scaling and cracking of lips (cheilitis) is commonly seen in acute febrile illness. It may be one of the signs of Kawasaki disease.
- Angular chelosis is characteristic of riboflavin deficiency. If it is associated with fungal infection, it is seen bluish in sunlight, called as perlèche.
- Moist lesions radiating from corners of mouth (rhagades) are characteristic of syphilis.
- *Philtrum:* The philtrum may be short (DiGeorge syndrome) or long (Hurler syndrome, Cornelia de Lange syndrome **(Fig. 11)**, fetal alcohol syndrome, and fetal hydantoin syndrome).
- *Buccal mucosa:*
  - Look for hydration, ulcers, inflammation, and color.
  - White curd like plaques, difficult to scrape off may be deposited on oral mucosa in candidiasis or thrush.
  - Oral mucosa may be erythematous along with tongue and lips in Kawasaki disease.
  - Grayish white spots surrounded by reddish hue may be seen in oral cavity opposite to the lower molar teeth in measles, called as Koplik spots.
  - Petechiae and bullae on oral mucosa along with extensive involvement of skin and conjunctiva are seen in a case of Stevens–Johnson syndrome.

- *Gums:* The gum hypertrophy may be due to some drugs like phenytoin or leukemia. Ulcerations and bleeding over gums may be due to scurvy or leukemia.
- *Palate:*
  - Look for cleft palate, small cleft palate is easy to miss, if not examined properly.
  - High arched palate is associated with several conditions like Down syndrome, Ehlers–Danlos syndrome, Marfan syndrome, etc.
  - Epstein pearls (benign epithelial swelling) are common on palate in midline in the neonates.
- *Tongue:*
  - Look for color of tongue (pallor, cyanosis, and strawberry red) **(Figs. 20A and B)**, fissures, ulcers **(Fig. 21)**, follicles, symmetry, and its movements. Frequent changes in shapes over dorsum of tongue is characteristic of geographic tongue **(Fig. 22)**.
  - Pale tongue is seen in anemia. Pale and bald tongue is seen in iron deficiency anemia. Blue tongue is seen with cyanosis. Strawberry tongue is seen in scarlet fever, Kawasaki disease, etc. Black tongue may be seen in fungal infection. Magenta color (purplish red) tongue is characteristic of riboflavin deficiency.
  - Macroglossia is seen in congenital hypothyroidism, mucopolysaccharidosis, Pompe disease, Beckwith–Wiedemann syndrome, Down syndrome, hemangioma, lymphangioma, angioneurotic edema, etc.

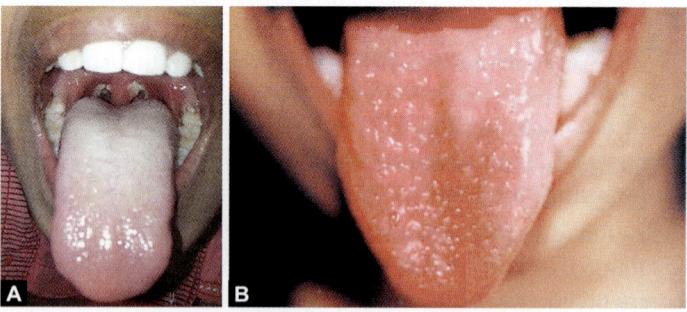

Figs. 20A and B: White and red strawberry tongues.

General Physical Examination

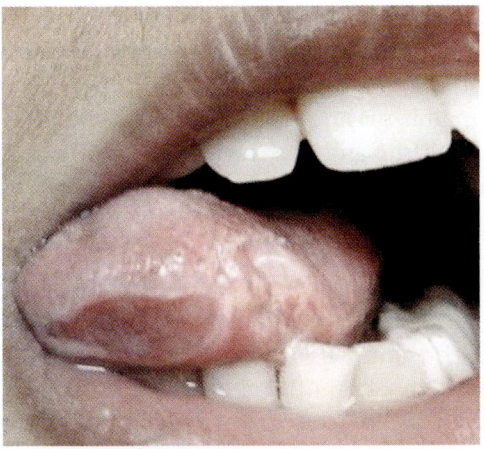

Fig. 21: Traumatic ulcer on tongue.

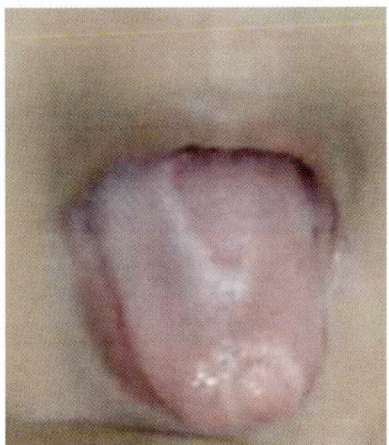

Fig. 22: Geographic tongue.

- Microglossia may be seen in lesions of hypoglossal and facial nerves.
- A thread-like structure seen on ventral aspect of tongue should not be mistaken as tongue tie. Rarely, it requires surgical intervention.
- Fasciculations of tongue are characteristic of Werdnig–Hoffman disease in a floppy infant.

- **Mandible and chin:**
  - Look for a small mandible (micrognathia) or a receding chin (retrognathia).
  - Retrognathia may be associated with cleft palate.
  - Micrognathia and glossoptosis leading to difficulty in breathing are classical features of Pierre-Robin syndrome.
  - Lock jaw is the classical feature of tetanus.
- *Teeth:*
  - Sometimes a newborn may have teeth as birth (natal teeth).
  - Absence of teeth is seen in ectodermal dysplasia **(Fig. 12)**.
  - Count the number of teeth. Primary teeth appear from 6 months to 24 months of age while secondary or permanent teeth usually start appearing from the age of 6 years.
  - Black staining of teeth occurs in children receiving oral iron preparations.
  - Yellow staining of teeth is seen in children receiving tetracycline.
  - Children with porphyria may have pink teeth.
  - Bluish line along the gum with bluish ending to the teeth known as Burton line is characteristic of lead poisoning.
  - Look for dental caries.
  - Peg-like incisors are seen in congenital syphilis.
- *Pharynx:* Ask the child to open the mouth and protrude his tongue, depress the tongue with spatula, and see the pharynx with torch light.
  - Look for any congestion of pharynx or bulge in the posterior pharyngeal wall (retropharyngeal abscess).
  - Check the uvula, central or deviated to one side. Deviation of uvula may occur in palate palsy, drawn toward normal side. Bifid uvula **(Fig. 23)** is rare malformation.
  - Examine for gag reflex.
  - Look for hyperplasia of lymphoid tissues.
  - If epiglottitis is suspected, do not attempt examination of pharynx unless facilities for intubation and mechanical ventilation are available.
- *Tonsils:* Ask the child to open the mouth and say "Aah", use the spatula to see the tonsils.
  - Examine the tonsils for their size, color, and presence of any membrane.

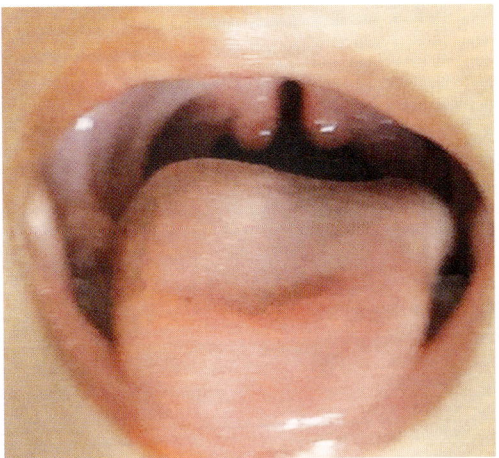

Fig. 23: Bifid uvula, a rare malformation.

- A gray or yellow membrane may be seen in diphtheria, streptococcal infection, and infectious mononucleosis.
- In case of quinsy (peritonsillar abscess), tonsil may be displaced to one side.

Neck

- *Length and position:*
    - Short neck is seen in Klippel–Feil anomaly, platybasia, Hurler syndrome, Morquio syndrome, Turner syndrome, etc.
    - Wry neck or torticollis (inclination of head on one side) may be due to sternomastoid tumor or any painful condition like an abscess.
- Neck stiffness may occur in meningitis, tetanus, caries of cervical spine, Arnold–Chiari malformation, acute poliomyelitis, etc.
- Look for any swelling in neck like thyroid swelling **(Fig. 24)**, thyroglossal cyst or fistula, branchial cyst, sternomastoid tumor, cystic hydroma, enlarged lymph node, etc.
- Observe prominence of neck veins in congestive cardiac failure. Check carotid pulsations.
- Acanthosis nigricans **(Fig. 25)** seen at back of neck is characteristic of polycystic ovarian disease (PCOD).

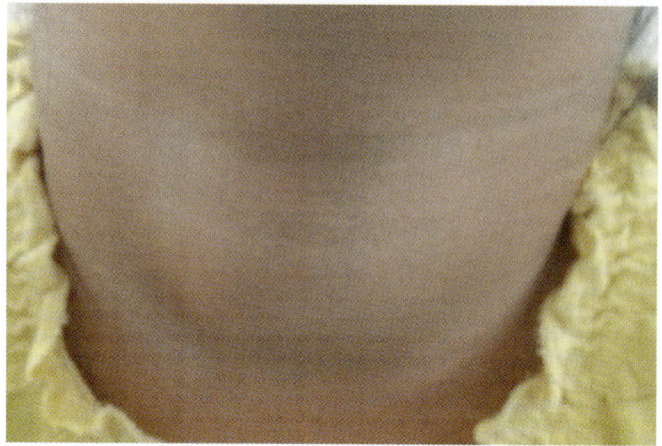

Fig. 24: Midline neck swelling, moving on deglutition in adolescent girl—thyroid swelling.

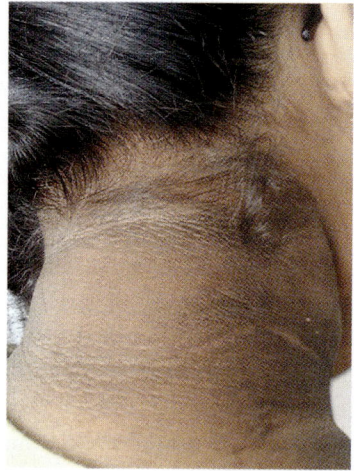

Fig. 25: Acanthosis nigricans on the back of neck in a girl with obesity and polycystic ovarian disease.

Hands, Feet, and Limbs

- *Size and shape:* Abnormalities of fingers and toes are shown in **Figures 26A and B**. Look for foot anomalies like (club foot) congenital talipes equinovarus, rocker bottom foot (Edward syndrome) **(Figs. 27A and B)**, etc.

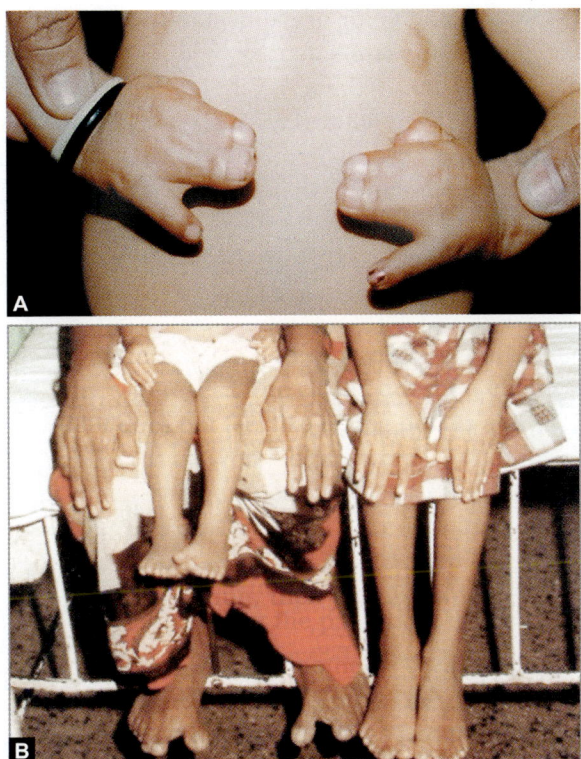

Figs. 26A and B: Abnormality of fingers. (A) Club fingers; (B) Polydactyly and syndactyly.

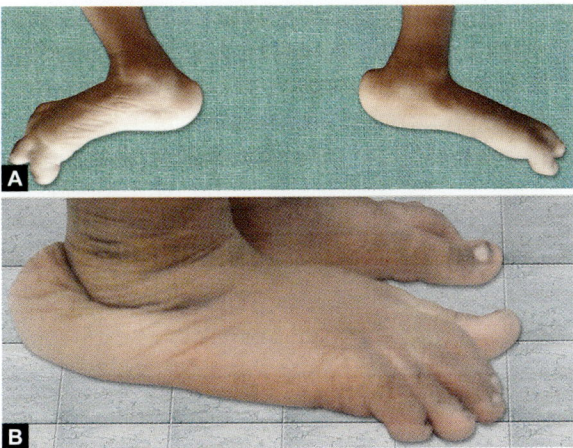

Figs. 27A and B: Rocker-bottom feet in Edward syndrome.

- *Color:* Observe the color of palms and soles. Pallor indicates anemia. Pale palms and sole may be due to sympathetic over activity like shock. Palmar erythema with liver disease is characteristic of liver failure. Bluish hue may be due to cyanosis or Raynaud phenomenon. Acrocyanosis (blue palms and soles) may be due to hypothermia in newborn.
- *Rash:*
  - Macules (Erythema multiforme)
  - Papules (Papular urticaria, scabies)
  - Vesicles [scabies, staphylococcal scalded skin syndrome (SSSS) **(Fig. 28)**, congenital syphilis]
  - *Nodules (Osler nodules in bacterial endocarditis over fingers and pulps):* Erythema nodosum on shin of tibia
  - Petechiae and purpura [Henoch–Schönlein purpura **(Figs. 29A and B)**, meningococcemia **(Fig. 30)**, rickettsia].
- *Nails:* Look for clubbing, platynychia, and koilonychia (spoon shaped nails) in iron-deficiency anemia, splinter hemorrhage (infective endocarditis), pitting discoloration of nails (paronychia), and dystrophy of nails (in recovery phase of hand–foot–month disease). Beau's lines **(Fig. 31)** in protein-energy malnutrition (PEM) and Kawasaki disease.
- *Bones and joints:* Observe for length of bones, their proportion, posture, and position of limbs and range of movements. Look for any joint swelling, tenderness, and erythema. Look for evidence of rickets like wrist widening, double malleoli. Look for genu valgus, genu varus, etc. Check for bony tenderness which may be seen in osteomyelitis, scurvy, syphilis, leukemia, etc.

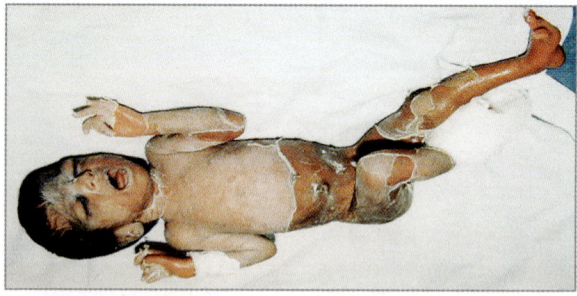

Fig. 28: Staphylococcal scalded skin syndrome (SSSS).

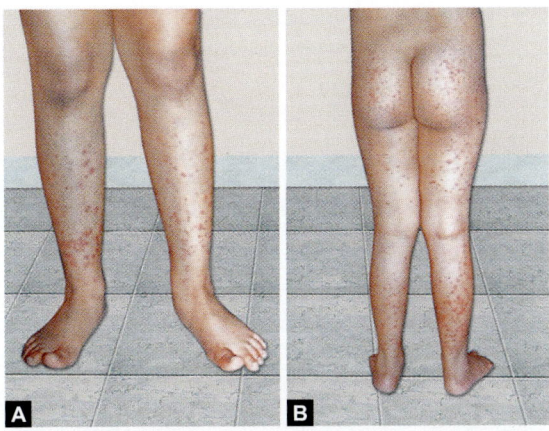

Figs. 29A and B: Petechial spots in a case of Henoch–Schönlein purpura.

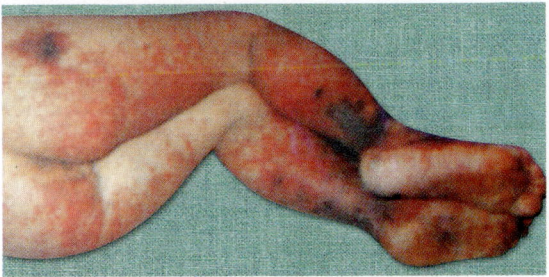

Fig. 30: Meningococcemia.

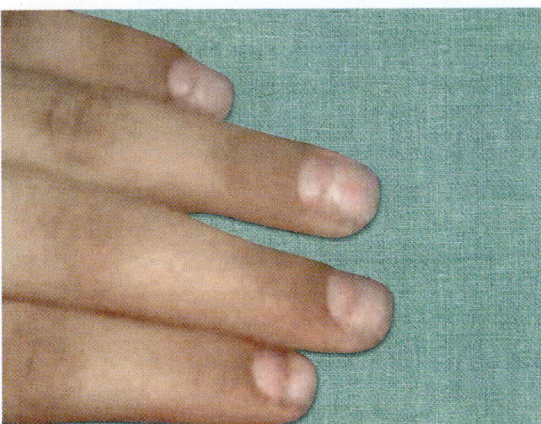

Fig. 31: Beau's lines.

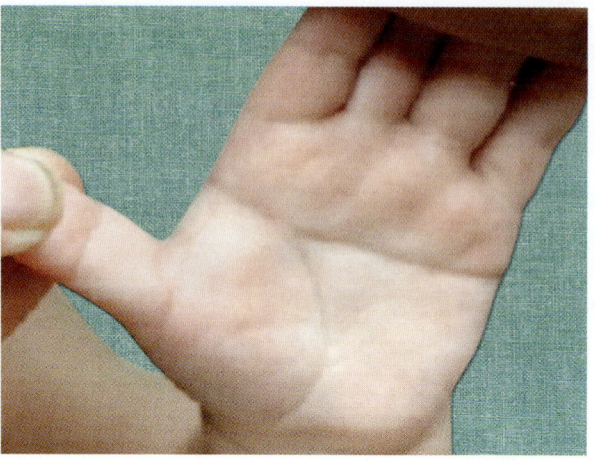

Fig. 32: Single transverse palmar crease (Simian crease).

- *Involuntary movements:*
  - Tremor (anxiety, hyperthyroidism, Wilson disease)
  - Chorea (rheumatic chorea, Huntington disease)
  - Carpopedal spasms (tetany)
- *Dermatoglyphics:*
  - Simian crease (single, transverse, palmar crease) **(Fig. 32)** in Down syndrome
  - Kennedy crease (plantar crease between great toe and second toe)
- *Limb length and proportions:*
  - Micromelia (shortening of entire limb)
  - Rhizomelia (shortening of proximal limb)
  - Mesomelia (shortening of middle segment)
  - Acromelia (shortening of distal segment)
  - Upper segment and lower segment ratio should be measured. Arm span should also be measured. Its detailed interpretations are discussed in chapter on anthropometry.

Skin

Skin should be examined for its color, texture, turgor, rashes, pigmentation, vesicles, pustules, subcutaneous nodules, scars, hirsutism, striae, nevi, xanthoma, dermographism, etc. Important skin lesions are shown in **Box 7**.

- Dry, scaly, coarse skin (phrynoderma) **(Fig. 33)** may be due to vitamin A and vitamin E deficiency, deficiency of essential fatty acids, hypothyroidism, etc. is seen over back of elbow.
- *Skin turgor:* On pinching the skin, failure of skin fold to go back to normal quickly suggests dehydration.
- Look for various skin rash, its character, distribution, symmetry, involvement of palms and soles, blanching, etc.

Box 7: Important skin lesions.

- *Macule:* Nonpalpable area of altered color
- *Papule:* Elevated lesions up to 5 mm in diameter
- *Nodule:* Palpable, solid lesions >5 mm in diameter
- *Vesicle:* Fluid-filled blister <5 mm in diameter
- *Bulla:* Fluid-filled blister >5 mm in diameter
- *Pustule:* Blister contains pus
- *Petechiae:* Subdermal bleed <3 mm in diameter (pin head)
- *Purpura:* Subdermal bleed 3–6 mm in diameter
- *Ecchymosis:* Subdermal bleed >6 mm
- *Hematoma:* Bleeding in muscles

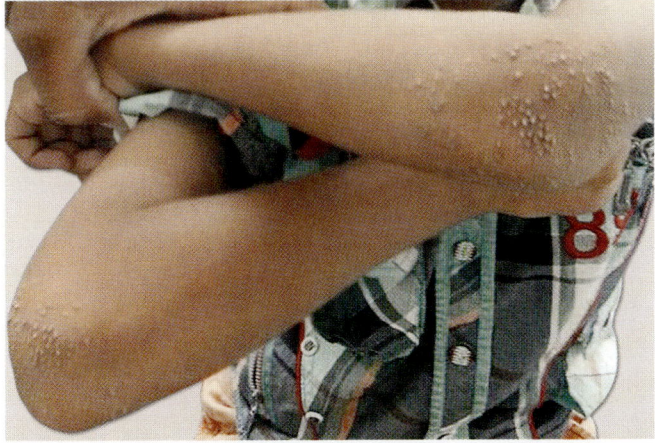

Fig. 33: Phrynoderma (follicular hyperkeratosis) on extensor aspect of elbows due to vitamin A deficiency.

- Look for neurocutaneous markers like café-au-lait spots, ash leaf macules, adenoma sebaceum, angiofibroma, subungual fibromas, etc.
- Look for spider nevi, palmar erythema, etc.

Nails

The changes in the nails may be primary where the disease is affecting nails or secondary to a systemic disease.
- Look for clubbing **(Fig. 34)**, platynychia or koilonychia **(Figs. 35A and B)**.
- Pitting in nails may be due to psoriasis or lichen planus.
- Beau's lines **(Fig. 31)** are transverse lines and furrows at the nail lunula, which are seen in PEM and Kawasaki disease.
- Nail biting is a common habit in children.

Genitalia

This is crucial point of examination in every child and is often missed. Before examination of genitalia, the child and parents should be explained regarding the procedure and its significance. Adolescent girls should be examined in the presence of a female attendant.
- Boys:
  - Orchidometer **(Fig. 36)** is used to measure the size of testis. It is measured in volume (mL). The normal testicular

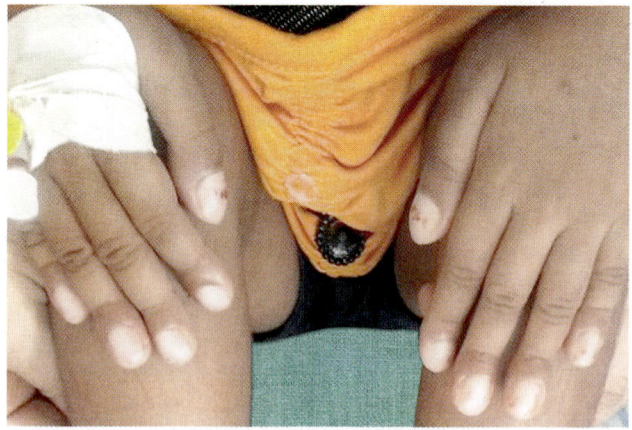

Fig. 34: Digital clubbing.

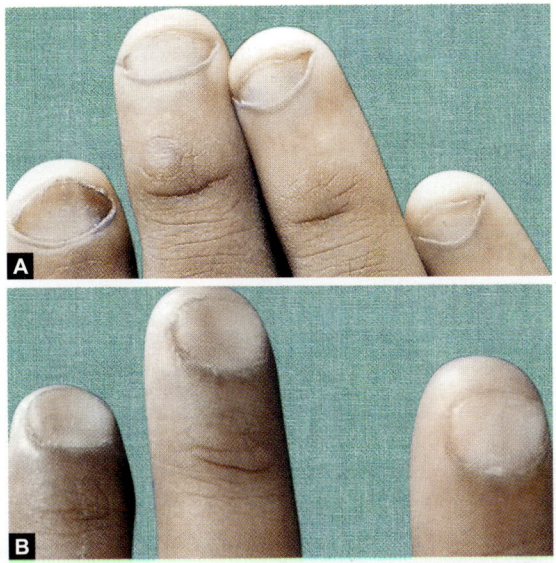

Figs. 35A and B: Platynychia and koilonychia in iron deficiency anemia.

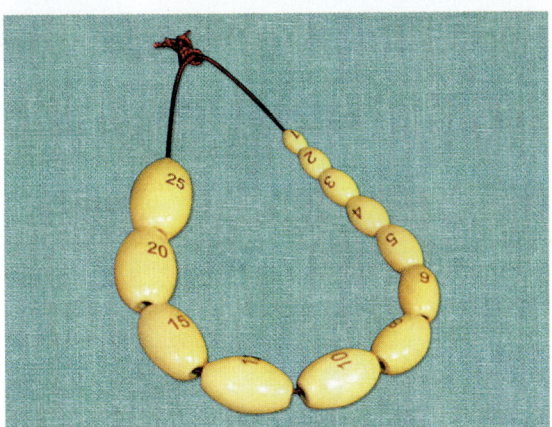

Fig. 36: Orchidometer to measure the size of testis in volume.

volume at infantile age is 2 mL, prepubertal 3.5–4 mL and adult 17–20 mL.
- Look for hypospadias, epispadias, hydrocele, hernia, etc.
- Look for presence of testes in scrotum (present in scrotum/retractile/undescended). In a case of undescended testis,

the scrotum on that side is underdeveloped (**Figs. 37A and B**). Epididymo-orchitis can also cause the pain.
- In a case of acute, severe lower abdominal pain, look for torsion of testis.
- Large size of testis may be a sign of fragile X syndrome or testicular tumor.
- Look for other anomalies like bifid scrotum.
- Forceful retraction of preputial skin may cause paraphimosis (**Fig. 38**).

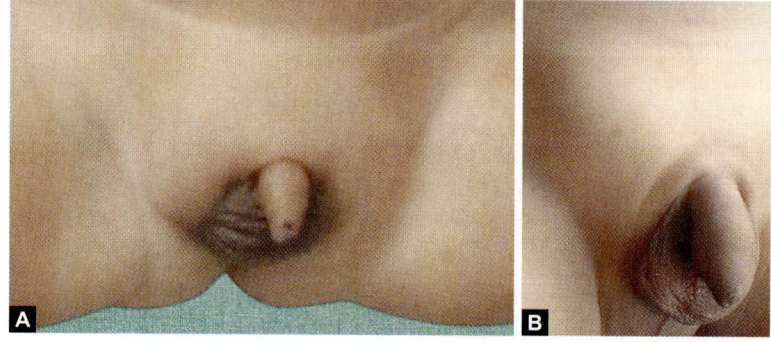

Figs. 37A and B: (A) Undescended testes: Scrotum on both the sides are empty and under developed; (B) Right side undescended testis. Note right side scrotum empty and inguinal swelling indicating presence of testis.

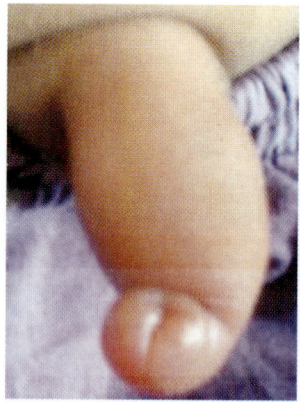

Fig. 38: Paraphimosis.

- *Girls:*
  - *Examination of breasts:*
    - Size, shape, galactorrhea, premature thelarche, etc.
    - See the distribution of axillary and pubic hairs.
    - Sexual maturity may be delayed in hypothyroidism, hypopituitarism, and Turner syndrome. It may be early (precocious) as in polycystic ovarian disease, McCune–Albright syndrome, teratoma, CNS tumors like hamartoma, hydrocephalus, etc.
    - In newborns, check for ambiguous genitalia. It may be due to congenital adrenal hyperplasia and other causes.

GENERAL MARKERS OF DISEASE
Pallor

Pallor means pale appearance of skin and mucous membrane, usually due to anemia and decreased perfusion (shock).
- Look for pallor at lower palpebral conjunctive, dorsum of the tongue, oral mucosa, palm, and nails.
- Pallor may be graded as mild to moderate and severe. In moderate pallor, mucosa appears pale, but palmar creases pink. In severe pallor, even the palmar creases become faint and pale.
- Pallor should not be mistaken as anemia in a case of poor perfusion (shock) as pallor in such cases may be due to vasoconstriction following sympathetic over activity. In nephrotic syndrome and hypothyroidism, there may be general appearance of pallor.
- *Look for associated signs for clinical clue to diagnosis:*
  - Tachycardia (congestive cardiac failure)
  - Edema (congestive heart failure, nephrotic syndrome)
  - Low pulse volume (shock)
  - Platynychia or koilonychia in iron deficiency anemia
  - Hyperpigmentation of knuckles (megaloblastic anemia)
  - Petechial spots and sick child (leukemia)
  - Lymphadenopathy and hepatosplenomegaly (infective, malignancy, infiltrative disease).

Jaundice (Icterus)

It is defined as yellow discoloration of sclera, mucous membrane, and skin. Usually, jaundice becomes clinically apparent as serum level exceeds 2 mg/dL in older children and at more than 5 mg/dL in neonates.
- Look for icterus at sclera, palate, undersurface of tongue, tip of nose, palms and soles (in neonates).
- For assessment of jaundice in neonates, press the skin against a bony surface (sternum) for 5 seconds to blanch the skin and observe the skin color. Due to physiological polycythemia in newborn, blanching is required to appreciate yellow color of the skin. It can also be examined over forehead and tip of nose.
- A lemon yellow color indicates underlying cause as hemolysis, while dark yellow with scratch marks indicates obstructive jaundice.

Cyanosis

Cyanosis is defined as bluish discoloration of skin and mucous membrane due to reduced hemoglobin more than 5 g/dL. Therefore, in severely anemic children (Hb <5 g/dL), cyanosis may not be apparent in spite of hypoxemia. Apparent clinical presence of cyanosis indicates oxygen saturation less than 85%.
- It is classified as follows according to its distribution:
  - *Acrocyanosis:* In newborns, due to hypothermia or hypoglycemia
  - *Central:* Cyanosis of lips, tongue (mucosa), and fingers and toes (extremities)
  - *Peripheral:* Cyanosis of fingers only
  - *Differential:* The fingers are pink but toes are blue, it is called as differential cyanosis. It indicates PDA with pulmonary hypertension in great arteries normally connected to respective ventricles. If the fingers are blue but the toes are pink, it is called as reversed differential cyanosis. It suggests PDA with pulmonary hypertension with transposition of great arteries. The common causes of cyanosis in children are shown in **Box 8**.

> **Box 8:** Common causes of cyanosis.
> - *Central cyanosis:*
>   - Tetralogy of Fallot
>   - Transposition of great arteries
>   - Tricuspid atresia
>   - Truncus arteriosus
>   - Total anomalous pulmonary venous return
>   - Ebstein anomaly
>   - AV fistulas
>   - Methemoglobinemia
>   - Severe bronchial asthma
>   - Respiratory failure
> - *Peripheral cyanosis:*
>   - Cold exposure
>   - Raynaud phenomenon
>   - Congestive cardiac failure

Clubbing

Clubbing is thickening of the terminal phalanges of fingers and toes. It is due to excessive growth of the connective tissues. It is described in details in chapter on respiratory system.

Lymphadenopathy

Lymph nodes are normally small oval or bean-shaped and located along the course of lymphatic vessels, to filter lymph on its way to the bloodstream. The primary function of lymph nodes is to filter microorganisms and abnormal cells, collected in lymph fluid.

Palpable lymph nodes are common in children. Lymph node enlargement (lymphadenopathy) occurs in response to antigenic, infectious or neoplastic stimuli.

- *Cervical lymph nodes:* For palpation of cervical lymph nodes, examiner should stand behind the child and flex the neck. Alternatively, neck can also be flexed from the front with the head tilted to side being examined. The superficial cervical lymph nodes must be examined from above downward: submental, submandibular, tonsillar, cervical (upper, middle and lower), posterior auricular, and occipital.
  - The lymph nodes should be palpated with pad of your index and middle fingers. The sequence of examination of various groups should be as shown in **Box 9**.

Box 9: Sequence of examination of cervical lymph nodes.
- Preauricular (in front of ear)
- Postauricular (behind the ear)
- Occipital (at base of skull)
- Tonsillar (angle of jaw)
- Submandibular (under the jaw on the side)
- Submental (under the jaw in midline)
- Superficial anterior cervical (over in front of the sternomastoid muscle)
- Posterior cervical (along anterior margin of trapezius)
- Deep cervical (palpate behind the sternomastoid with thumb and finger)
- Supraclavicular (in the angle of the sternomastoid and the clavicle)

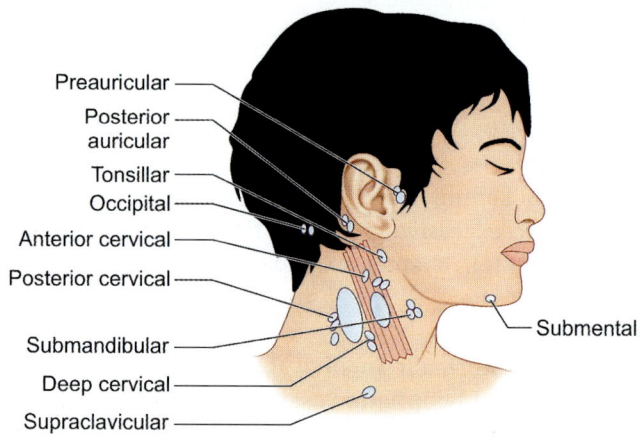

Fig. 39: Anatomical location of cervical lymph nodes.

- Deep cervical lymph nodes should be palpated, one side at a time. Gently bend the child's head forward and roll your fingers over the deeper muscles along the carotid artery.
- To palpate the scalene nodes, roll your fingers gently behind the clavicles.

  Figure 39 shows location of different cervical lymph nodes.
- *Axillary lymph nodes:* Axillary lymph nodes should be examined by inserting the fingers in the axillae with the patient's arm slightly abducted. The apical, anterior, posterior, medial, and lateral groups are examined. You can examine apical, anterior, medial, and lateral groups of axillary lymph nodes

while standing in front of the child, while the posterior group is examined, standing behind the patient.
- *Right anterior axillary lymph nodes:* These nodes should be palpated by palmar surface of your left hand. Abduct the child's arm slightly, flex the elbow, and passively place his forearm on your right palm. Now with your left hand palpate the pectoralis major muscle forming the anterior axillary fold and the lymph nodes on its posterior surface.
- *Right apical axillary lymph nodes:* In the same position by depressing the child's shoulder with your right hand, palpate the right apical group by insinuating your fingers of left hand, deeper into the axilla.
- *Right medial axillary lymph nodes:* Palpate the right medial group with your left hand against the upper lateral chest wall.
- *Right lateral axillary lymph nodes:* These nodes are palpated using your right hand against the upper medial humerus, after abducting the child's shoulder with your left hand on the elbow.
- *Right posterior axillary lymph nodes:* You should stand behind the patient. Abduct the child's shoulder and ask to place his right hand over the opposite shoulder. Now, using your right hand, palpate the posterior axillary fold formed by the latissimus dorsi muscle and the posterior group on the anterior surface. For the opposite side, the given steps should be performed with the opposite hand.
- *Is the mass lymph node in cervical region?:* Solitary enlarged lymph node in the neck may raise the question, is it lymph node or something else? The nonlymphoid masses in neck should be kept in mind like thyroid tumors, congenital cyst and sinuses, cyst hygroma, and sternomastoid tumor.
- *What is significant lymphadenopathy?:* Usually, lymph nodes are not palpated in newborns, if they are palpable, search for etiology. In older children, cervical and axillary lymph nodes >1 cm and inguinal lymph nodes >1.5 cm in size are considered as significant lymphadenopathy. Epitrochlear, supraclavicular, and popliteal lymph nodes of any size should be considered always significant and it warrants to decide the cause of it.

- *What are the characteristics of lymphadenopathy?:*
  - Localized (regional) lymphadenopathy indicates infection in the involved node and/or its drainage area. Enlarged left axillary lymph node in an infant may be due to BCG adenitis **(Fig. 40)**. Inguinal lymphadenitis **(Figs. 41A and B)** is very common due to bacterial infection, tuberculosis and HIV.
  - Generalized lymphadenopathy is defined as enlarged lymph nodes of >2 noncontagious regions. It denotes

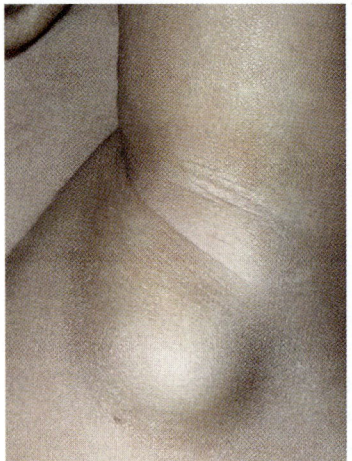

Fig. 40: Left axillary BCG adenitis.

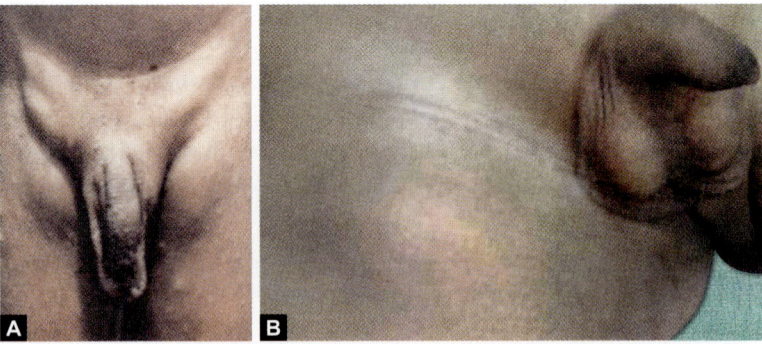

Figs. 41A and B: Inguinal lymphadenitis.

usually systemic disease and often it is accompanied by abnormal physical findings in other systems.
- *Location signifies likely pathology:*
    - *Anterior cervical LN:* Pharyngitis, tonsillitis, and acute otitis media. Most common organisms are *Streptococcus* and *Staphylococcus aureus*.
    - Reactive LN due to pediculosis and seborrheic dermatitis.
    - Cervical and supraclavicular most commonly due to lymphoma
    - Anterior cervical group involvement is common in Kawasaki disease.
    - Suboccipital and postauricular enlarged LN may be due to rubella.
    - Epitrochlear LN enlargement is commonly seen in congenital syphilis.
- Size
- Single/multiple
- Rubbery (lymphoma)
- Soft (infection/inflammation)
- Firm [tuberculosis, systemic lupus erythematosus (SLE)]
- Hard and fixed (malignancy)
- Matted/draining sinus (tuberculosis)

Edema

Edema is clinically examined by applying pressure against a bony prominence to look for presence of depression. In ambulatory patients, it is examined at ankle above the medial malleolus or at shin of tibia. The pressure is applied with the examiner's thumb for 30 seconds. If pitting edema is present, a pit or depression is seen at the site. In very sick and bed-ridden patients, edema is examined at the most dependent part, sacrum. Nonpitting edema is seen in hypothyroidism, Turner syndrome, filariasis, and lymphangiectasis. Localized edema is seen in cellulitis, insect bite, urticaria, and angioneurotic edema cases. One should differentiate puffy face, massive edema face and steroid face due to steroid toxicity **(Figs. 42A to C)**.

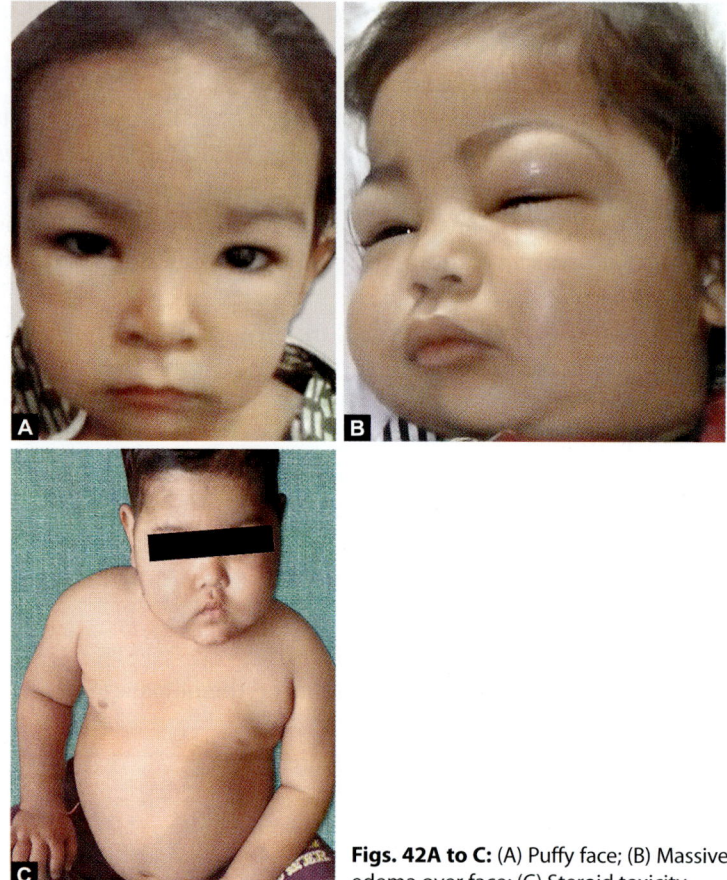

Figs. 42A to C: (A) Puffy face; (B) Massive edema over face; (C) Steroid toxicity.

The edema may develop due to following mechanism:
- Decreased plasma oncotic pressure due to hypoproteinemia in conditions like kwashiorkor, nephrotic syndrome, chronic liver diseases, and malabsorption, etc.
- Increased hydrostatic pressure like congestive heart failure, constrictive pericarditis, acute glomerulonephritis, hypertension, Budd–Chiari syndrome, etc.
- Increased capillary permeability such as in angioneurotic edema and vasculitis (dengue fever, SLE, etc.)

- Impaired lymphatic drainage like filariasis, lymphangiectasis, etc.
- Occasionally, some drugs also can cause edema. Common causes of edema are listed in **Box 10**.

Clinical Signs of Micronutrient Deficiency

During general physical examination of the child, one should attentively look for signs of micronutrient deficiency. Some of them may be very specific, almost diagnostic of a particular micronutrient deficiency as shown in **Box 11**.

- *Vitamin A deficiency:* Vitamin A deficiency is characterized by night blindness and xerophthalmia. WHO classification of vitamin A deficiency is shown in **Box 12**.
- *Vitamin B deficiency:*
  - *Vitamin B_1:* Dry beriberi—irritability, fatigue, emotional disturbances, edema, tender calf muscles, and diminished deep tendon reflex (DTR). Wet beriberi—congestive heart failure.
  - *Vitamin B_2:* Cheilosis, circumcorneal vascularization and keratinization, photophobia, hyperesthesia, glossitis, etc.

Box 10: Common causes of edema.

- *Nutritional:* Kwashiorkor, marasmic kwashiorkor
- *Cardiac:* Congestive cardiac failure, anemia, beriberi
- *Renal:* Acute glomerulonephritis, nephrotic syndrome, hypertension
- *Hepatic:* Chronic liver disease, cirrhosis of liver
- *Endocrine:* Hypothyroidism, Cushing syndrome, steroid therapy
- *Lymphatic causes:* Filariasis, lymphangiectasis

Box 11: Diagnostic signs of micronutrient deficiency.

- *Cheilosis (angular stomatitis) (dry scaling and fissuring at angle of mouth):* Riboflavin deficiency
- *Bitot spots (dirty white spots on temporal side of eye):* Vitamin A deficiency
- *Hyperpigmented knuckles:* Folate and vitamin B_{12} deficiency
- *Rachitic rosary:* Vitamin D deficiency (rickets)
- *Scorbutic rosary:* Vitamin C deficiency (scurvy)
- *Phrynoderma (Toad like skin due to follicular hyperkeratosis):* Essential fatty acids and vitamin A and vitamin E deficiency

> **Box 12:** WHO classification of vitamin A deficiency.
>
> *Primary signs:*
> - *X1A:* Conjunctival xerosis
> - *X1B:* Bitot spot
> - *X2:* Corneal xerosis
> - *X3A:* Corneal ulceration, <1/3 of cornea
> - *X3B:* Corneal ulceration (>1/3 of cornea)
>
> *Secondary signs:*
> - *XN:* Night blindness
> - *XF:* Fundal changes
> - *XS:* Corneal scarring

- *Niacin:* Dermatitis (pigmented, scaly, cracked skin on exposed parts, casal necklace, hyperpigmentation of hands and feet), diarrhea, and dementia.
- *Pyridoxine:* Pallor, hyperacusis, and convulsions.
- *Vitamin B_{12}:* Megaloblastic anemia, mild icterus, loss of position, and proprioception.
- *Vitamin C deficiency (scurvy):* Bleeding tendency, mucosal bleeds, gum swelling, pallor, bone pains, pseudoparalysis, scorbutic rosary, and conjunctival and subperiosteal hemorrhage.
- *Vitamin D deficiency (rickets):* Frontal and parietal bossing, craniotabes, rachitic rosary, pigeon chest, Harrison sulcus, widening of wrists, double malleoli, cubitus/genu valgum, hypotonia, short stature, visceroptosis, tetany, etc.
- *Vitamin E deficiency:* Phrynoderma (rough, scaly skin), ataxia, and pallor.

Dysmorphism and Congenital Anomalies

Dysmorphism refers to abnormal morphology which can result from various mechanisms as follows:

- *Malformation:* Birth defect arising because of poor tissue formation
- *Deformation:* Birth defected caused by disruption of morphogenesis
- *Disruption:* Breakdown of already formed normal tissues
- *Dysplasia:* Abnormal organization of cells in the tissue
- *Association:* It is the nonrandom tendency of some malformations to occur together than expected by chance. For example, VATER which includes vertebral defects, anal atresia, tracheo-esophageal fistula with esophageal atresia, and renal dysplasia.

- *Sequence:* When a single defect in morphogenesis leads to a cascade and subsequent defects, the pattern of structural defect is called as sequence. It may be of four types:
  1. *Malformation sequence:* A single localized poor formation of tissues leading to a chain of subsequent defects. As for example, Pierre Robin sequence occurs when micrognathia leads to glossoptosis, which results in cleft palate.
  2. *Deformation sequence:* There is no defect in the embryo or fetus, but mechanical forces like uterine constraint result in altered morphogenesis. For example, oligohydramnios/Potter deformation sequence due to chronic leakage of amniotic fluid or renal agencies, leading to decreased amniotic fluid, which results in intrauterine compression of the fetus and leads to limb anomalies, flattened facies, and pulmonary hypoplasia.
  3. *Disruption sequence:* The normal fetus is subjected to a destructive problem and its consequences. Amniotic band disruption sequence is characterized by varied clinical manifestations ranging from partial amputations to major craniofacial and limb defects, as a consequence of early amnion rupture and vascular disruption events.
  4. *Dysplasia sequence:* The primary defect is a lack of normal organization of cells into tissues. Neurocutaneous melanosis sequence is due to lack of migration of melanoblastic precursors from neural crest which results in melanocyte hamartomas of the skin in conjunction with similar changes in the pia and arachnoid.

Syndromes

When multiple structural defects occur together that cannot be explained on the basis of a single initiating defect and its consequences, but are due to multiple defects in one or more tissues, the recurrent patterns of maldevelopment are called malformation syndromes. For example, William syndrome is characterized by Elfin facies, supra valvular aortic stenosis, peripheral pulmonary stenosis, and hypercalciuria.

Dermatoglyphics

Dermatoglyphics refers to the dermal ridge, patterns which can be seen on the palm, soles, fingers, and toes of an individual.

- *Fingertip patterns:* The various patterns seen on fingertips include whorls, loops (ulnar and radial), and arches. Some characteristic patterns are seen in certain dysmorphic syndrome like ulnar loops on most fingers in Down syndrome (trisomy 21), mostly arches in Edward syndrome (trisomy 18), etc.

> **Box 13:** Examination of a dysmorphic child.
>
> - *Head:*
>   - Shape and size
>   - Microcephaly/macrocephaly
>   - Sutures closed/open
>   - Measurement of occipital frontal circumference (Head o)
> - *Eyes:*
>   - Spacing normal/abnormal
>   - Hypertelorism/hypotelorism/normal
>   - Microphthalmia
>   - Look for palpable fissures, epicanthic folds, synophrys, coloboma, ptosis, corneal clouding, blue sclera
>   - Prominent eyeballs (exomphalos)
> - *Ears:*
>   - Low set
>   - Shape, size
>   - Preauricular skin tags
> - *Face:*
>   - Hypoplasia of mandible/maxilla
>   - Hypertrophy of gums
>   - Cleft lip and palpate
>   - Pallor
>   - Cyanosis
>   - Macroglossia
>   - Teeth number and caries
>   - Pigmentation
> - *Hands:* Look for simian crease, clinodactyly, polydactyly, syndactyly, arachnodactyly, and broad or absent thumb hypoplastic radii
> - *Skin:* Look for alopecia, hirsutism, café-au-lait spots, neurofibroma, hypo- or hyperpigmentation
> - *Genitalia:* Look for ambiguous genitalia, cryptorchidism, hypospadias, epispadias, micropenis

- *Flexion creases:* Usually, there are three flexion creases present in palm.
  - *Simian crease:* It is a single transverse midpalmar crease which occurs when the two distal palmar creases are fused, characteristically present in Down syndrome. It may be seen in some normal persons.
  - *Sydney crease:* It occurs when the proximal crease runs through the entire palm while the distal crease is normally present.
- *Tri-radii:* The ridges in the palms meet at certain points which are called tri-radii. The tri-radii in each palm are called as a, b, c and d. The angle formed at tri-radii and by joining a, t, and d is called ATD angle which is usually about 40°. In Down syndrome, Turner syndrome, the ATD angle is obtuse as the proximal triradius is shifted distally. The dysmorphic child should be examined methodologically as shown in **Box 13**.

CHAPTER 4

Infant and Young Child Feeding

Bakulesh Chauhan, Baldev Prajapati

INTRODUCTION

Optimum nutrition is essential for child survival and quality of life. Breast milk is the natural food for an infant and it is species specific. The concept of Infant and Young Child Feeding (IYCF) was introduced in 2002. The fetal and infant nutrition is the foundation for growth, development, intelligence, emotional well-being and immunity. The period of first 1000 days (270 days in uterus + 730 days postnatal) (Fetal life + first 2 years of life), is considered very crucial for nutritional programming. The five key facts and 10 steps of IYCF proposed by UNICEF are very important in this reference.

The Five Facts

1. Indian children have growth and development potential as all children worldwide.
2. Child malnutrition remains one of the greatest developmental challenges of India.
3. Student children have stunted bodies, stunted brains and stunted lives.
4. Child under nutrition starts early in life to make a lifelong lasting difference.
5. No need to discover new vaccines or new drugs: *We know what works.*

The Ten Key Interventions

1. Timely initiation of breastfeeding within 1 hour of birth.
2. Exclusive breastfeeding during first 6 months of life.
3. Timely introduction of complementary foods at 6 months.

4. Age appropriate food for children 6 months to 2 years.
5. Hygienic complementary feeding practices.
6. Immunization and biannual vitamin A supplementation with deworming.
7. Appropriate feeding for children during and after illness.
8. Therapeutic feeding for children with severe acute malnutrition.
9. Adequate nutrition and support for adolescent girls to prevent anemia.
10. Adequate nutrition and support for pregnant and breastfeeding mothers.

BREASTFEEDING

Breastfeeding is the most natural way of feeding young ones. Since the introduction of the "Baby Friendly Hospital Initiative (BFHI)" in 1992, exclusive demand feeding is accepted as the only mode of early infant feeding. World Breastfeeding Week (WBW) is celebrated from August 1st to 7th every year to bring the awareness among the people regarding importance of breast feeding.

The BFHI is a global program organized by UNICEF. It was launched in 1992 and adopted by India in 1993. In order to actively protect, promote and support breastfeeding, every facility providing maternity services and care for newborn infants should practice the following ten steps:

1. Have a written breastfeeding policy that is routinely communicated to all healthcare staff.
2. Train all healthcare staff in skills necessary to implement policy.
3. Inform all pregnant women about the benefits and management of breastfeeding.
4. Help mothers to initiate breastfeeding within an hour of birth.
5. Show mothers how to breastfeed and how to maintain lactation even if they are separated from their infants.
6. Give newborn infants no food or drink other than breast milk, unless medically indicated.
7. Practice rooming in and allow mothers and infants to remain together 24 hours a day.
8. Encourage breastfeeding on demand.

9. Give no artificial teats or pacifiers (also called dummies or soothers) to breastfeeding infants.
10. Foster the establishment of breastfeeding support groups and refer mothers to them on discharge from the hospital or clinic.

On the basis of these ten steps, the hospital policies are formulated and exhibited. The ten policies are as follows:
1. Our hospital has an official policy to protect, promote and support breastfeeding.
2. All maternity and child care health staff in the hospital receive training in the skills to promote breastfeeding.
3. All mothers, both antenatal and postnatal, are informed about the benefits of breastfeeding.
4. We assist mother in the early initiation of breastfeeding, within half an hour of birth for a normal delivery and within 4 hours of birth of cesarean section.
5. All mothers are shown in how to breastfeed and how to maintain lactation even if they should be temporarily separated from their infants.
6. We give newborns no food or drink other than breast milk. Infant foods and breast milk substitutes are prohibited in this institution.
7. We practice, "rooming-in" by allowing the mothers and babies to remain together 24 hours a day.
8. We encourage all mothers to breastfeed on demand.
9. We strictly prohibit the use of artificial teats, pacifiers, soothers and feeding bottles.
10. We provide follow-up support to mothers for exclusive breastfeeding up to 6 months after birth and continued breastfeeding up to 2 years of age. We enlist the cooperation of visiting family members to support breastfeeding mothers. Mothers are also advised on whom to contact for assistance in overcoming any problems in breastfeeding.

Preparing the Mother for Breastfeeding

The antenatal mother should be motivated and prepared for breastfeeding. It should be routine to examine breast for retracted or cracked nipples in the last trimester of pregnancy. Antenatal mother should take extra 300 kcal and 15 g protein and lactating mother should take extra 500 kcal and 25 g protein.

Initiation of Breastfeeding

The baby must be put to breast within half an hour after normal delivery and within 4 hours after cesarean section operation. Prelacteal feeds like water, honey, distilled water, glucose, etc. should not be given. In the first 4 days, small quantity of colostrum (10–40 mL) is secreted and that is sufficient for the child. It is rich in protein and immunoglobulins.

Rooming-in, keeping the mother and baby in same room, Bedding-in, keeping the mother and baby in same bed and mothering-in, keeping the baby on the abdomen of mother are measures to ensure mother–infant bonding and skin to skin contact. Skin to skin contact, eye-to-eye contact and mother–infant bonding lead to successful breastfeeding and emotional adjustment.

The mother and baby should be relaxed and in comfortable position during breastfeeding. Initially, somebody should help them. The baby's head may be resting on the elbow of the mother and she should also support the breast between the index finger and middle finger of the opposite hand during feeding.

The different comfortable positions to mother and baby can be adopted as shown in **Figures 1 to 3**.

Sucking should be continued as long as the baby wants to suck so that baby is satisfied and hind milk becomes available. Hind milk is more nutritious and rich in fat, providing satiety to the baby. When the baby sucks only for few minutes, it will get only the foremilk. Foremilk is rich in lactose and water which will satisfy the thirst of baby. It is better to suckle from both the breasts and usually it takes about 20–30 minutes.

ANATOMY OF BREAST

The breast consists of 15–20 lobes with multiple lobules which contain clusters of acini or alveoli. Lactiferous ducts are arranged in a radial fashion, originating from each lobe and commencing toward nipple. The space between the alveoli and lactiferous ducts is packed with stroma containing fat, muscle fibers, blood vessels, nerves and connective tissues. The main lactiferous ducts widen to form ampulla under areola, storing the milk and opening into the tip of nipple **(Fig. 4)**.

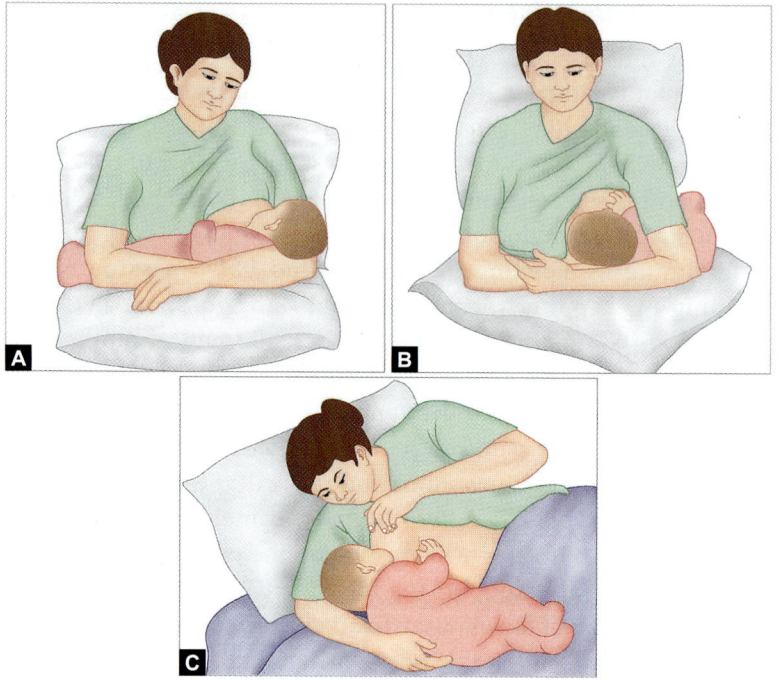

Figs. 1A to C: Normal various feeding positions for newborn.

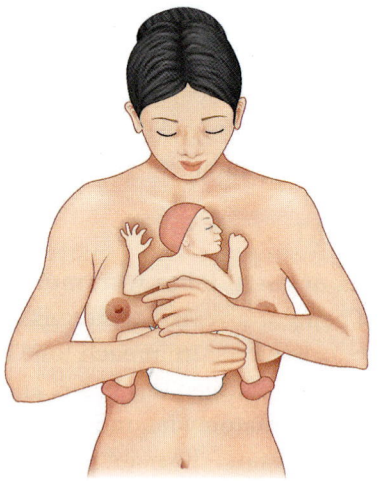

Fig. 2: Kangaroo mother care.

Infant and Young Child Feeding

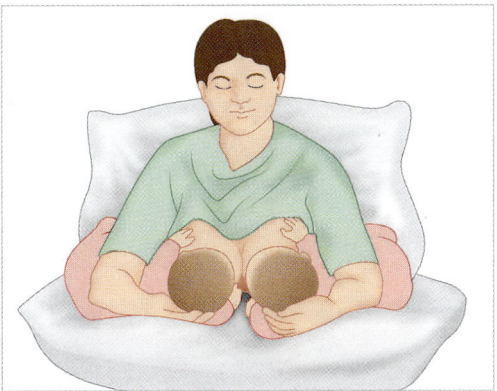

Fig. 3: Football holding method for feeding twins.

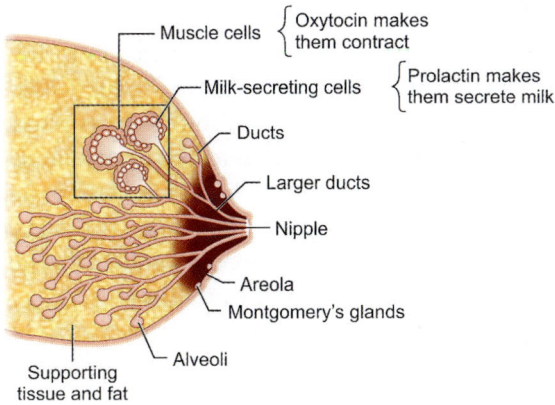

Fig. 4: Anatomy of breast.

PHYSIOLOGY OF LACTATION

Three reflexes, rooting, sucking and swallowing help the baby in breastfeeding. When breast nipple touches the cheek of baby, it will open the mouth and takes the nipple in mouth and starts sucking. This is rooting reflex. Sucking and swallowing become coordinated by 34 weeks of gestation.

- *Prolactin (Milk production) reflex* **(Fig. 5):** The milk is produced as a result of interaction between hormones and reflexes.

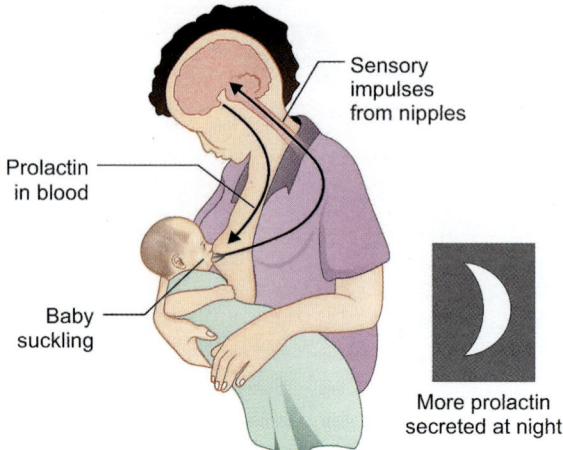

Fig. 5: Prolactin reflex (milk production reflex).

Prolactin, a hormone, produced by the anterior pituitary stimulates glandular tissues of breast to produce milk. When the baby sucks, the nerve endings in the nipple carry messages to the anterior pituitary which is turn releases prolactin in the blood. The more the baby sucks at the breast, greater is the stimulus for milk production by release of prolactin. The earlier the baby is put to breast, sooner the reflex is established. The greater is the demand for milk, more milk is produced.

- *Oxytocin (let-down reflex) (milk ejection reflex)* **(Fig. 6):** The ejection of milk is facilitated by let-down reflex which is mediated through the release of oxytocin from posterior pituitary. Oxytocin is released in response to stimulation of the nerve endings in the nipple by sucking as well as by thought, sight, smell or sound of the baby. Oxytocin causes contraction of myoepithelium around the glands leading to ejection of milk from the glands into the lacteal sinuses and lacteal ducts. This reflex is affected by mothers' emotions, a relaxed, comfortable and stress free atmosphere helps in milk ejection reflex. On the other hand, a tense, apprehensive, worried mother or pain and discomfort during breastfeeding slows down the milk flow. Effective attachment and emptying of breast during each feeding is associated with enhanced milk production **(Figs. 7A and B)**.

Infant and Young Child Feeding

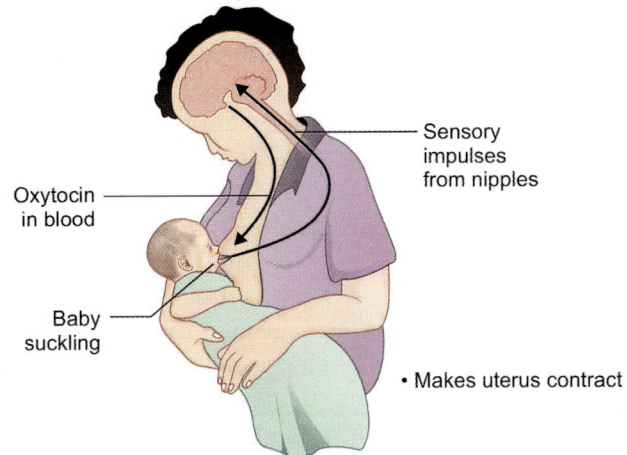

Fig. 6: Oxytocin reflex (milk ejection reflex).

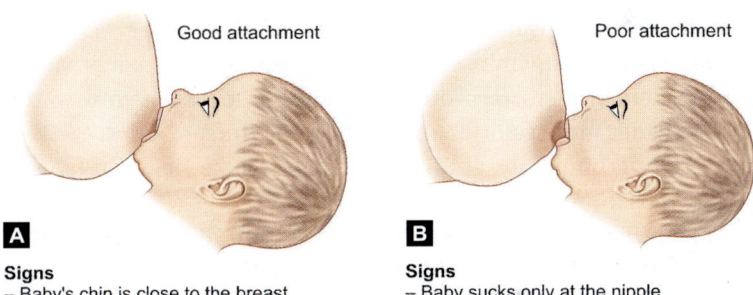

Signs
– Baby's chin is close to the breast
– Baby's tongue is under the lactiferous sinuses and nipple against the palate
– Baby's mouth is wide open and the lower lip turned outwards
– More areola is visible above the baby's mouth than below it
– No pain while breastfeeding
– Baby's cheeks are full, not hollow
– Regular, slow, deep sucks

Signs
– Baby sucks only at the nipple
– Mouth is not wide open and much of the areola and thus lactiferous sinuses are outside the mouth
– Baby's tongue is also inside the mouth and does not cup over the breast tissue
– Chin is away from the breast
– It is painful while breastfeeding

Figs. 7A and B: Good attachment and poor attachment during breastfeeding.

TYPES OF BREAST MILK

The composition of breast milk is changing at different stages of lactation to suit the need of the baby. Breast milk is not only species specific, it is baby specific!

- *Colostrum:* Colostrum is the milk secreted during the first 3–4 days after delivery. It is thick and yellow, contains more

antibodies, protein and WBCs. Though it is secreted in small quantity (10–40 mL/day), it is sufficient as the baby needs. It should never be discarded.
- *Transitional milk:* It is the breast milk secreted during the following 2 weeks. It is the stage between the colostrum and mature milk.
- *Mature milk:* It follows the transitional milk. It is thinner and watery but contains all the nutrients essential for optimal growth of the baby. It gradually increases till 6 months after delivery and later remains same. Average quantity of breast milk is 500–800 mL/day. Prolactin being secreted more at night, night feeding is important for continuing breastfeeding.
- *Preterm milk:* The milk of mother who delivers prematurely contains more calories, higher concentration of fat, proteins and sodium which are need by the preterm baby. The concentration of lactose, calcium and phosphorus are lower as compared to milk produced by mother of term infants.
- *Fore milk:* It is the milk secreted at the start of a feed. It is watery and rich in lactose, proteins, vitamins, minerals and water. It provides more calories and satisfies the thirst of baby.
- *Hind milk:* It comes at the end of feed and is richer in fat and provides more energy and satiety.

For optimum growth, the baby needs both fore and hind milk and therefore, the baby should be allowed to empty the breast completely before putting him to the opposite breast.

COMPOSITION OF HUMAN MILK AND COW'S MILK

There are several biochemical, nutritional and physiological differences between human's and cow's milk **(Table 1)**. The major differences are as follows:
- The whey protein in human milk is easily digestible.
- Human milk lipase promotes fat digestion.
- Higher content of certain amino acids (cystine and taurine), long chain fatty acids like arachidonic acid and docosahexaenoic acid (DHA) and lactase in human milk promotes faster development, maturation and myelination of human brain. DHA content of human milk is 30 times more compared to cow's milk.
- The bioavailability of iron is better in human milk.

Infant and Young Child Feeding

Table 1: Composition of human and cow milk.

Item	Human milk	Cow milk
Nonprotein nitrogen	0.2 g	0.03 g
Protein	1.1 g	3.0 g
Casein: Whey	40:60 (β casein, lactalbumin and lactoferrin)	80:20 (α casein, β lactoglobulin)
Lactose	7 g	4.5 g
Fat	3.8 g	3.7 g
EFA	13%	2%
P/S ratio	1.2:1	1:2
Ash/minerals	0.25 g	0.75 g
Ca:P ratio	2:1	<2
Sodium	0.7 mEq	2.2 mEq
Potassium	1.4 mEq	3.5 mEq
Vitamin K	0.2 µg	0.60 µg
Vitamin E	0.2 mg/IU	0.1 mg/IU
Osmolality	260 mOsm/kg	260 mOsm/kg
Energy: protein ratio	70:1	25:1
Calories	67 kcal	67 kcal

- The nutrients available in human milk are more readily absorbed and better utilized due to higher biological efficiency.
- The presence of epidermal growth factor and peptides in human milk enhance physical growth.

Immunological Components of Human Milk

Human milk is not only best suited and specific for nutritional needs but it also boosts the host defense mechanism of the newborn. It contains immunoglobulins, cellular elements and nonspecific humoral protective factors **(Table 2)**.

COMMON PROBLEMS DURING BREASTFEEDING

- *Flat or inverted nipples:* The size of the resting nipple is not important. It is just a guide to show where the baby has to take the breast. The areola and the breast tissue beneath should

Table 2: Immunological components of human milk.

S. No.	Components
1.	*Immunoglobulins*: Secretory IgA, IgG, IgM
2.	*Cellular elements*: Lymphoid cells, polymorphs, macrophages, plasma cells
3.	Opsonic and chemotactic activities of C_3 and C_4 complement system
4.	Unsaturated lactoferrin and transferrin
5.	Lysozyme
6.	Lactoperoxidase
7.	Oligosaccharides
8.	*Specific inhibitors (nonimmunoglobulins)*: Antiviral and antistaphylococcal factors
9.	Growth factors for lactobacillus bifidus
10.	Para-aminobenzoic acid may afford some protection against malaria

be capable of being pulled out to form the teat. If the nipple goes deeper into the breast on attempting to pull out, it is true inverted nipple. Nipple protractility test should be done during pregnancy. The nipple becomes more protractile (capable of being pulled out) as pregnancy advances and the mother should be reassured that she would be able to breastfeed successfully.

- *Inverted syringe technique:* Usually, the nipple gets corrected in due course of time as the baby suckles. Few cases may require inverted syringe technique **(Fig. 8)**.
    - Cut the nozzle end of a disposable 10–20 mL syringe.
    - Introduce the piston from the cut end side.
    - Ask the mother to apply smooth side of the syringe on the nipple and gently pull out piston and let her wait for a minute or so.
    - Nipple would protrude into the syringe. Ask the mother to release the suction and put the baby to the breast. It helps the nipple to erect out and baby is able to suckle in the proper position.
    - After feeding, the nipple may retract back, but doing it each time before feeding over a period of few days, the problem will be solved.

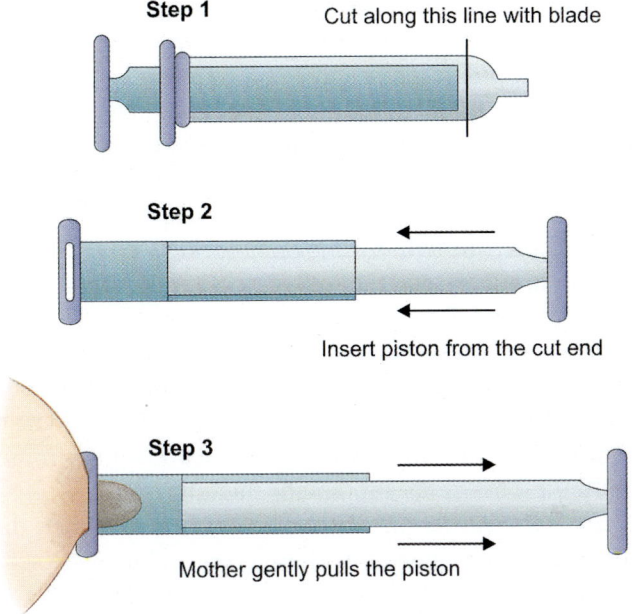

Fig. 8: Inverted syringe technique.

- *Engorgement of the breast:* Fullness of the breast is a frequent problem. Still, milk flow continues and the baby can feed normally. If enough milk is not removed, it may result in engorgement of breast. The engorged breast becomes full, tender and lumpy. The common causes of engorgement of the breast are giving prelacteal feed and thereby delayed initiation of breastfeeding, bottle feeding and any restriction of breastfeeding. Due to pain, the mother avoids feeding, leading to inadequate emptying of breast, decreased production of milk and sometimes infection. Once the engorgement of breast develops, the baby should be breastfed frequently followed by expression of breast milk. Application of moist heat, gentle massage and stroking the breast toward the nipple, expression of breast milk, frequent breastfeeding, etc. may solve the problem in a day or two. Mother should be relaxed and may take paracetamol for pain.

- *Sore nipple and cracked nipple:* If the baby is not attached to the breast (poor attachment) **(Figs. 7A and B)**, it sucks only the nipple. It is the most common cause of sore nipple. If feeding is continued in a poor position, it may lead to cracked nipple becomes trauma and later on mastitis or breast abscess. Proper technique and correct positions **(Figs. 7A and B)** will prevent soreness and cracking of the nipple.
- *Blocked duct:* If the baby does not suckle well on a particular segment of the breast, the milk blocks the lactiferous duct to a painful, hard swelling, usually no fever.
- *Mastitis and breast abscess:* If the blockage of the duct or engorgement of breast persists, infection may develop leading to red, hot, tender, swollen breast (mastitis). It should be treated promptly and the measures include counseling, removal of milk, antibiotics and symptomatic therapy.
- *Schedule of breastfeeding:* Exclusive demand feeding is the ideal schedule for breastfeeding. There is no "tailor-made schedule". On an average, baby should be fed *eight* times in a day for 15–20 minutes for each feed.
- *Burping after feeding:* A lot of air is sucked in by a baby during feeding. It will lead to abdominal distention, regurgitation, colic, etc. To get rid of this, burping should be done. The baby should be put on the shoulder of the mother and head is supported, the opposite arm supports the buttocks. Gently pat on the back of baby. The air comes out slowly and baby becomes comfortable. The baby can also be kept in the mother lap in prone position and gently pat the back. Keeping the baby in the right lateral position is also useful.
- *Points indicating adequacy of breast milk:*
    - Baby goes to sleep after taking breast milk.
    - Gaining the weight.
    - Passing pale colored urine for more than five times in a day.

How Long to Breastfeed?

It is recommended to breastfeed till 2 years of age of the baby, the period of maximum brain growth and myelination. By 6 months of age, complementary foods should be started in addition to breastfeeding.

Breastfeeding and Maternal Illness
- Breastfeeding can be continued during most of common maternal illnesses such as viral fever, malaria, UTI, mastitis, breast abscess, etc.
- If the mother is open case of tuberculosis, she should continue ATT and baby should be put on chemoprophylaxis (INH 10 mg/kg/day for 6 months). One should confirm that the baby is not suffering from the disease. Cough hygiene and other measures are also important. If the mother is suffering from MDR-TB, follow the standard protocol for the baby.
- If mother is suffering from hepatitis B, the baby should receive hepatitis B immunoglobulin on one thigh and hepatitis B vaccine on opposite thigh. Complete the vaccine schedule and follow the standard protocol.
- In HIV-positive mother, breastfeeding may be continued along with other measures. If top feeding can be managed satisfactorily, it is the next option instead of breastfeeding.

CONTRAINDICATIONS TO BREASTFEEDING
- Galactosemia
- Congenital lactose intolerance
- Mother is on antithyroid, antimalignant drugs
- Postpartum psychosis.

COMPLEMENTARY FEEDING PRACTICES
Complementary feeding after 6 months of age is extremely important due to risk of micronutrient deficiencies and malnutrition. It is the systemic process of introduction of suitable food at the right time in addition to breastfeeding in order to provide needed nutrients to the infant. It is said that weaning is the second step for self-existence, the first step is cutting the umbilical cord. The term complementary feeding is now preferred because weaning implies abrupt stoppage of breastfeeding to some mothers.
- *Time of complementary feeding:* Birth weight doubles by 4 months of age and the nutritional demands gradually increase, the calcium and iron stores get depleted. The breast milk supply increases till 6 months and then it plateaus off. The baby is biologically ready to accept semisolids by 6 months of age.

Early introduction of complementary foods may cause allergy problems and infections, while late leads to growth faltering and malnutrition.

- *Continuation of breastfeeding:* Breastfeeding should be continued for as long as feasible, preferably till 2 years of age.
- *Complementary foods:* Complementary food should be home made. It should be started with mono-cereals, followed by multicereals and cereals–pulse combination. Cereal such as rice is the best choice to start weaning as it is gluten free and easily digestible. Different combinations such as wheat, pulse, vegetables, etc. can be made. They should be locally easily available, economical and acceptable. Addition of jaggery for calories and minerals, milk for protein and oil for calories can make homemade food more nutrient denser.
- *Family feeding:* It is essential to switch over gradually to the usual family food.
    - *Around 6 months of age*: Cereal-based porridge (ragi, suji, rice, etc.) enriched with jaggery/sugar, oil/ghee and animal milk can be started. Start with small quantity and can be increased gradually in addition to breastfeeding. Fruit juices can also be started.
    - *6–9 months of age*: Mashed items from family pot enriched with jaggery/sugar and oil/ghee can be started. Mashed rice with pulses, mashed fruits, biscuits, egg yolk, etc. can be further added in addition to breast milk.
    - *9–12 months of age*: After 9 months, introduce soft food that can be chewed, avoiding hot spices. Chapatti and other hard items can be made soft by adding milk. A variety of food from family pot can be given 4–6 times a day, gradually increasing quantity. By 1 year of age, the child should be taking everything cooked at home. At 1 year of age, the child should eat half of what the mother eats.

    The calculation of calories according to weight of the child **(Box 1)**, amount of food to be served at different ages **(Table 3)**, daily requirement of vitamins and minerals **(Table 4)**, nutritive value of common foods **(Table 5)** and food value in house hold measures **(Table 6)** is very essential for every clinician to know.

Infant and Young Child Feeding

> **Box 1:** Calculation of calories according to weight of the child.
> - *Up to 10 kg:* 100 kcal/kg
> - *10–20 kg:* 1,000 kcal + 50 kcal for each kg above 10 kg
> - *Above 20 kg:* 1,500 + 20 kcal/each kg in excess above 20 kg

Table 3: Amount of food to be offered at different age.

Age	Texture	Frequency	Average amount of each meal
6–8 months	Start with thick porridge, well mashed foods	2–3 meals per day plus frequent Breastfeeding	Start with 2–3 table spoonful
9–11 months	Finely chopped or mashed food and foods that baby can pick up	3–4 meals plus breastfeed Depending on appetite offer 1–2 snacks	½ of a 250 mL cup/bowl
12–23 months	Family foods, chopped or mashed, if necessary	3–4 meals plus breastfeed Depending on appetite offer 1–2 snacks	3/4 to one 250 mL cup/bowl

Source: IAP. IYCF Guidelines 2010. Mumbai: Indian Academy of Pediatrics; 2010.

Table 4: Recommended daily allowances (RDAs) of vitamins and minerals.

The approximate RDA of vitamins and minerals

Vitamin A	1,500 IU/day (500 µg)
Vitamin D	400 IU/day (10 µg)
Vitamin E	5–15 IU/day (5–15 mg)
Vitamin B complex • B_1 (Thiamine) • B_2 (Riboflavin) • B_6 (Pyridoxine) • B_3 (Niacin) • B_{11} (Folic acid) • B_{12} (Cyanocobalamin) • Vitamin C	0.5–1.5 mg/day 0.5–1.0 mg/day 0.5–1.0 mg/day 5–15 mg/day 50–150 µ/day 0.5–1.5 µ/day 40 mg/day
Macronutrient • Calcium • Phosphorus • Magnesium	500–1,000 mg/day 800–1,000 mg/day 200–300 mg/day

Contd…

Contd...

The approximate RDA of vitamins and minerals	
• Iron	10–20 g/day
• Iodine	50–150 µg/day
• Copper	1–2 mg/day
• Zinc	5–15 mg/day
• Fluoride	1–5 mg/day
• Manganese	1–5 mg/day
• Selenium	100 µg/day
• Molybdenum	200–500 µg/day
• Chromium	10 µ/day

Source: Elizabeth KE. Nutrition and Child Development, 4th edition. Hyderabad: Paras Medical Publisher; 2015.

Table 5: Nutritive value of common foods/100 g.

Item	Protein (g)	Fat (g)	Fiber (g)	CHO (g)	Energy (Kcal)	Iron (mg)
Cereals/grains						
Rice	7	0.5	0.2	78	350	0.7
Ragi	7	1.3	3.6	72	330	3.9
Wheat	11	1.5	1.2	71	350	5.3
Maize	11	3.6	2.7	66	340	2.3
Pulses/legumes						
Bengal gram	17	5.3	3.9	60	360	4.6
Black gram	24	1.4	0.9	60	350	3.8
Green gram	24	1.3	4.1	57	340	4.4
Red gram	22	1.7	1.5	58	340	2.7
Soya bean	43	19.5	3.7	20	430	10.4
Leafy vegetables						
Agathi	8	1.4	2.2	12	93	3.9
Amaranth	4	0.5	1.0	6	45	3.5
Cabbage	2	0.1	1.0	5	27	0.8
Drumstick	6	1.7	0.9	12	92	0.9
Spinach	2	0.7	0.6	3	26	1.1
Roots and tubers						
Arrowroot	0.2	0.1	–	83	340	1.0
Beetroot	1.7	0.1	0.9	9	43	1.2
Carrot	0.9	0.2	1.2	10	50	1.0
Onion (Big)	1.2	0.1	0.6	11	50	0.6
Potato	1.6	0.1	0.4	22	100	1.2
Sweet potato	1.2	0.3	0.8	28	120	0.2

Contd...

Contd…

Item	Protein (g)	Fat (g)	Fiber (g)	CHO (g)	Energy (Kcal)	Iron (mg)
Nuts and oils						
Almond	20	58	1.7	11	655	5.0
Cashew	21	47	1.3	22	600	5.8
Coconut (fresh)	4.5	41	1.0	13	444	1.7
Coconut (dry)	6.8	62	6.6	18	660	7.8
Groundnut	25	40	3.1	26	560	2.5
Fruits						
Amla	0.5	0.1	3.1	14	58	1.2
Apple	0.2	0.5	1.0	13	59	0.6
Banana	1.2	0.3	0.4	27	116	0.4
Dates	2.5	0.4	3.9	75	317	7.3
Grapes	0.6	0.4	2.8	13	58	0.5
Guava	0.9	0.3	5.2	11	50	0.3
Jackfruit	1.9	0.1	1.1	20	88	0.6
Lemon	1.0	0.9	1.7	11	57	0.7
Sweet lime	0.8	0.3	0.5	9	43	1.3
Mango	0.6	0.4	0.7	17	75	7.9
Watermelon	0.2	0.2	0.2	3	16	0.3
Orange	0.7	0.2	0.3	10	48	0.3
Papaya	0.6	0.1	0.8	7.2	32	0.5
Pineapple	0.4	0.1	0.5	10.8	46	2.4
Tomato	0.9	0.2	0.8	3.6	20	0.6
Meat group						
Fish	20–60	1–10	–	0–5	100–300	1–50
Beef	8	10	0.5	0.2	400	18
Egg	13	13	–	–	173	2
Chicken	26	0.6	–	–	109	2.5
Mutton	20	13	–	–	194	–
Pork	18	4.4	–	–	114	2.5 2.2
Milk and milk products						
Cow's milk	3.2	4.1	–	4.4	67	0.2
Buffalo's milk	4.3	6.5	–	5	117	0.2
Human milk	1.1	3.4	–	7.4	65	0.3
Cheese	24	25	–	6.3	348	2.1
Skimmed milk powder	38	0.1	–	51	357	1.4

Source: Elizabeth KE. Nutrition and Child Development, 4th edition. Hyderabad: Paras Medical Publisher; 2015.

Table 6: Food values of household measures.

Items	Protein (g)	Energy (kcal)
Cow's milk 1 glass (200 mL)	6	120
Cooked rice 1 cup	4	175
Cooked dhal 1 tsp	0.5	10
Egg	6	80
Fish 1 oz (10 cm piece)	6	80
Mutton 1 oz (8 bits)	6	50
Bread 1 oz (1 slice)	2	70
Dosa 1	2	70
Idli 1	2	50
Chapatti 1	2	70
Puri	1	35
Vada 1	1	50
Upma 1 cup	6	250
Sugar 1 tsp	–	20
Jaggery 1 tsp	–	20
Ghee/butter 1 tsp	–	36
Groundnuts 10	1	20
Biscuit 1	0.5	20
Coffee 1 cup	1.8	80
Tea cup 1	1.0	60

Source: Elizabeth KE. Nutrition and Child Development, 4th edition. Hyderabad: Paras Medical Publisher; 2015.

- *Bridging calories and other nutrient gap:* The calorie gap can be met by using oil/ghee and sugar selecting high density food items. Cereal-pulse combinations, root and tubers, vegetables, especially green leafy vegetables, seasonal fruits, milk products, egg, fish, meat, etc. given to the baby will bridge the nutrient gap. Frequently feeding is desirable as it aids in good acceptance by the infant. Sprouting or germination will enhance vitamin content and make it amylase rich food and will decrease the bulk on cooking. Fermentation enhances vitamin C and digestibility, e.g., curd/yogurt.
- *Developing readiness for family foods through varied textures and tastes:* Introducing new tastes with addition of vegetables, fruits, etc., will expose the baby to healthy eating practices. It is essential to practice the child toward good nutrition and healthy eating habits, right from complementary feeding period.

- *Preparation and storage of weaning foods:* Hygienic preparation and storage of complementary food is important. Hand washing with soap and water should be practiced before cooking and feeding. The food should be freshly prepared.
- *Careful feeding practices:* In thick consistency, the mother should not add more water to feed as it might lead to dilution of nutrients, which will lead to malnutrition.
- *Complementary bridge and safety net to prevent malnutrition:* Most of the children fall into category of malnutrition during weaning and postweaning period. Continued breastfeeding, introduction of vegetable protein and animal protein are important components of it.
- *Responsive feeding:* It refers to mother and child interactions during feeding which has a great impact.
- *Toddlers (1-3 years of age):* A toddler needs more than half the food that the mother eats. This should be given in frequent servings. Eating while playing, group eating and eating from a special vessel may be good methods.
- *Preschool children (3-6 years):* A preschool child should eat half the quantity that the father eats. Their interest is group play and in exploring and mastering the environment. They enjoy variety in food items.
- *School-going children:* They should eat three-fourths of food that the father eats. They should take a balanced diet and should not miss meals, especially breakfast which is the brain's food.
- *Feeding during and after illness:* Breastfeeding and feeding of easily digestible soft food items should be continued during illness. Starvations should be avoided unless medically advised.
- *Monitoring growth and development:* Monitoring growth chart is important. It will bring to our notice regarding flat curve, downward curve, or growth faltering which may require further necessary investigations.

TEN COMMANDMENTS IN NUTRITION

1. Be baby friendly. Initiate breastfeeding soon after birth, preferably within an hour.
2. Exclusive breastfeeding for first 6 months of age.

3. Continue breastfeeding as long as possible, preferably till 2 years of age.
4. Complementary feeding should be started at the age of 6 months.
5. Slowly switch over to family pot feeding by 1 year of age.
6. Small, frequent feeds prevent malnutrition.
7. Ensure balanced diet that includes various food items and nutrients.
8. During adolescence, pregnancy, lactation ensures extra nutrition.
9. Ensure micronutrients and antioxidants by including green leafy vegetables and fruits.
10. Ensure quality of survival and overall development by non-nutritional interventions such as good sanitation, safe water supply, vaccination, family harmony, etc.

Anthropometry and Assessment of Growth

CHAPTER 5

Vikram Bhaskar

INTRODUCTION
The growth assessment is crucial in childcare to assess the nutritional status and for the identification of growth failure. Assessing the growth of a child requires taking some measurements at regular intervals, approximately at the same time of the day, and seeing their trend. The measurements thus obtained are then compared with standard references.

WEIGHT
An electronic scale or a balance-beam scale should be used, that is accurate to 0.01 kg (<2 years) and 0.1 kg (>2 years). Spring type scales are not recommended because their accuracy cannot be assured after repeated use.

According to WHO, weighing machine should allow "tared weighing", which means that the scale can be reset to zero ("tared") with the person just weighed still on it.

Infants: 0–2 years
- Before measurements are taken, zero calibration of the scale must be done.
- The infant must be placed in the middle of the scale, without any clothes or diaper. If a diaper is worn, the weight must be corrected by subtracting the weight of the diaper.
- Before a reading is taken, wait for the baby to lie still. The baby must not hold onto anything for support.
- An average of three readings is taken and measurements are read to the nearest 0.01 kg.
- The above method is also used in children (up to 20 kg) who are unable to stand.

Children: 2–18 years

- Before measurements are taken, zero calibration of the scale must be done.
- Weigh without shoes and only light clothing must be worn.
- The subject must stand still with the weight equally distributed on both feet. The child must not hold onto to anything for support.
- An average of three readings is taken and measurements are read to the nearest 0.1 kg.
- In nonambulatory patients, one can also weigh the child with the parent/caregiver and then subtract this amount from the parent/caregiver's weight to obtain the child's estimated weight.

Growth Based on Weight

- An average normal newborn weighs 2.5–3 kg at birth, loses up to 10% of birth weight by 7 days and regains it by 10th day of life.
- On an average, infants gain 30 g/day for first 3 months of life and 20 g/day between 3 and 6 months.
- A child usually doubles the birth weight by 5 months, triples the birth weight by the end of 1 year and quadruples it by 2 years of age.
- From the 2nd year onwards, the child gains 2–2.5 kg per year till the onset of pubertal growth spurt.
- The pubertal acceleration of growth occurs in girls (10–12 years) and later in boys (12–14 years).
- The expected weight can be calculated by Weech's formula **(Table 1)**.

Table 1: Weech's formula.	
3–12 months	$\dfrac{X+9}{2}$ (X = Age in months)
1–6 years	$2X + 8$ (X = Age in years)
7–12 years	$\dfrac{7X-5}{2}$ (X = Age in years)

LENGTH OR HEIGHT

Depending on a child's age and ability to stand, measure the child's length or height.
- If a child is less than 2 years old, measure recumbent length.
- If a child is aged 2 years or older and able to stand, measure standing height.

In general, standing height is about 0.7 cm less than recumbent length. Therefore, it is important to adjust the measurements if length is taken instead of height, and vice versa.
- If a child less than 2 years old will not lie down for measurement of length, measure standing height and add 0.7 cm to convert it to length.
- If a child aged 2 years or older cannot stand, measure recumbent length and subtract 0.7 cm to convert it to height.

Equipment needed to measure length is called infantometer **(Fig. 1)**, which should be placed on a flat, stable surface such as a table. To measure height, use a height board, also called a stadiometer **(Fig. 2)**, mounted at a right angle between a level floor and against a straight, vertical surface such as a wall or pillar.

Before measuring the length or height, ensure that the child's shoes, socks, and hair ornaments have been removed.

Whether measuring length or height, the mother is needed to help with measurement and to soothe and comfort the child. Explain to the mother the reasons for the measurement and the steps in the procedure. Answer any questions that she may have. Show her and tell her how she can help you.

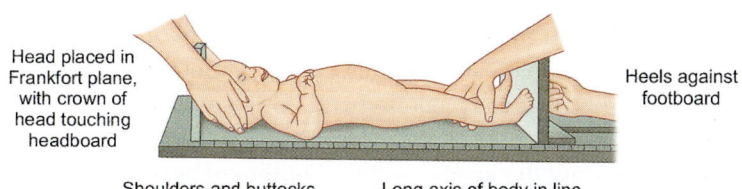

Fig. 1: Measuring length on an infantometer.

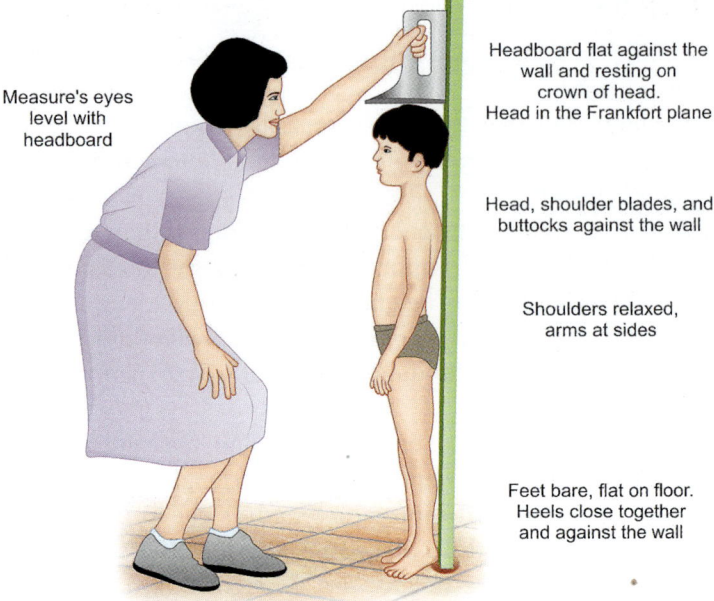

Fig. 2: Measuring the height with stadiometer.

Measuring Length

- When the mother understands your instructions and is ready to assist, ask her to lay the child on his back with his head against the fixed headboard, compressing the hair.
- Check that the child lies straight along the board and does not change position. Shoulders should touch the board and the spine should not be arched.
- The child's eyes should be looking straight up.
- Hold down the child's legs with one hand and move the footboard with the other. Apply gentle pressure to the knees to straighten the legs as far as they can go without causing injury. (If a child is extremely agitated and both legs cannot be held in position, measure with oneleg in position.)
- While holding the knees, pull the footboard against the child's feet. The soles of the feet should be flat against the footboard, toes pointing upward.

- Read the measurement and record the child's length in centimeters to the last completed 0.1 cm.
- An average of three readings is taken and recorded in growth record.

Measuring Height

- Help the child to stand on the baseboard with feet slightly apart. The back of the head, shoulder blades, buttocks, calves, and heels should all touch the vertical board.
- Position the child's head so that a horizontal line from the ear canal to the lower border of the eye socket runs parallel to the baseboard (Frankfort plane).
- Still keeping the head in position, pull down the headboard to rest firmly on top of the head and compress the hair.
- To avoid errors of parallax, the measurer's eyes should be at level with the headboard.
- Read the measurement and record the child's height in centimeters to the last completed 0.1 cm.
- An average of three readings is taken and recorded in growth record.

Growth Based on Height

- A full-term newborn measures 45–50 cm at birth and attains a length of 65 cm at 6 months, 75 cm at 1 year, 87.5 cm at 2 years and 100 cm at 4 years. Thereafter, till the onset of puberty, children gain 5 cm/year.
- The formula used to calculate the expected height between the age of 2 and 12 years is, Expected height (cm) = (Age in years × 6) + 77. As an example, for a 5-year-old child, the expected height would be (5 × 6) + 77 = 107 cm.

HEAD CIRCUMFERENCE

- A flexible, nonstretchable measuring tape must be used with 1 cm increments.
- Infants can be measured whilst sitting in the caregivers lap and older children can be measured while standing.

- Headgear or any objects, e.g., hairpins must be removed.
- The tape is positioned just above the eyebrows (i.e., supraorbital ridges), above the ears, and around the back of the head (i.e., occiput) **(Fig. 3)** so that the maximum circumference is measured.

The tape should be on the same plane on both sides of the head and tight enough to compress the hair. An average of three readings is taken and measurements are read to the nearest millimeter.

Rate of increase in head circumference from birth to 5 years of age is shown in **Table 2**.

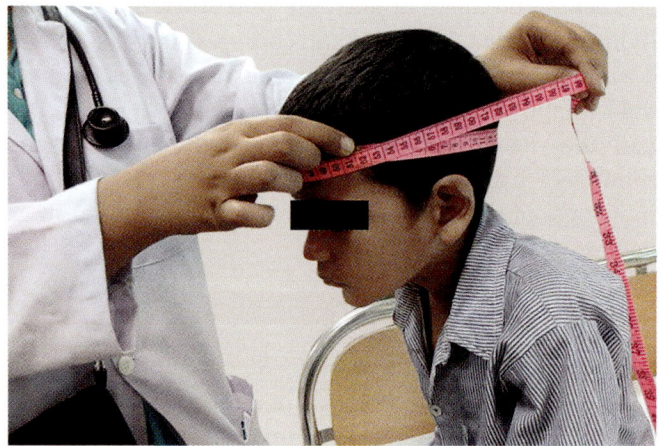

Fig. 3: Measuring the head circumference.

Table 2: Rate of Increase in head circumference from birth to 5 years of age.

Age	Increase in head ⌀	Measured head ⌀
0–3 months	2 cm/month	40 cm at 3 months
3–6 months	1 cm/month	43 cm at 6 months
6–12 months	0.5 cm/month	46 cm at 1 year
1–3 years	2 cm/year	50 cm at 3 years
3–5 years	1 cm/year	52 cm at 5 years

MID-UPPER ARM CIRCUMFERENCE

- A nonstretchable measuring tape is used.
- Measurement is taken on the nondominant arm at the midpoint of the arm.
- The arm is bent at the elbow to form a 90° angle. The palm of the hand faces upward. The reading is taken midway between the acromion process of the scapula and the olecranon process of the ulna **(Figs. 4A and B)**. This point is called midpoint of arm.

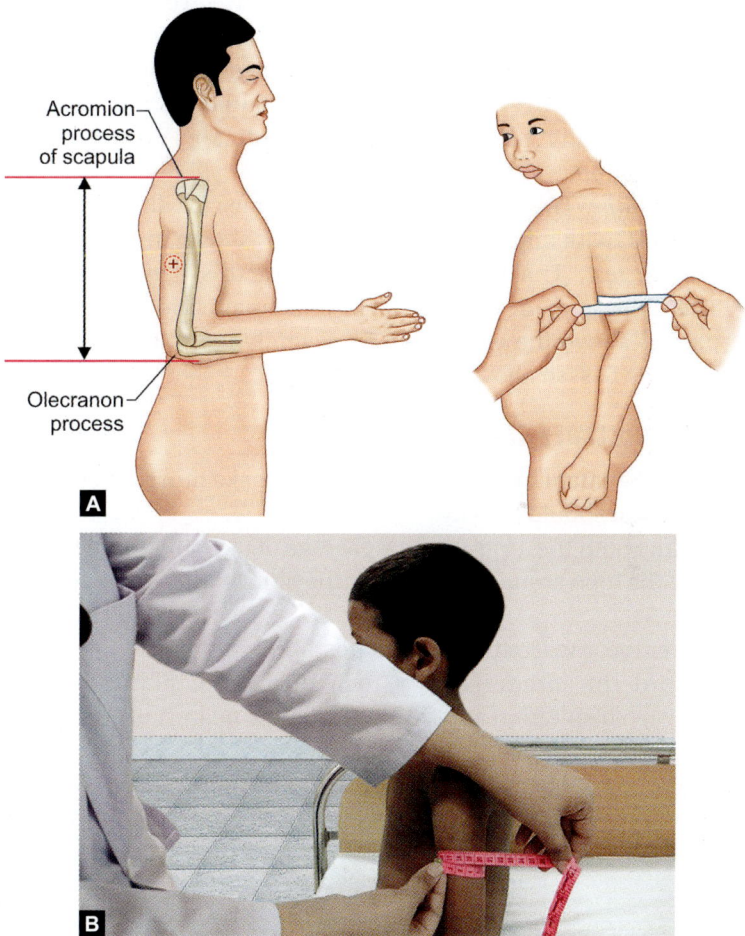

Figs. 4A and B: Measuring the mid arm circumference.

- Patient now stands with arms relaxed at the side and with the palm facing toward the thigh.
- The measuring tape is placed at midpoint, perpendicular to the long axis of the arm.
- The tape must not cut into the flesh. The reading is taken to the nearest millimeter.

MID UPPER ARM CIRCUMFERENCE AND ASSESSMENT OF NUTRITION

- Mid upper arm circumference (MUAC) remains nearly constant between the ages of 1 and 5 years. It is also an age-independent anthropometric criterion for the assessment of malnutrition. MUAC less than 12.5 cm indicates malnutrition, while reading less than 11.5 cm indicates Severe Acute Malnutrition.
- *Shakir tape:* This tape has three color zones for different values of MUAC with different interpretations as shown in **Table 3**.
- *Bangle test:* The internal diameter of this bangle is 4 cm. The child is made to wear it. In a normal child, it cannot be passed above the elbow, but in severely malnourished child, it can be passed above the elbow.

CHEST CIRCUMFERENCE

- Place the infant in the lap of mother, or make him stand straight. The chest should be bare.
- Abduct both the arms to allow passage of tape around the chest.
- Pass the tape around the chest of the child at the level of nipples **(Fig. 5)**.
- Lower the arms to their natural position.
- Record the circumference in a horizontal plane, midway between inspiration and expiration, to the nearest of 0.1 cm.

Table 3: Measurements on Shakir tape and its interpretations.

Color zone	Measured value	Interpretation
Red	<12.5 cm	Wasted
Yellow	12.5–13.5 cm	Borderline
Green	>13.5 cm	Normal

Anthropometry and Assessment of Growth

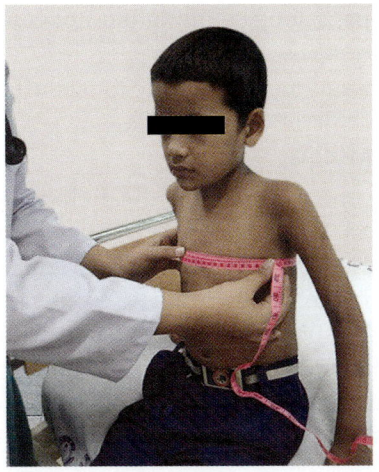

Fig. 5: Measuring the chest circumference.

Chest circumference is less than the head circumference (HC) at birth; however it exceeds the HC by 1 year of age.

WAIST CIRCUMFERENCE
- Ask the child to stand straight and remove the clothes from the upper torso.
- Lower the pants slightly to palpate the iliac crest.
- Mark a horizontal line at the highest point of iliac crest on both sides.
- Place a measuring tape around the trunk passing through both horizontal lines.
- Ensure that tape is fitting snuggly but not compressing the skin.
- Record the measurement at minimal respiration to the nearest 0.1 cm.

HIP CIRCUMFERENCE
- Ask the child to stand straight. The child should be wearing briefs only.
- Stand at the back of the child and place the measuring tape around the hips.
- Place the tape horizontally at the maximum convexity of hips.

- Ensure that tape is snuggly fitting but not compressing the skin or soft tissue.
- Record the measurement from side to nearest 0.1 cm.

SKINFOLD THICKNESS

All skinfolds are measured with the help of skinfold calipers (Lange, Holtain, or Harpenden). WHO used Holtain calipers in their growth study. The measurements are taken on left side of body. It is preferable to mark the site to be measured. The skinfold (skin and subcutaneous tissue) is grasped with the thumb and index finger of left hand above the mark. The caliper tips are placed perpendicular to the length of the fold, and measurements are taken to the nearest 0.1 mm on the Harpenden or 0.5 mm on the Lange caliper.

Triceps Skinfold

- Let the arm hang relax by the side.
- Stand behind the child and grasp the skinfold 1 cm above the midpoint marked over triceps muscle, along the long axis of arm.
- Apply the caliper jaws over the mark, perpendicular to skinfold.
- Gently release the caliper handles and allow the jaws to close on the fat fold for 2 seconds, while maintaining the grip on skinfold.
- Record the reading as described above.

Subscapular Skinfold

- Ask the child to sit or stand with shoulder relaxed.
- Palpate and mark the inferior angle of left scapula.
- Grasp the skinfold 1 cm below and medial to the mark.
- The skinfold runs at a 45° angle directed down and toward left side.
- Apply the caliper at the mark, perpendicular to skinfold.
- Record the measurements as described above.
  Skinfold measurements are not reliable when edema is present.

BODY PROPORTIONS

Body proportions like upper segment to lower segment ratio and arm span may give valuable information regarding growth disturbances.

Upper Segment to Lower Segment Ratio

Lower segment is measured from symphysis pubis to the heel. Upper segment is calculated by subtracting lower segment from total length or height. The ratio of upper segment to lower segment is 1.7 at birth. It decreases to 1.3 by 3–4 years of age. The ratio equalizes at around 7–10 years of age (ratio 1:1). High upper/lower segment ratio indicates short limb dwarfism, while low ratio indicates spinal pathologies.

Sitting Height

- It denotes the upper segment length.
- The child sits on a stool with his back and buttocks in contact with the wall.
- Place the head in Frankfort's horizontal plane. The knees should be directed straight ahead with the arms and hands at the sides.
- Ask the child to sit tall, take a deep breath, and then bring the horizontal bar down snugly to the head.
- Measure the distance between the sitting board of the stool and the horizontal head board to the nearest 0.1 cm.

Arm Span

- Ask the child to stand erect against a wall and outstretch both the arms at 90° to the body with palm facing outward.
- The arms and the back of the palms should also be in contact with the wall.
- Mark the points corresponding to the tips of middle fingers of opposite hands on the wall.
- Measure the distance between the two points.

Arm span is less than the stature by 1–2 cm by 10 years of age. Thereafter, arm span exceeds the height but the difference always stays less than 3–5 cm.

INDICES

An index is a combination of two measurements or one measurement plus the person's age. These indices are essential for the interpretation of measurements. It is evident that a value of

Table 4: Age-independent methods of assessment of nutrition.

Name of index	Method to obtain	Normal range	Undernourished
Mid upper arm circumference (MUAC)	Taken between age 1 and 5 years	>13.5 cm	<12.5 cm
Dugdale's index	$\frac{\text{Weight in kg}}{(\text{Height in cm})^{1.6}} \times 100$	0.88–0.97	<0.79
Rao's index	$\frac{\text{Weight in kg}}{(\text{Height in cm})^2} \times 100$	0.15–0.16	<0.14
Kanawati index	$\frac{\text{MUAC (cm)}}{\text{Head circumference (cm)}}$	0.32–0.33	≤0.25

body weight alone has no meaning unless it is related to an individual's height or age. Following are some useful indices:

- *Ponderal index:* It is calculated for newborn as birth weight (g)/length (cm)^3 × 100. A ponderal index of <2 indicates asymmetrical growth retardation.
- *Waist-hip ratio:* It is calculated as waist circumference/hip circumference and is an indicator of obesity.
- *Weight-for-age:* It is calculated as observed weight/expected weight (50th centile of reference) × 100.

Some anthropometric indices do not vary significantly with age. These indices are useful in situations where exact age of child is not known. These are called age-independent indices and are shown in **Table 4**.

BMI

Body mass index (BMI) is calculated as weight (kg)/height (m^2). It is an important indicator of body composition of an individual. Age-related standards are used to compare with observed values and are interpreted as shown in **Table 5**.

Interpretation of Anthropometric Indices

The anthropometric indices can be expressed in terms of Z-scores, percentiles, or percent of median, which can then be used to

Table 5: BMI and nutritional status.

BMI for age	Nutritional status
<5th percentile	Underweight
5th–84th percentile	Normal
85th–94th percentile	Overweight
≥95th percentile	Obese

(BMI: body mass index)

compare a child with a reference population. These reporting indices are as follows:

Percentile: The rank position of an individual on a given reference distribution, stated in terms of what percentage of the group, the individual equals or exceeds. The median lies at 50th percentile, on either side of which lies half of the observation.

Z-score: The deviation of the value for an individual from the median value of the reference population, divided by the standard deviation for the reference population:

$$\text{Z-score} = \frac{\text{(Observed value)} - \text{(Median reference value)}}{\text{Standard deviation of reference population}}$$

Percent of median: The ratio of measured value in the individual to the median value of the reference data for the same value, expressed as percentage.

If the distribution of reference values follows a normal distribution, percentiles, and Z-scores are related through a mathematical transformation. The commonly used –3, –2, and –1 Z-scores are respectively the 0.13th, 2.28th, and 15.8th percentile. Similarly, the 1st, 3rd, and 10th percentile corresponds to, respectively the –2.33, –1.88, and –1.29 Z-scores. It can be seen that the 3rd percentile and the –2 Z-score are very close to each other.

How to Use Growth Charts?

Growth charts are tool to monitor a child's physical growth. The WHO growth charts are international standards that show how healthy children should grow. The standards describe the growth of children living in six countries in environments believed to support optimal growth. One of the several criteria defined for optimal growth is breastfeeding. Following steps should be used to interpret the growth charts:

- *Obtain accurate measurements:* Measure the growth parameters as described above by using the equipment that are well maintained.
- *Select appropriate growth chart:* Select the growth chart to be used based on the age and sex of the child being weighed and measured. Determine the accurate age of child from health records.
- *Record data:* After selecting the appropriate chart, enter the patient's name, record number, age, and parent's stature on growth chart.
- *Plot measurements:*
  - Find the child's age on the horizontal axis. Use a straight edge or ruler to draw a vertical line from this point.
  - Find the appropriate measurement (weight, length, BMI) on the vertical axis. Use a straight edge or ruler to draw a horizontal line from this point.
  - Make a small dot where the two lines intersect.
  - *Interpret the plotted measurements:* In a WHO growth chart, there are curved lines representing either percentiles or Z-scores. There are usually five percentiles lines corresponding to 3rd, 15th, 50th, 85th, and 97th percentile (from below to up). In Z-score charts however, the lines corresponds to –3 Z, –2 Z, 0, 2 Z, and 3 Z-scores. Child's growth is interpreted based on the position of dot in relation to above references. A normal child remains between 15th and 85th percentiles **(Figs. 6 to 8)**.

Assessment of Nutritional Status by Anthropometry

The term "malnutrition" means both undernutrition and overnutrition ranging from severe nutrient deficiencies to extreme obesity. Anthropometric measurements can give a fair idea about the nutritional status of a child. Several classification systems are used to categorize the grade of malnutrition in a particular child.

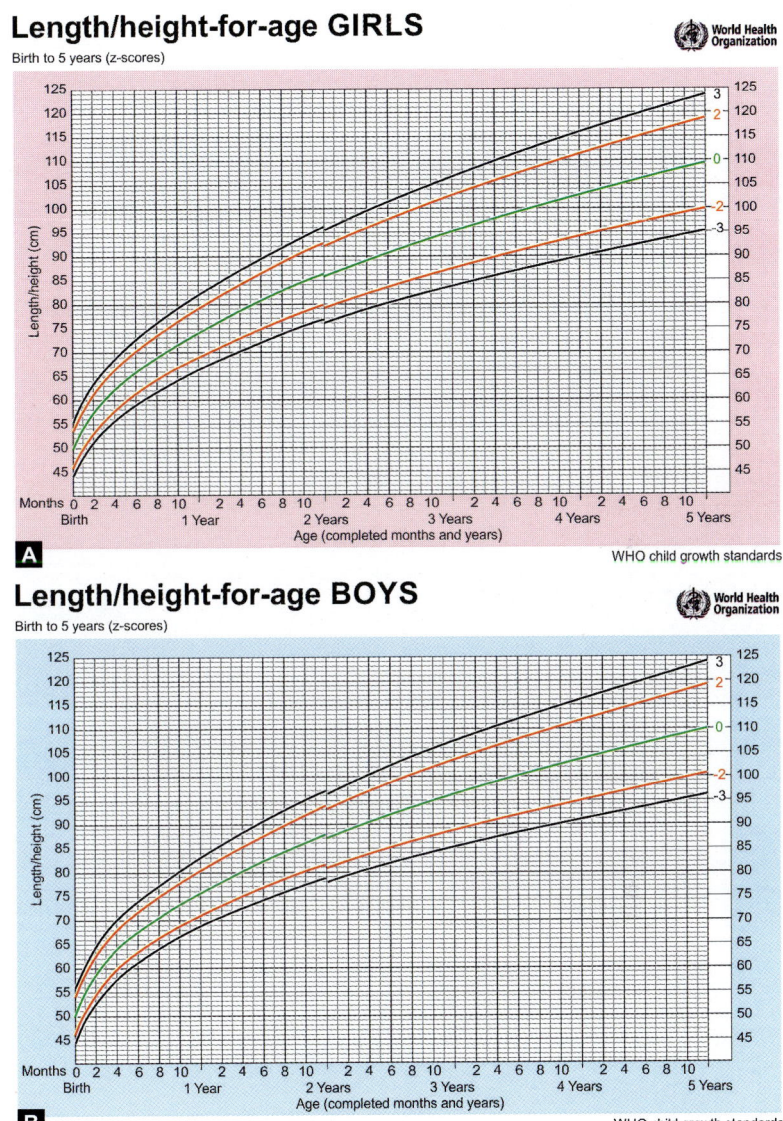

Figs. 6A and B: Length/height-for-age.
(A) Girls; and (B) Boys from birth to 5 years (percentile).

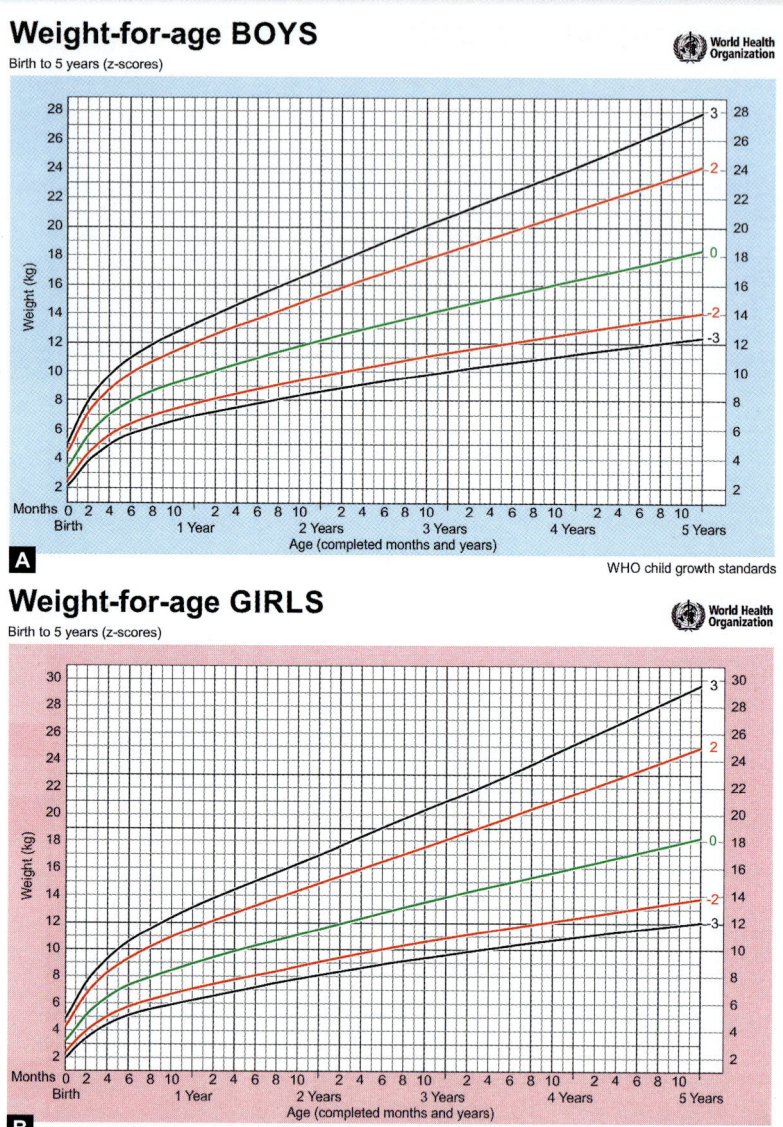

Figs. 7A and B: Weight-for-age.
(A) Boys; and (B) Girls from birth to 5 years (percentiles).

Anthropometry and Assessment of Growth

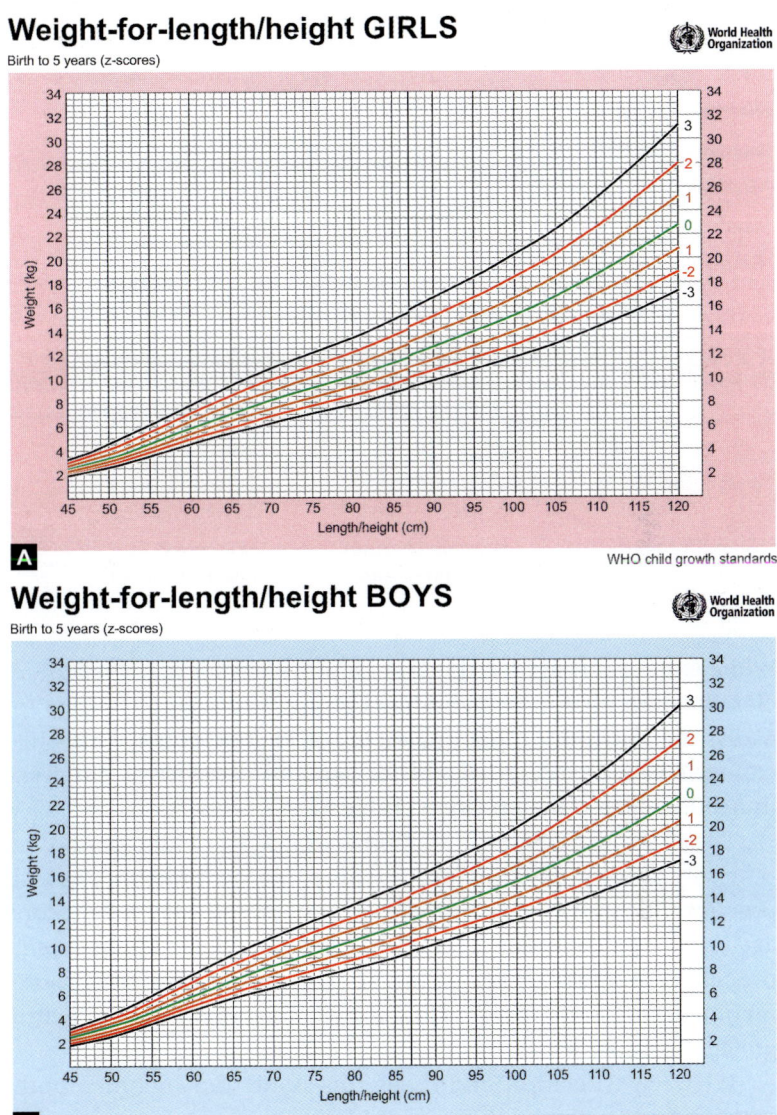

Figs. 8A and B: Weight-for-length/height.
(A) Girls; and (B) Boys from birth to 3 years (percentile).

Table 6: Indian Academy of Pediatrics classification of malnutrition.

Grade of malnutrition	Weight-for-age of the standard (median) %
Normal	>80
Grade I	71–80
Grade II	61–70
Grade III	51–60
Grade IV	<50

Table 7: WHO classification for undernutrition.

	Moderate malnutrition	Severe malnutrition
Symmetrical edema	No	Yes
Weight-for-height	SD score (Z-score) between −2 and −3	SD score < −3 Severe wasting
Height-for-age	SD score (Z-score) between −2 and −3	SD score < −3 Severe stunting

While Gomez introduced the criteria of weight-for-age, Wellcome classification also included edema along with weight-for-age to assess malnutrition. Indian Academy of Pediatrics (IAP) classification is also based on weight-for-age and categorizes children into four grades of malnutrition **(Table 6)**.

The drawback of above method is that age of child should be precisely known, which is not possible many a times in clinical practice. Secondly, it has now been understood that weight-for-age is in fact a compound parameter or two virtually independent processes, namely stunting (low height for age due to chronic malnutrition) and wasting (low weight for height due to acute growth retardation).

WHO classification addresses this issue and includes both stunting and wasting as shown in **Table 7**.

# Developmental Assessment

CHAPTER 6

Rhishikesh Thakre, Archana Kadam

INTRODUCTION

The first years of life are crucial for lifelong learning and development. Close monitoring of development together with coordination of treatment for any emerging problems is referred to as developmental follow-up. The domains for developmental assessment are motor (gross motor and fine motor), cognitive (thinking, memory learning, and problem solving), communicative (understanding and production of meaningful symbolic communication with gestures and talking) and social or emotional (emotional reactions to events and interactions with others), and self-help skills. Evaluating a child in all domains of development helps in early identification of developmental delay. The components of developmental surveillance are depicted in **Box 1**.

PRINCIPLES OF DEVELOPMENT

- Development is a continuous process from conception to maturity.
- The rate of development may vary in individual child, but the sequence of development is same in all children.
- The development always proceeds in a cephalocaudal direction. A child will learn first to hold his head, followed by sitting

Box 1: Components of developmental surveillance.
- Identifying risk factors and high-risk infants
- Documenting and maintaining developmental history
- Eliciting and attending to parents' concern regarding the child's development
- Make accurate observations of the child
- Maintaining accurate record of findings
- Identifying protective factors

and then walking. This sequence from head to toe will always remain the same, though the age at which each milestone is achieved may differ.
- Development is related to maturation, myelination of the nervous system. The normal development needs an intact anatomical and functionally normal central nervous system (CNS). Anatomical CNS malformations like anencephaly, meningomyelocele are commonly associated with developmental problems. A child who had any CNS insult like hypoxic ischemic encephalopathy, CNS infection, kernicterus, hypoglycemia or any other metabolic cause may have delayed development. Such insult during first 5 years of life (while brain is growing) may play an important role in its development.
- It is important that certain primitive reflexes are lost before voluntary functions are achieved. For example, the grasp reflex should be lost (by 3–4 months of age) before the infant can learn to reach for objects and grasp them voluntarily (by 4–5 months of age). Similarly, asymmetric tonic neck reflex has to be lost before a child learns to turn over in bed.

  Persistence of primitive reflexes beyond the age at which they should have disappeared, indicates abnormal development. Moro's reflex disappears by 3 months of age, but presence of Moro's reflex in 7 months of child is suggestive of abnormal development.
- The development in one field may not be parallel to that in other fields and this is termed as developmental dissociation. It helps to decide anatomical localization of the pathology.
- Developmental delay should be differentiated from developmental regression in which there is loss of milestones which already the child had achieved.

DOMAINS OF DEVELOPMENT

Development is usually assessed in terms of achieving the mile stones in four separate domains. They are:
1. Gross motor
2. Fine motor

3. Language (speech and hearing)
4. Personal–social milestones

The gross motor skills and activities like head control and sitting are the most obvious initial areas of the child development while personal social development is a spectrum of the psychological developmental process. If one domain of development is affected, it may have an impact on the other domains. For example, if a child has hearing deficit, it can also affect language as well as personal and social development.

The development of a child is an outcome of the interaction between hereditary and environmental factors. The hereditary factors would determine the potential of how the child develops and the environmental factors like physical, social and emotional would influence the extent to which the potential achieved.

The following points should be taken into consideration while evaluating development of the child:
- Has the child achieved his age appropriate development in each domain?
- Is the sequence of developmental process normal? Is there any skipping of the milestones?
- Is the developmental progress in each domain similar?
- How does the development of the child relate to the chronological age?
- Is the development normal or abnormal? If it is delayed, whether it is global delay or there is a dissociation between the various domains of development. For example, a child with hearing deficit resulting in speech delay can have normal motor milestones.
- Is it developmental delay or regression? In some cases, the child may have acquired initial milestones appropriate for age and after certain age there is delay in development. It can be due to neurological insult, severe acute illness or severe acute malnutrition. The regression of milestones may be due to neurodegenerative disorders.

Gross Motor Milestones

Gross motor milestones are those concerned with locomotion and control of body like head control, sitting, standing, walking, running, jumping, etc. It depends upon the maturation of muscular, skeletal and nervous system. The major gross motor milestones are listed in **Table 1**.

In the neonatal period, the baby lies supine in flexed and symmetrical posture and has a marked head lag on being pulled up **(Fig. 1)**. The motor development for the young infant in the first 3 months is tested by following methods:

Ventral Suspension

The child is held in ventral suspension in the prone position with the examiner's hand under the abdomen. At 6 weeks, the baby momentarily holds the head in a horizontal position in the plane of the trunk and by 12 weeks, the head is held above the horizontal plane **(Figs. 2A and B)**. This indicates development of gradual head control with increasing myelination and muscle tone.

Prone Position

The child lifts the chin up momentarily at 4 weeks, face is lifted at 45° by 8 weeks and child can bear weight on forearms with chin off

Table 1: Gross motor milestones.

Age	Milestones
3 months	Head control/neck holding
5 months	Rolling over (turning from supine to prone and prone to supine)
6 months	Sitting with support
7 months	Sitting without support
9–10 months	Standing with support
12–13 months	Standing to rise and walking without support
18 months	Running
2 years	Climbing upstairs using two feet per step. Kicking a ball
2.5 years	Jumping
3 years	Riding a tricycle. Standing on one leg momentarily
4 years	Hopping on one foot. Climbing up and downstairs with one foot per step
5 years	Skipping and jumping

the couch and face lifted up to 90° **(Fig. 3)**. The baby learns to roll over, first from prone to supine and then from supine to prone at 5 months of age.

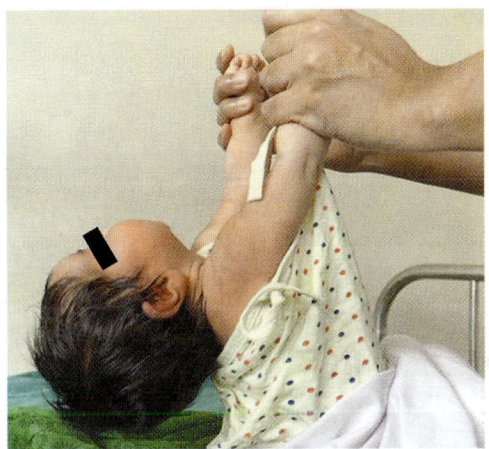

Fig. 1: Head lag in newborn on being pulled up.

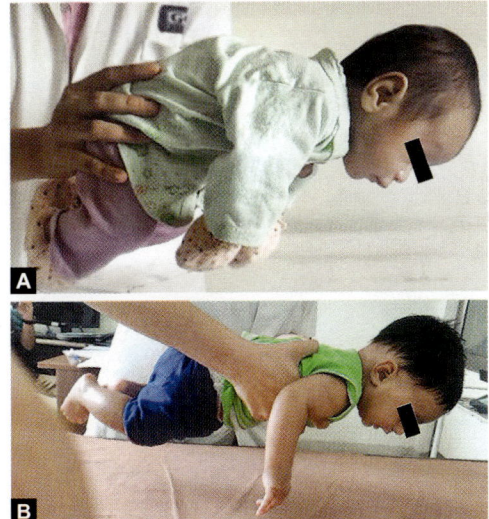

Figs. 2A and B: (A) Ventral suspension at 6 weeks: head momentarily held in the same plane as the body; (B) Ventral suspension at 12-week-old baby: head held above the horizontal plane.

Sitting

The infant learns to sit with support at 6–7 months of age. Initially, the child sits with support of hands forwarded with a rounded back. Later, at the age of 7–8 months, the baby sits with a straight back without any support **(Fig. 4)**.

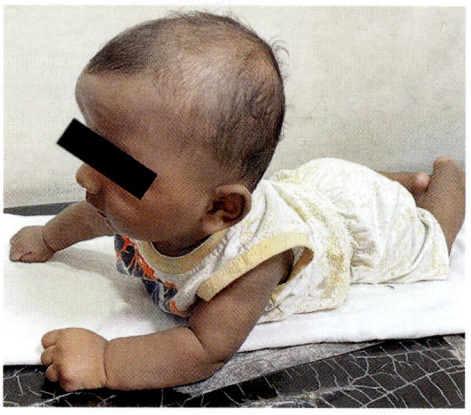

Fig. 3: Prone position at 12 weeks: bearing weight on forearms and lifting face at 90°.

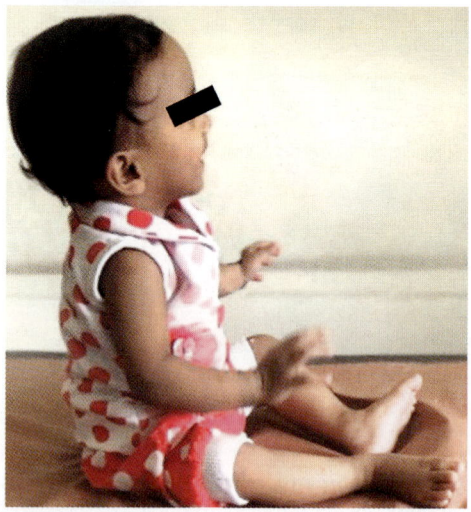

Fig. 4: Sitting at 7–8 months with straight back and without any support.

Crawling

The child learns crawling on hands and knees at 9 months of age **(Fig. 5)**. Most of children crawl before they walk, but few may not crawl and straight away learn to stand and walk. This may be due to not putting them on hard surface by the parents.

Standing and Walking

Most infants learn to stand and walk, holding a chair or couch **(Fig. 6)**. Then, they learn walking without support, initially unsteadily with hands apart and broad gait by the age of 11–12 months. They walk alone steadily by 14–15 months of age **(Fig. 7)**.

Fine Motor Development

Fine motor development mainly involves body movements, coordination and manipulation skills. Hand regard is an important milestone seen in an infant between the age of 3 and 5 months. There is observation of hands by the infant when he is lying supine **(Fig. 8)**. Subsequently, the baby learns holding the object. Persistence of hand regard beyond 5 months is abnormal.

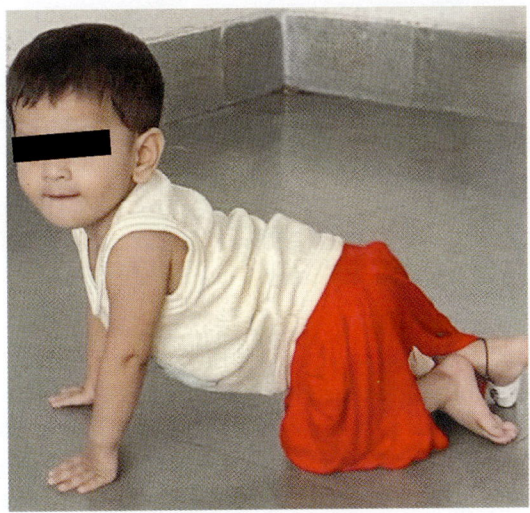

Fig. 5: A 9-month-old infants crawling on hands and knees.

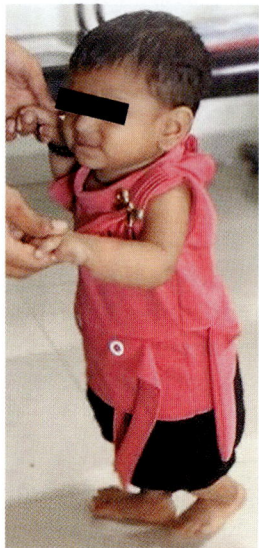

Fig. 6: A 10-month-old infant walking with support.

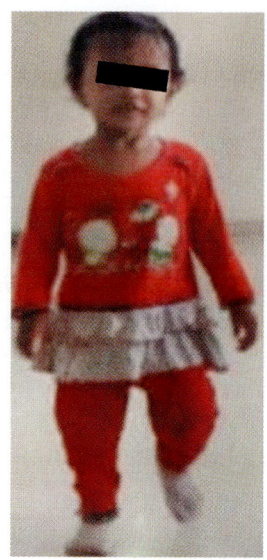

Fig. 7: A 14-month-old child walking independently and steadily.

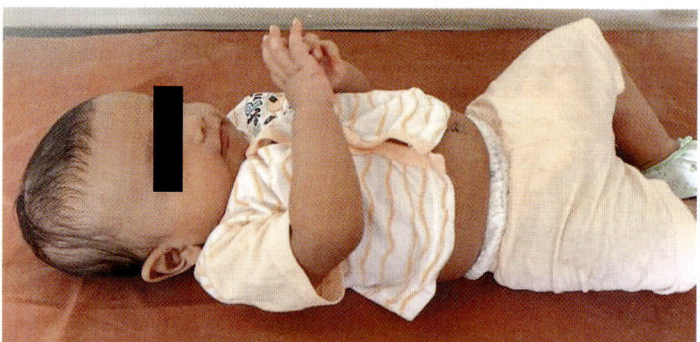

Fig. 8: Hand regard in 4-month-old infant.

Subsequently, the baby learns holding the object. Grasp is assessed by giving the cubes. Initially, the grasp is bidextrous that changes to unidextrous and then to pincer grasp. Holding an object between index finger and thumb is called pincer grasp and it matures at 12 months **(Fig. 9)**. By 6 months of age, the baby starts putting everything that is in his hand into the mouth, called as hand-to-mouth reflex. It disappears by age of 1 year. The child learns to draw a circle at 3 years of age, square at 4 years of age and triangle at 5 years of age. The important fine motor milestones are listed in **Table 2**.

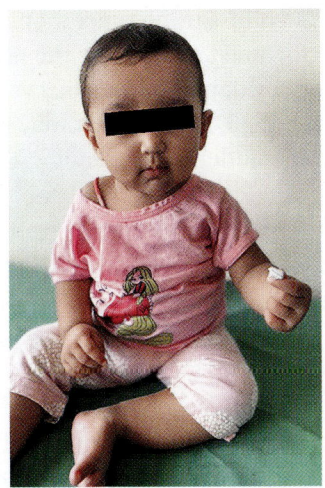

Fig. 9: Pincer grasp in 9-month-old infant.

Table 2: Fine motor milestones.

Age	Milestones
6 weeks	Follows face in midline and turns head towards moving object
4 months	Reaches for toy or red ring or rattle in front with both hands
6 months	Reaches for objects by one hand only (palmar grasp)
7 months	Transfers objects from one hand to another
9 months	Pincer grasp (picks up a pellet with thumb and index finger)
12 months	Casting (throwing the object away)
15 months	Able to feed himself with spoon without spilling
18 months	Builds tower of three cubes and scribbles
2 years	Vertical and circular strokes
3 years	Copies a circle
4 years	Copies a square and cross
5 years	Draws a triangle

Personal and Social Development

Cognitive development and understanding is reflected by attainment of milestones in this domain. The main personal and social milestones are listed in **Table 3**.

Toilet training is an integral part of development. By the age of 10–12 months, the child can be placed on the baby toilet seat and is usually ready for toilet training by the age of 15–18 months. The child becomes dry by day by the age of 2 years and dry by night by the age of 3 years. Still, 5% of children may not be toilet trained by this age but achieve bladder control later.

Language Development

The infant has several ways of preverbal communication. The newborn and infant communicate by crying, smiling or frowning. Thus, language development is the progressive development of infant's ability to use language from simple sound production to fluency of words. During the first 3 months, the language development is observed by his ability to vocalize and recognize mother's voice and respond to human voice. The main language milestones are shown in **Table 4**.

Table 3: Personal and social development.

Age	Milestones
4 weeks	Alert to sound
2 months	Social smile (response with smile to social contact)
3 months	Recognizes mother
6 months	Smiles at reflection in the mirror
9 months	Waves 'Bye Bye'
12 months	Plays simple ball games
15–18 months	Holds spoon and feeds without spilling
18–24 months	Copies parent's tasks
3 years	Shares toys and knowns name and gender. Dry by night
4 years	Attends the toilet alone
5 years	Helps in household works, dresses and undresses

Table 4: Language development.

Age	Milestones
4 weeks	Turns head to sound
3 months	Vocalizes and cooing sounds
6 months	Speaks monosyllables (ma, ba)
7–8 months	Turns to soft sound out of sight
9 months	Speaks bisyllables (mama, baba)
12 months	Two words with meaning
18 months	Ten to fifteen words with meaning. Shows two parts of body
2 years	Uses 2–3 words to make phrases
3 years	Speaks in sentences, tells short stories

SCREENING VERSUS ASSESSMENT

Developmental screening refers to detection of unsuspected deviations from normal development that would not otherwise be identified in routine pediatric practice.

The purpose of developmental screening is to identify children who are at increased risk of delay and warrant additional testing. It is not diagnostic of developmental delay. It is performed by the pediatrician or parents **(Fig. 10)**.

Assessment is a formal in-depth evaluation for developmental delay using standardized developmental tools by a trained personnel or developmental pediatrician. The purpose is to create a profile of the child's strengths and weaknesses and to plan intervention accordingly.

TIMING OF EXAMINATION

Developmental surveillance is a periodic assessment of a child's developmental progress and is one of the fundamental evaluations in pediatric practice. Each meeting between the pediatrician and a child is an opportunity to assess developmental and behavior. If the visit does identify developmental issues, focused developmental screening may be recommended. One of the best times to

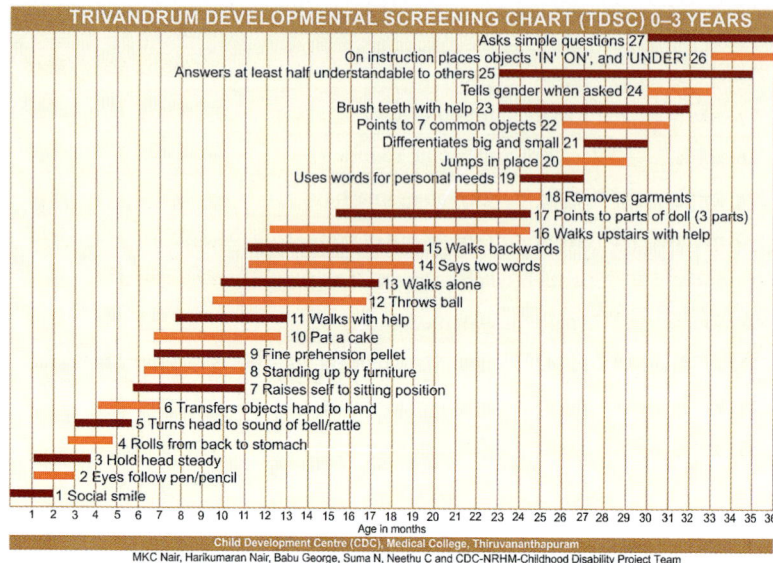

Fig. 10: Indian tests used for developmental screening—TDSC (Trivandrum development screening chart). This is a development screening tool. Note the age of the infant on X axis. Draw a vertical line for age. Each milestone has a range. For a particular age, the infant should be able to achieve milestones on the left for that age. For example at 3 months, the infant should achieve the milestones on left, i.e., have social smile and follow objects. Inability to do so is an indication for formal developmental assessment.

examine the infant is between feeds. The infant is assessed in a quiet room, when he or she is not hungry, sleepy, irritable, or sick. For optimum evaluation, first assessment should be done at 3 months of age. In children with high risk for delay follow-up should be 6 months, 9 months, 12 months, 18 months, and 6 monthly till 3 years and annually till 2 years after school entry. Low-risk child should be screened at 9 months, 18 months, 24 months, and 36 months visit. The high-risk children for developmental screening are—(1) NICU graduates, (2) parents express concerns of development, (3) babies with surgical conditions, major malformations, hypocalcemia, and inborn errors of metabolism, (4) babies having a syndrome that has a high probability of resulting in delay (e.g., Down syndrome), and (5) suboptimal family environment.

Place of Examination
Developmental surveillance is offered through public or private agencies and can be provided in a variety of settings, including a child's home, clinic, or child care center.

Correction for Prematurity
One needs to correct for prematurity till the age of 24 months while assessing development. Corrected age is the sum of chronological age in weeks minus the difference between gestational age at birth and 40 weeks' gestation. The chronological age is not taken into consideration while assessing milestones.

Common Tools (Figs. 11A and B)
- Red ball for visual assessment
- Pooja bell for hearing
- A red rattle and red pencil to test manipulation, voluntary reach, and transfer of objects
- Raisin or rice puff (murmura) to test for pincer grasp
- A doll—social imitation
- A paper and crayon to see for scribbling at one year

Assessing Development
- *Step 1: Evaluate for risk factors*—identify risk factors on history. Assess the feeding, growth, sleep patterns medical, social, economic, and psychological background of the child and family. Elicit and attend to parents' concern regarding the child's development.
- *Step 2: Red flags*—a red flag means the child is not doing what 90% children can perform for the given age. These red flags are a quick guide for a busy pediatrician to simplify the task of early detection and referral but are not screening or diagnostic tools **(Tables 5 and 6)**.
- *Step 3: Observing the infant*—Make accurate observations of the child. Note the baby's posture, arousal, alertness, and responsiveness.
  - *Posture:* Alignment of head, neck, body, asymmetric tonic neck reflex (ATNR) spontaneous, and if correctible,

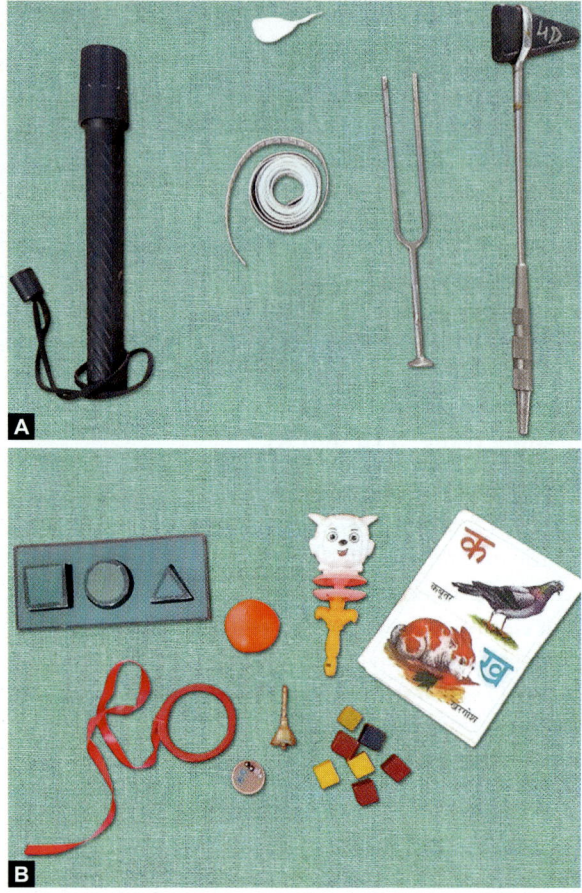

Figs. 11A and B: Common tools for assessment of development.

Table 5: Red flags—motor/fine motor.			
Gross motor	Age	Fine motor	Age
No head control	4½ months	Persistent fisting most of the time	3½ months
No roll over	6 months	Not holding rattle	4–5 months
Not sitting without support	9 months	Not transferring	5–6 months
Not standing while holding	10 months	No pincer grasp	10–11 months
Not walking	15 months	Not holding crayon	12 months
Bottom shuffling, W sitting		Handedness	<18 months

Table 6: Red flags—language and social.

Receptive	Age	Expressive	Age	Social	Age
Not turning to sound	6 months	No responsive vocalization	4 months	No social smile	3 months
Not responding to name	9 months	No attempt for sound	6 months	Not laughing in playful situations	6–8 months
Not following simple commands	12 months	Not babbling	12 months	Hard to console, stiffens when approached	12 months
Not locating or pointing to 5 objects	15 months	Not gesturing need	12 months		
		No bye bye or three words with meaning	15 months		

see movements—voluntary patterns, involuntary movements, abnormal patterns of movement like rolling for movement, bottom shuffling, toe walking, and symmetry (hemiplegia).

- *Eyes:* Look for pupil milky appearance (leukocoria—cataract), look for fix and follow—check with red hanging ring or red ball and face (normal) delay occurs in developmental immaturity or vision difficulty—cortical or in the eye. Nystagmus normally absent but present in cortical vision involvement or Down syndrome or cerebellar abnormality.
- *Hearing:* Use bell or rattle out of sight—see if child quietens and turns to sound—normal, no quieten (immaturity or hearing loss).
- *Check the spine:* Look for dysmorphic features. Look for features of hypothyroidism. Look at the umbilicus and inguinal region for hernia. Note the spontaneous movement, involuntary movements, cutaneous markers physical growth status, hygiene, skin, hair, teeth, and family interaction.

- *Step 4: Assess play and cognition*
  - Check social smile present—normal; absent (delay or vision abnormality)
  - Look for hand reach and hand play and hand to mouth, check transfer by giving another object in the same hand that the first toy was given, check for hidden object for memory, check imitation of tasks like pat doll to sleep; is as per age expectation is normal if not could suggest delay or motor or vision abnormality.
  - See if baby responds to name, tries to locate familiar people or objects, follows simple commands, babbles, and expressive jargon; if as per age expectations, is normal, if not, evaluate for delay.
    - *3 months normal:* Eyes fix and follow. Baby quietens to sound and may turn to sound and may occasionally vocalize when talked to. Baby brings hands to midline with hand-to-hand and hand to mouth, may watch hands and has a fidgety rhythm.
    - *6 months normal*: Reach for toys consistently; transfer of objects from one hand to another, banging toys holds two objects in two hands at one time. Turns to sound and vocalizes.
    - *9 months normal*: Can clap hands in midline, rings rattle and bell purposively, responds to name, babbles
    - *12 months normal:* Pincer grasp, scribbles, locates familiar objects and people, waves bye, and starts indicating needs with gestures and expressive jargon.
- *Step 5: Head examination*
  - *Size:* Head circumference <3rd centile poor brain growth; >3rd centile (macrocephaly or hydrocephalus). Monitor growth trajectory.
  - *AF:* Open, pulsatile (normal); small (slow brain growth); and tense nonpulsatile (raised intracranial pressure)
  - Sutures—normal and overriding suture (microcephaly especially squamotemporal sutures).
- *Step 6: Assess tone* **(Figs. 12 and 13)**
  - *Passive tone:* Tone is assessed on inspecting the posture, passive tone assessed by extensibility measured as angles

Developmental Assessment

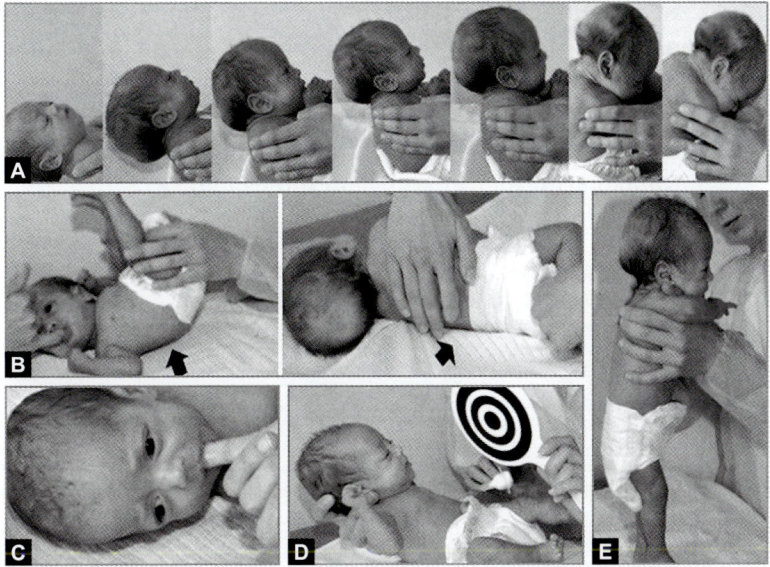

Figs. 12A to E: Neurologic assessment. (A) Axial tone (active tone): Raise to sit, head forward and backward; (B) Axial tone (passive tone): Ventral and dorsal incurvation; (C) Feeding autonomy and suckling; (D) Fix and track; (E) Righting reaction (active tone).

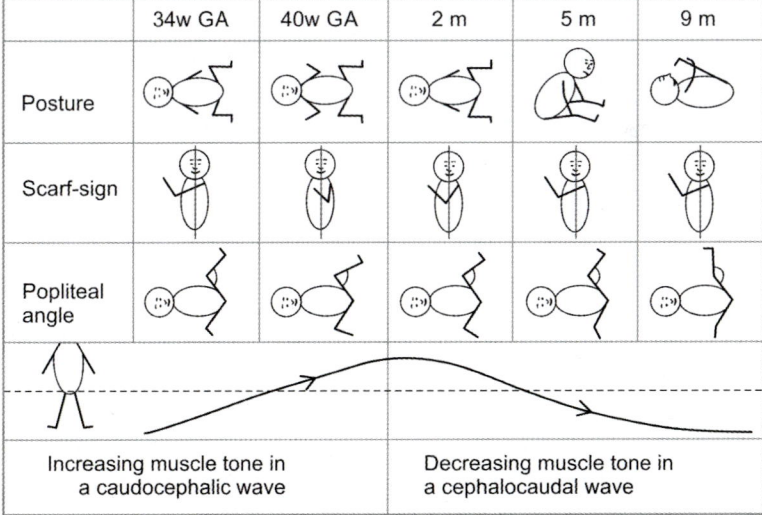

Fig. 13: Evolution of tone.

estimated but not measured or in association with certain landmarks like scarf sign. Observing the range of motions and comparing for symmetry and resistance to passive movement.

In first year of life, passive tone is formally assessed by estimating the following angles **(Tables 7 and 8)**.

Table 7: Assessment of passive tone.

Test	Procedure	Observe
Posture	Note the position of upper and lower limbs in relation to trunk. Note the degree of flexion at elbow and knee	Note for symmetry, relationship of upper with lower limb
Heel to ear	With the infant on back, raise both heels together with head in midline, not raising the pelvis, and try to move feet towards the head	Note the degree of movement, resistance and the angle formed between the heels with the ground
Popliteal angle	With the infant on back, pelvis flat, flex the thigh at the hip to achieve a knee chest position. Holding the thigh in this position, lift the lower segment of the leg and note the angle formed with the thigh. Note the angle in both legs simultaneously	Note for symmetry, resistance, and degree of movement
Dorsiflexion of feet	Try to flex the feet at ankle	Note the degree of flexion at the ankle
Scarf sign	With the infant on back, head in midline, gently hold the hand at elbow and try to move inward toward the opposite shoulder. Note the range of movement, resistance, and symmetry, ability to reach or cross the midline. Perform on other hand	Note for symmetry, resistance, and degree of movement
Adductor angle	With the infant lying on bed, head in midline, pelvis stable, grasp the knees with index finger along the thigh, and try to move the thigh outward	Note the resistance, symmetry, and the hip adductor angle

Table 8: Assessment of tone by Amiel–Tison method.

Age (months)	Adductor angle	Popliteal angle	Dorsiflexion angle	Scarf sign
0–3	40–80	80–100	60–70	Elbow does not cross the midline
4–6	70–110	90–120	60–70	Elbow crosses midline
7–9	110–140	110–160	60–70	Elbow goes beyond axillary line
10–12	140–160	150–170	60–70	

Note:
- A limitation of angles indicates hypertonia and wide angles indicate hypotonia.
- Does not replace developmental scales as mental development is not assessed.
- Predictive value at 3 months for normal development at 12 months is >93%.

- *Active tone (Figs. 14 to 18):* Hold the infant in different postures and note the position of head, limbs, and curvature of spine. Place the infant in prone position. Note the ability to lift the head and trunk. Hold the infant with both hands in axilla and note for floppiness or stiffness. On pulled to sit, note the ability of the head to reach the midline and curvature of spine. On ventral suspension, note the position of head with spine, limb position, and spine curvature. On pulled to stand, note the ability of weight bearing, position of feet and symmetry in legs.
- Step 7: *Evaluate for primitive reflexes (Table 9):*
  - *Moro reflex (Figs. 19A to C):* This is a vestibular reflex. It appears at 28 weeks of gestation and fully develops by term age. It disappears by 4–5 months of age. The infant should be held in supine over the right hand and the forearm. The flexed head is suddenly allowed to drop by 30. (A) A positive response consists of rapid abduction and extension of upper limbs and opening of hands (B) followed by slower adduction and flexion or embrace equivalent. The infant may cry. The Moro reflex may be incomplete in preterm babies. Asymmetric Moro response may suggest brachial palsy or fracture of clavicle or humerus.

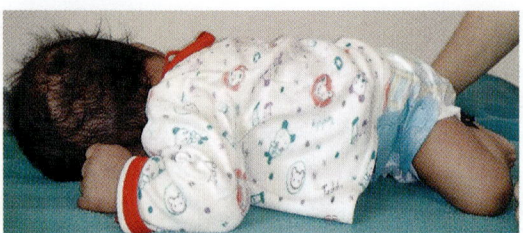

Fig. 14: Prone position. Head is moved to one side and the pelvis is raised in a newborn baby.

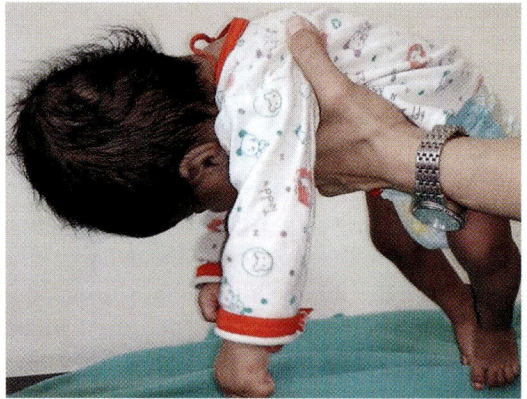

Fig. 15: Head is momentarily lifted up on ventral suspension in a 4-week-old infant.

The response may be depressed or absent in infants with cerebral depression. The exaggerated response may be obtained in cases of cerebral irritability.

- *3 months normal:* Baby has partial head holding; props on forearm in prone position; primitive reflexes like the ATNR are diminishing, and can be overcome spontaneously. Hand unfisted 50% of the time.
- *3–5 months* **(Figs. 20 and 21)**: A hand regards is key milestone seen between 3 and 5 months. It occurs when the infant is lying supine. There is observation of hands by the infant. Persistence beyond 5 months is abnormal.
- *6 months normal:* Head control achieved, roll over both sides achieved—normal, primitive reflexes absent or integrated.

Developmental Assessment

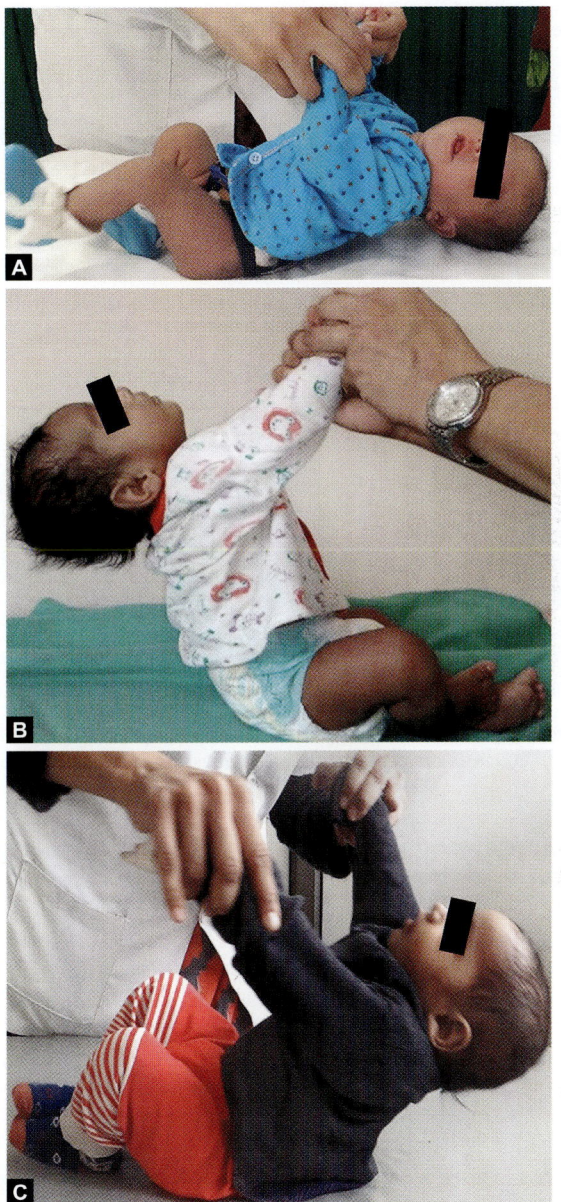

Figs. 16A to C: Traction response: Infant is being pulled from supine to sitting position by holding at forearms. (A) There is complete head lag in a newborn baby; (B) Head is momentarily maintained at around 6–8 weeks; (C) No head lag at 12 weeks.

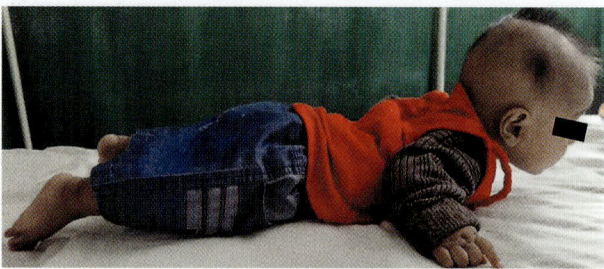

Fig. 17: Prone position. Pelvis is not raised and head is lifted off the couch momentarily at around 6 weeks of age.

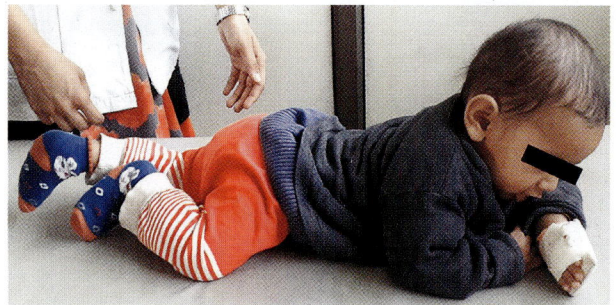

Fig. 18: Prone position. Chest is maintained of the couch and body is supported on forearms at 16–20 weeks of age.

Table 9: Neonatal reflexes.			
	Technique	*Assess*	*Disappearance*
Palmar grasp	Place your finger or an object on the infants palm and stroke	Infants fingers close and grasp the object/finger	3 months
Rooting reflex	Stroke the cheek or corner of the mouth by your finger	Infants head turns toward the side of stroking and opens the mouth	4 months
Sucking reflex	Place your finger in baby mouth	Infant starts sucking on the finger	By 4 months becomes a voluntary activity

Contd…

Contd...

	Technique	Assess	Disappearance
Moro reflex: Moro is the last item in the assessment as the baby may cry and not cooperate later	One hand supports the head in midline and the other the back. Raise infant to 45° and when baby is relaxed let the head fall through 10°	The legs and head extend while the arms jerk up with the fingers extended followed by adduction of both the upper limbs, clenching of fist and cry	6 months
Stepping reflex	Touch the shin across the edge of the table. Test each side separately the table	The infant raises the opposite foot as if trying to walk	2 months
Asymmetric tonic neck reflex	With the baby in supine, turn the head to one side	The arm on the side stretching out and the opposite arm bends at the elbow	6 months

- *9 months (Fig. 22):* Come to sit, come to fours, lateral propping, and forward extension emerges.
- *12 months (Fig. 23):* Come to stand, momentary standing unsupported.

ENDPOINT OF EVALUATION

- If the child fails a developmental screen, refer for a formal developmental assessment. Evaluations and assessments consist of informal and formal testing; use of standardized tests like the DASII (Developmental Assessment Scales for Indian Infants) and observations made by parents, caregivers, and medical or child development professionals.
- Identify if there is delay, deviation, or dissociation [Condition mimicking cerebral palsy **(Box 2)** should be identified]. *Global developmental delay* is identified, if the developmental quotient (DQ) is <70 in one or more domains. *Deviation* is identified, if the child develops skills out of the usual sequence, e.g., hand preference by 12 months. This is characteristic of cerebral palsy. Check for other markers of cerebral palsy **(Box 3)**.

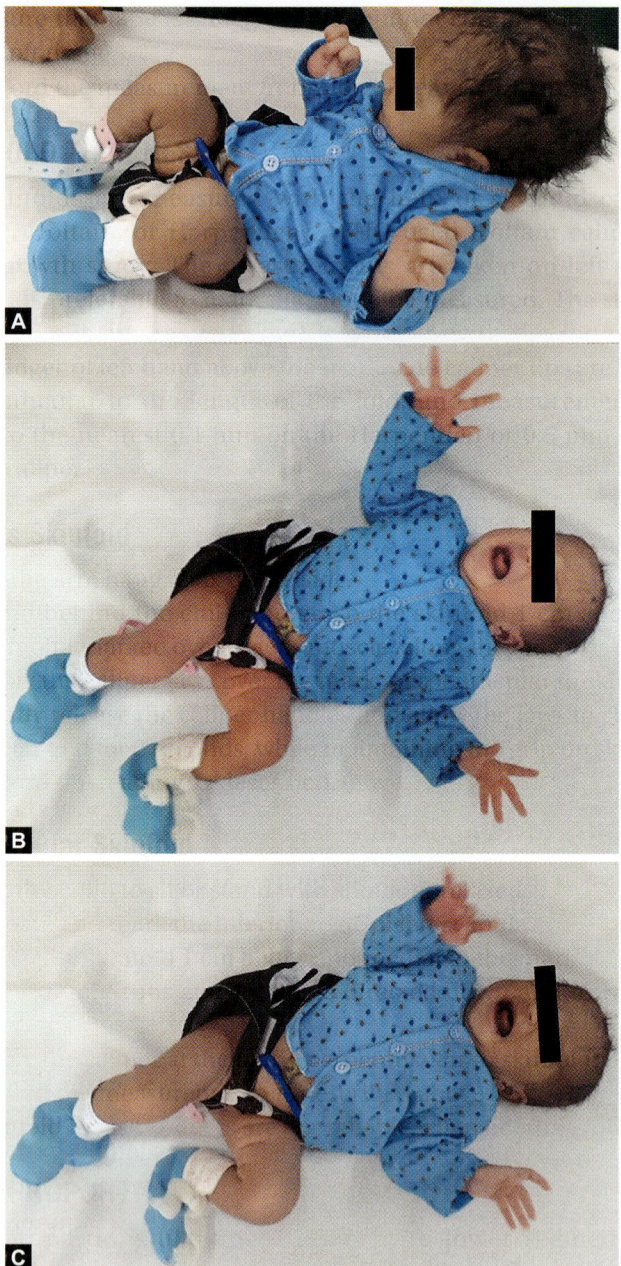

Figs. 19A to C: Moro reflex.

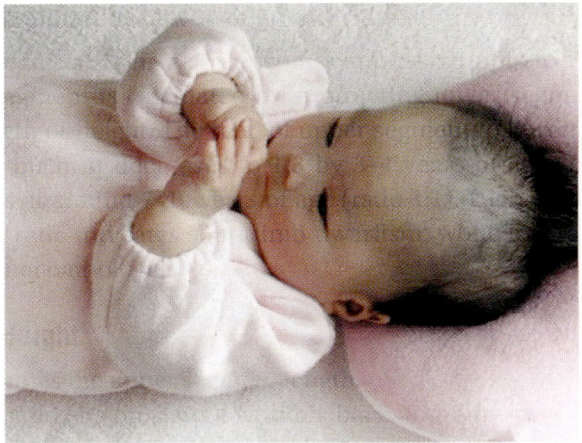

Fig. 20: Hand regard. A key milestone seen between 3 and 5 months. It occurs when the infant is lying supine. There is observation of hands by the infant. Persistence beyond 5 months is abnormal.

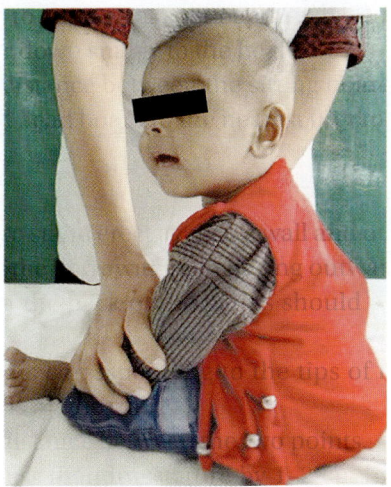

Fig. 21: Sitting with support at around 4–5 months of age.

Dissociation is identified if the development is different in different developmental spheres, e.g., autism. The assessment results determine the child's strengths and weaknesses and help to direct the intervention or specialized services the child will receive.

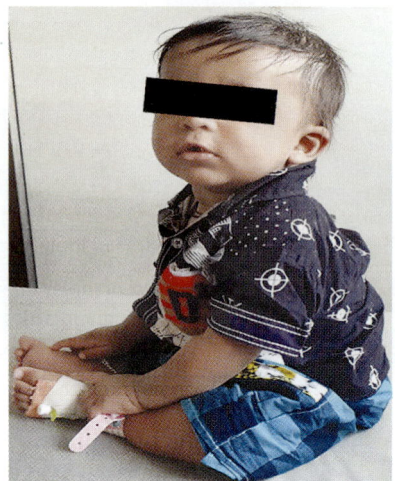

Fig. 22: Sitting without support and maintaining straight back at around 7–8 months of age.

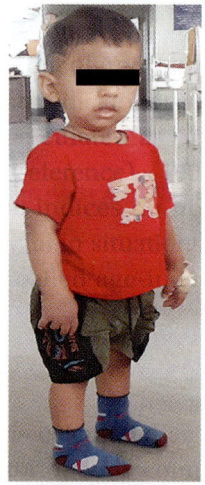

Fig. 23: Standing without support and walking at around 1 year of age.

- The assessment results direct the intervention or specialized services the child will receive.
- Lay down the plan with family to help them and their child.

Developmental Assessment

Box 2: Conditions mimicking developmental delay.

- Transient tone abnormalities
- Less environmental stimulation
- Vision and hearing loss
- Epilepsy
- Autism
- Child with chronic illness
- Muscular disorders
- Neurodegenerative disorders
- Space occupying lesions of brain
- Hydrocephalus
- Metabolic disorder
- Genetic syndromes

Box 3: Markers for cerebral palsy in infancy.

- Acquire handedness before 1 year of age
- Cross midline to pick up a toy
- Persistent fisting after 4 months of age
- Log roll rather than segmental roll
- Leg scissoring when picked up
- Persistent primitive reflexes

Table 10: Grading of developmental quotient (DQ).

DQ	Implications
>85	Considered as within normal limits
<70	In two or more streams are considered as global developmental delay
<70	In any stream warrants serious consideration of the cause and early intervention
<50	Evaluate for an organic etiology

- Refer to early intervention specialists so that the family is taught activities, games, and exercises they can do to provide a stimulating environment to their child and discuss the family's needs.
- While assessment results provide partial evidence of a child's abilities and needs, intervention activities are planned to fill in the gaps, providing for specific needs, and at the same time building on a base of the child's abilities rather than disabilities.

Table 11: Interpreting the observations.

Test/observation	Optimal response	Interpretation
Head circumference	Appropriate for age	Adequate brain growth
Cranial sutures	Edge to edge	
Fix, follow, response to object	Present	No central nervous system (CNS) depression
Social interaction	Present	
Sucking reflex	Efficient	
Raised to sit and reverse	Active flexor muscles	Upper motor control integrity
Passive axial tone	More flexion than extension	
Passive tone in limbs	Symmetrical and appropriate for gestation	
Fingers and thumb	Independent movements and abduction of thumbs	
Autonomic control during assessment	Stable color, heart rate, and respiration	Abnormality suggest autonomic instability
Primitive reflexes	Persistence beyond age	Significant brain insult

- Determine the developmental quotient (DQ)

$$DQ = \frac{\text{Developmental age}}{\text{Chronological age}} \times 100$$

- Grading of DQ **(Table 10)** should be decided.
- Interpretation of observations **(Table 11)** is very crucial as it may indicate the pathology and likely condition.

The Alimentary System and Abdomen

CHAPTER 7

Baldev Prajapati

INTRODUCTION

It is conventionally called as the gastrointestinal (GI) system, but the abdomen is occupied by the GI system, hepatobiliary system, and genitourinary system. Therefore, examination of abdomen is complex. In addition to the primary disorder related to intra-abdominal organs, abdomen may be secondarily involved in which primary disease is related to other systems.

SYMPTOMS RELATED TO ABDOMEN

Careful and detailed evaluation of symptoms related to the abdomen is necessary as sometimes these symptoms could be manifestations of extra-abdominal pathology. The parents may misinterpret symptoms such as excessive crying due to abdominal pain in a young child. A child less than 3 years of age may not be able to complain about pain in abdomen at all, but the parents may falsely interpret crying due to abdominal pain. Therefore, very careful approach is necessary and the symptoms should be evaluated in details with reference to associated complaints. Common symptoms related to abdomen are enlisted in **Box 1**.

Abdominal Pain

Abdominal pain can be acute, chronic or recurrent. The acute abdominal pain may be sudden or of few days in duration. The chronic abdominal pain is described as intermittent or constant that has been present for at least 2 months. The criteria of recurrent abdominal pain are:
- ≥3 episodes of abdominal pain
- Pain sufficiently severe to affect activities

> **Box 1:** Common symptoms related to abdomen.
> - Abdominal pain
> - Vomiting
> - Diarrhea
> - Constipation
> - Alterations in appetite
> - Distention of abdomen
> - Failure to thrive
> - Jaundice
> - Hematemesis
> - Melena
> - Bleeding per rectum
> - Urinary symptoms
> - Hematuria
> - Scrotal swelling

- Episodes occur over a period of ≥3 months
- No known organic cause.

One should remember that even in the absence of pain in abdomen, there may be serious disease, e.g., chronic liver disease, hydronephrosis, malignancy, massive splenomegaly, chronic renal failure, etc.

Medical conditions presenting as abdominal pain should be kept in mind like diabetic ketoacidosis, sickle cell crisis, Henoch-Schönlein purpura, abdominal migraine, abdominal epilepsy, acute intermittent porphyria, lead poisoning, etc.

- *Site of pain:* The knowledge of relevant anatomy and the location of intra-abdominal organs are essential in deciding site of pain and the organ of origin.

  Anatomically, the abdomen is divided into nine quadrants **(Fig. 1)** by two vertical lines from the midclavicular points on each side and two horizontal lines, the upper one connecting the two lowermost points of costal margins and the lower line connecting the iliac crests on each side. The contents of each abdominal quadrant are shown in **Table 1**.
  - *Right hypochondrium:* Liver is the main organ in this area. Due to inflammation of liver, there is stretching of hepatic capsule giving rise to pain. Acute hepatitis, liver abscess, congestive hepatomegaly in a case of congestive

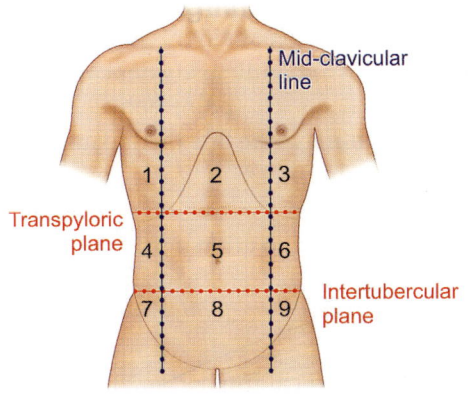

Fig. 1: Abdominal quadrants.

Table 1: Abdominal quadrants (regions) and their contents.	
Right hypochondrium	Liver, gallbladder
Epigastrium	Stomach, pancreas, left lobe of liver
Left hypochondrium	Spleen, colon
Right lumbar region (Rt flank)	Right kidney, colon
Umbilical region	Small intestines
Left lumbar region (Lt flank)	Left kidney, colon
Right iliac region (Rt groin)	Ileocecal junction, appendix, large intestines
Left iliac region (Lt groin)	Large intestines
Suprapubic (Hypogastrium) region (Pubic)	Urinary bladder

cardiac failure, cholecystitis, and right side pleurisy are main causes for pain in right hypochondrium.
- *Epigastrium:* The most common cause of pain in epigastrium is gastritis. Pancreatitis is another cause for pain in epigastric region, although it is not common in children.
- *Left hypochondrium:* Splenic infarct, splenic abscess, and left-sided pleurisy can cause pain in left hypochondrium.
- *Periumbilical region:* It is the most common site of pain in abdomen in children and mostly functional in nature.

However, organic conditions involving small bowel and acute appendicitis may give rise to pain in this area.
- *Right iliac fossa:* The pain of appendicitis is typically felt at McBurney's point in right iliac fossa (point between lateral one-third and medial two-thirds of the line joining umbilicus and anterior superior iliac spine).
- *Lumbar regions/Flanks:* Pain in this region is usually of renal origin and there may be loin to groin radiation.
- *Suprapubic (Hypogastrium) region:* Causes related to urinary bladder such as cystitis and bladder calculus can give rise to suprapubic pain.
- *Left iliac fossa:* Constipation, fecal impaction, and inflammatory bowel disease are common causes for pain in left iliac fossa.
- *Referred pain:* The pain is said to be referred pain when it is felt at some other region having same segmental innervations as the site of lesion. The pain of appendicitis is referred to umbilicus. The pain of diaphragmatic irritation is referred to shoulder on the same side as diaphragm is supplied by phrenic nerve (C_3 and C_4). The pain of pleurisy may be referred to upper abdomen.
- *Radiation of pain:* The pain may radiate to a different site as seen in renal colic where the pain originates in lumbar region and radiates to the groin (loin to groin) and the inner thigh. Pain due to pancreatitis radiates to the back and gallbladder pain radiates toward the tip of right scapula.
- *Timing of pain:* Episodes of pain in children at school going time may be due to anxiety or a reason for not going to school. Pain during day time and never during night or sleep indicates functional abdominal pain. The pain at night awakening the child from sleep is mostly due to underlying organic cause. Pain occurring on empty stomach and getting relieved by meals indicates acid peptic disease.
- *Character/Nature/Type of pain:*
  - *Colicky:* Sharp, intermittent, gripping pain suggests spasm of any tubular hollow organ. It may be due to obstruction like ureteric calculus, bowel obstruction, and dysmenorrhea in adolescent girls.

Table 2: Associated symptoms with abdominal pain and their correlates.

Symptoms	Clinical relevance
Diarrhea	Gastroenteritis, inflammatory bowel disease, celiac disease
Blood in stool	Dysentery, inflammatory bowel disease
Hematemesis	Esophageal varices, peptic ulcer, drug-induced gastritis
Bilious vomiting	Small bowel obstruction
Jaundice	Hepatic, biliary disease
Joint swelling	Henoch-Schönlein purpura, inflammatory bowel disease
Hematuria/Dysuria	Urinary tract infection

- *Dull aching:* It indicates diffuse inflammation of intestine.
- *Burning:* Burning pain in epigastric region or retrosternal area may be due to gastritis or esophagitis. It can cause irritation, excessive crying, and arching in infants with gastroesophageal reflux disease (GERD).
- *Piercing:* It is characteristic of vasculitis like mesenteric artery syndrome.
- *Associated symptoms:* The associated symptoms with abdominal pain and their clinical correlates are shown in **Table 2**.

Vomiting

Vomiting should be differentiated from regurgitation.

Regurgitation is passive expulsion of contents of stomach. It is a normal phenomenon in infants due to poor lower esophageal sphincter tone. As the tone improves with the age, the regurgitation decreases and disappears. It may be due to aerophagy, ingestion of air while feeding, especially in bottle-fed babies. The child does not develop dehydration, gains the weight, and remains playful with regurgitation. It does not require any investigation or medicine. The parents should be reassured.

Vomiting is a forceful expulsion of contents of stomach, usually associated with contraction of abdominal wall muscles. Vomiting requires more details to decide the cause.

- *Age:* Infants with congenital hypertrophic pyloric stenosis typically present at age of 3–4 weeks. Vomiting develops after

each feed and it may cause metabolic alkalosis, electrolyte disturbances, and failure to thrive.
- *Contents of vomiting:*
  - Vomiting soon after taking feed and containing only food particles, nonbilious, indicates obstruction before second part of duodenum, e.g., congenital hypertrophic pyloric stenosis.
  - Bilious vomiting is seen in obstruction distal to ampulla of Vater at second part of duodenum. Bilious vomiting should be considered as significant complaint, suggesting surgical conditions like duodenal atresia, annular pancreas, and intestinal obstruction.
  - History of blood in vomiting should be noted. It indicates hematemesis.
- *Type of vomiting:* It can be projectile or nonprojectile. Projectile vomiting is forceful where vomitus falls away. It is classically seen with raised intracranial pressure and pyloric stenosis.
- *Vomiting and acute diarrhea:* Most children develop vomiting initially, followed by diarrhea. Vomiting may subside before diarrhea is controlled. Usually, it takes about a week for recovery.
- *Associated symptoms:* Associated other symptoms with vomiting may indicate various conditions. These include loose stool (acute gastroenteritis), jaundice (hepatitis), headache and irritability or convulsions (raised intra cranial pressure), constipation (intestinal obstruction), abdominal pain (renal calculus), urinary symptoms like burning and frequency of micturition (UTI), weight loss, polyuria, and acidotic breathing (diabetic ketoacidosis), etc.
- Post-tussive vomiting is common in children with pertussis. The common causes of vomiting are listed in **Table 3**.

Diarrhea

Generally, diarrhea is defined as passage of three or more loose or watery stools in a 24-hour period. However, for practical purpose, it is the recent change in consistency and character of stool and its water content rather than the number of stools

Table 3: Common causes of vomiting.

Medical conditions	Surgical conditions
• Overfeeding (Faulty feeding) • Gastroenteritis • Gastroesophageal reflux (GER) • Drug induced • Hepatitis • Urinary tract infection • Raised intracranial pressure • (CNS infections, hydrocephalus, space occupying lesions) • Diabetic ketoacidosis • Uremia • Inborn error of metabolism • Post-tussive vomiting in pertussis and bronchial asthma • Psychogenic	• Congenital hypertrophic pyloric stenosis • Intestinal obstruction • Appendicitis • Intussusception • Peritonitis • Renal colic

(CNS: central nervous system)

that is important. The following information is more useful to decide its etiology:

- *Onset and category:*
  - *Acute diarrhea:* An episode of diarrhea which lasts for less than 14 days is termed as acute diarrheal disease (ADD). Most common cause of ADD is viral infection or cholera.
  - *Persistent diarrhea:* Diarrhea for more than 14 days is defined as persistent diarrhea. It is followed by ADD and most common causes are infections and lactose intolerance.
  - *Chronic diarrhea:* Insidious onset and more than 14 days duration, loose, bulky, and foul smell stool are the characteristics. The most common causes are malabsorption syndromes and inflammatory bowel diseases.
- *Consistency and color of stool:* Watery (viral infection), rice watery (cholera), blood containing (dysentery), bulky, frothy and foul smell (malabsorption), and clay colored stool (cholestatic jaundice).
- *Related to food:* Food poisoning and milk protein allergy can be defined if associated.

> **Box 2:** Common causes of diarrhea.
> - Acute diarrheal disease
> - Food poisoning
> - Dysentery
> - Drug (antibiotic) induced diarrhea
> - Cow's milk protein allergy
> - Lactose intolerance
> - Giardiasis
> - Celiac disease
> - Inflammatory bowel disease
> - Parenteral diarrhea (AOM, UTI, pneumonia)
> - Hyperthyroidism
> - Irritable bowel syndrome
>
> (AOM: acute otitis media; UTI: urinary tract infection)

- *Associated symptoms:* Fever (infections causes like enteric fever, dysentery), abdominal pain (dysentery, inflammatory bowel disease), perianal excoriation (lactose intolerance), prolapse rectum (malnutrition, worms infestation), etc.
- *Tenesmus:* Tenesmus is commonly associated with amoebic dysentery.
- *Parental diarrhea:* Pneumonia, urinary tract infection, and acute otitis media are known causes in infants and young children to cause diarrhea.
- Frequency of stool and gastrocolic reflux should not be mistaken for diarrhea.

The common causes of diarrhea are listed in **Box 2**.

Constipation

Constipation is defined as passage of hard stool with straining and pain.

A normal child who is on exclusive breastfed may pass stool every 3rd or 4th day, but consistency of stool is normal, should not be mistaken as constipation.

- *Onset:*
  - Since birth (Hirschsprung disease)
  - Sudden or acute (Intestinal obstruction)
  - Insidious (Functional).

- *Duration:* Chronic (Hirschsprung disease, hypothyroidism, neurogenic)
- *Relation to flatus:* Obstipation (inability to pass flatus) indicates intestinal obstruction, peritonitis
- *Associated symptoms:* Pain and difficulty (dyschezia) during defecation (anal fissure, perianal excoriation), and abdominal distention (intestinal obstruction).

The common causes of constipation are listed in **Box 3**.

Abdominal Distention

The distention of abdomen may be physiological in infants (protuberant abdomen) due to poor muscle tone, it may be exaggerated after feeds. The most common causes of distention of abdomen in children are shown in **Box 4**.

Box 3: Common causes of constipation.

- Functional (Dietary)
- Hirschsprung disease
- Intestinal obstruction
- Peritonitis
- Hypothyroidism
- Cystic fibrosis
- Hypokalemia
- Anal stenosis
- Anal stricture
- Prolong drug therapy like calcium and magnesium

Box 4: Causes of distention of abdomen.

- Physiological (Protuberant abdomen in infants)
- Rickets
- Protein–energy malnutrition
- Ascites
- Hepatosplenomegaly
- Intestinal obstruction
- Hypokalemia
- Hypothyroidism
- Mucopolysaccharidosis
- Intra-abdominal lumps (Wilms tumor, neuroblastoma, cysts, etc.)

Jaundice

Severe pallor can cause yellow halo which is mistaken as jaundice by the parents, which should be clarified.

Commonly, the patient of jaundice presents with complaint of yellow eyes and urine. Apart from jaundice, dark colored urine may be due to concentrated urine in case of dehydration, high-grade fever, etc. It can also be due to some drugs like vitamin B complex, rifampicin, etc. Jaundice can be direct (conjugated) or indirect (unconjugated). Indirect jaundice occurs due to hemolysis, while direct jaundice occurs due to hepatic or posthepatic (obstructive) causes.

- As conjugated (direct) bilirubin is water soluble and gets excreted in urine, the urine turns dark yellow in color while it remains unchanged in unconjugated (indirect) hyperbilirubinemia.
- In case of obstructive cause of direct jaundice, the patient may have a history of passing clay colored or pale stool. Itching may be associated complaint with obstructive jaundice.
- Acute jaundice is commonly due to viral hepatitis (A, B, E, and C). The course of jaundice may be variable in different types of viral hepatitis. Unusual course of jaundice may be due to development of complications or associated conditions like chronic viral hepatitis, metabolic disorders such as Wilson's disease, autoimmune hepatitis, etc.
- Recurrent or waxing and waning jaundice can be due to several reasons like metabolic disorders (Wilson's disease, tyrosinemia, fatty acid oxidative disease, etc.), autoimmune hepatitis, sickle cell disease, etc.
- Persistent jaundice may be due to choledochal cyst, hereditary spherocytosis etc.
- History of hepatotoxic drugs like isoniazid, rifampicin, pyrazinamide, sodium valproate, etc. suggests drug-induced hepatitis.
- History of blood transfusion in past may be responsible for hepatitis B or C viral infections.

Gastrointestinal Bleeding

History of blood in vomiting (hematemesis), black colored stool (melena) or frank bleeding per rectum are indicators of bleeding

> **Box 5:** Common causes of bleeding from gastrointestinal tract.
> - Esophageal varices (Portal hypertension)
> - Gastritis, peptic ulcer (Drug induced, inflammation)
> - Cow's milk protein intolerance
> - Chronic liver disease (Coagulopathy)
> - Inflammatory bowel disease
> - Intussusception
> - Meckel's diverticulum
> - Colonic polyp
> - Dysentery
> - Anal fissure
> - Hemorrhoids

from GI tract. Bleeding from GI tract may be due to chronic liver disease (lack of synthesis of coagulation factors), esophageal varices (portal hypertension) or local mucosal bleeding due to various reasons. The common causes of bleeding from GI tract are shown in **Box 5**.

- *Hematemesis:* Presence of blood in vomiting is called hematemesis. It should not be confused with hemoptysis (blood in sputum). Hematemesis is most commonly due to portal hypertension. It can also be due to severe gastritis (drug induced), peptic ulcer, etc. Hematemesis can also be due to coagulopathy in a case of chronic hepatic disease or hepatic failure.
- *Melena:* Passage of black, tarry, sticky, and offensive stool is termed as melena. With bleeding from upper GI tract, hydrochloric acid in the stomach converts hemoglobin to acid hematin. Blood should enter the colon slowly, so that the colonic bacteria can convert the hematin to hemochromogens, which are black. It takes about 14 hours for blood to be broken down within the intestinal lumen. Therefore, if transit time is more than 14 hours, the patient will have melena. Melena can persist for 4–7 days after treating the source of bleeding. Blood in the intestine for longer periods of time leads to elevated blood urea levels. The minimum quantity of blood required to produce melena is 50 mL.

Following ingestion of iron and bismuth, the stools appear blackish, but the stools are well-formed, unlike melena.

The melena can be confirmed by stool examination for occult blood for 3 consecutive days. In case of iron therapy going on, iron should be stopped for 3–7 days before stool examination for occult blood.
- *Hematochezia:* Hematochezia is the passage of fresh blood with the stool. It is usually indicative of bleeding from the rectum and anus. However, 50% is due to proximal lesions that are profuse enough that they avoid remaining in the gut for >8 hours. The common causes for hematochezia in newborns are swallowed maternal blood and necrotizing enterocolitis and in children, intussusception, Meckel's diverticulum, inflammatory bowel diseases, etc.
- *Bleeding per rectum:* It is essential to differentiate whether the child has fresh bleeding per rectum or has mixed blood with stool.

Fresh bleeding per rectum can be due to rectal polyp, fistula, anal fissure or hemorrhoids due to portal hypertension. The recurrent jelly stool is the characteristic of intussusception.

Scrotal Swelling

Scrotal swelling is frequently found in boys. It can be acute or chronic, painful or painless. It should be attended immediately and evaluated. Acute and painful scrotal swelling may be due to testicular torsion or incarcerated inguinal hernia which requires urgent surgical intervention. Epididymo-orchitis also presents as painful swelling. Hydrocele is chronic swelling of the scrotum which may subside by its own or may require surgical intervention. Varicocele and testicular tumors are other cause of scrotal swelling.

Hematuria

Red-colored urine can be due to several reasons as shown in **Box 6**. The cause of red urine should be decided. Hematuria is the most common cause of red urine. It can be due to acute glomerulonephritis, renal calculus, urinary tract infection, cystitis, trauma, Wilms tumor or systemic causes like thrombocytopenia, disseminated intravascular coagulation (DIC) etc.

> **Box 6:** Causes of red-colored urine.
> - *Food items:* Beetroot, black berries, food coloring agents
> - *Drugs:* Pyridium, rifampicin, nimesulide, nitrofurantoin sulfasalazine, etc.
> - Hematuria
> - Hemoglobinuria
> - Myoglobinuria
> - Porphyria

Alteration in Appetite

Loss of appetite is common with chronic illness like tuberculosis, chronic liver or renal diseases, malignancy, etc. Acute loss of appetite is very common with viral hepatitis. Voracious appetite may be due to giardiasis worm infestation etc. In spite of increased appetite, weight loss is commonly seen due to diabetes mellitus and hyperthyroidism-like illness.

GENERAL PHYSICAL EXAMINATION: RELEVANT TO ABDOMEN (BOX 7)

- *Heart rate:* A child with jaundice may have bradycardia. Tachycardia may indicate serious conditions like shock, appendicitis, intestinal perforation, peritonitis, etc.
- *Respiratory rate:* Tachypnea and respiratory distress are very common with huge distention of abdomen.
- *Blood pressure:* A child with shock, intestinal perforation and peritonitis may have hypotension. Children with glomerulonephritis, renal failure, Wilms tumor, neuroblastoma, and pheochromocytoma can have hypertension.
- *Oral cavity:* Look for signs of vitamin B_{12} deficiency, oral thrush, pallor, gingival hypertrophy, and number of teeth. Cleft palate is often missed in infants unless specifically looked for.
- *Nutritional and growth assessment:* Anthropometry and plotting of readings on growth chart is important for assessment of growth and nutrition of the child. In chronic liver and renal disease, celiac disease, malabsorption, protein–energy malnutrition (PEM), growth, and nutrition are significantly affected.
- *Eyes:* Look for signs of vitamin A deficiency which can be present in a case of obstructive jaundice, malabsorption,

> **Box 7:** General examination relevant to abdomen.
> - Vitals
> - Assessment of nutrition and growth
> - Oral cavity
> - Eye examination
> - Jaundice
> - Pallor
> - Clubbing
> - Edema
> - Dehydration
> - Lymphadenopathy
> - Signs of hepatocellular failure
> - Bony tenderness

PEM, etc. Kayser–Fleischer ring may be seen with torch light in Wilson disease, but can be seen better with slit lamp examination. Check for icterus in upper part of sclera in day light.

- *Pallor:* Pallor can be associated with several conditions like malabsorption, PEM, chronic liver and renal diseases, worm infestations, hemolytic anemia, malaria, etc.
- *Edema:* Check for pedal edema, periorbital puffiness or generalized anasarca. Edema may be seen with chronic liver disease, nephrotic syndrome, glomerulonephritis, congestive cardiac failure etc.
- Signs of dehydration should be checked in a case of ADD.
- *Clubbing:* Presence of clubbing indicates celiac disease, ulcerative colitis, Crohn's disease, and chronic liver diseases.
- *Lymphadenopathy:* Generalized lymphadenopathy may be present in children with leukemia, lymphoma, HIV, tuberculosis, etc.
- Bony tenderness is an important marker for leukemia.
- Signs of liver cell failure should be checked as shown in **Box 8**.

EXAMINATION OF THE ABDOMEN

- Younger children (<2 years) should be examined in mother's lap so that child is comfortable and allowing for proper examination **(Fig. 2)**. If the baby is crying or irritable, she can be put to the mother's breast to pacify. In some very irritable and over anxious children, it may be impossible to pacify the child and

> **Box 8:** Signs of hepatocellular failure.
> - Persistent fever, vomiting, abdominal pain
> - Progressive jaundice
> - Altered sensorium
> - Decrease in liver size
> - Ascites
> - Bleeding tendency
> - Hepatic encephalopathy
> - Fetor hepaticus
> - Palmar erythema
> - Spider angioma
> - Parotid swelling (in chronic liver disease)
> - Gynecomastia and testicular atrophy in adolescents (in chronic liver disease)

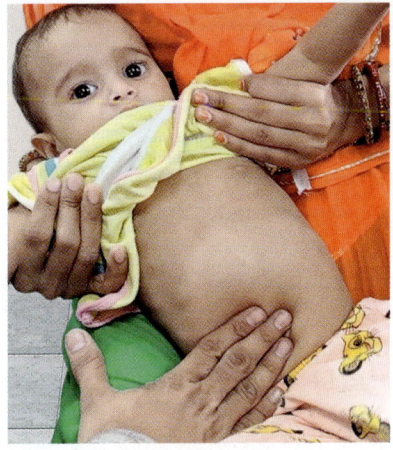

Fig. 2: Examination of young children (<2 years) in the mother's lap.

it may be wise to wait till the child falls asleep and abdominal muscles are relaxed.
- A toddler is afraid of lying down on the couch. Examination of a resisting and crying child is not fruitful. Taking the child in the confidence by talking to him softly, offering a toy and keeping him engaged and presence of parents make the task easy.
- An older child and adolescents can be examined in lying down position or standing position **(Fig. 3)**. Talking to the child throughout the examination diverts his attention and abdominal muscles are relaxed and our job becomes easier.

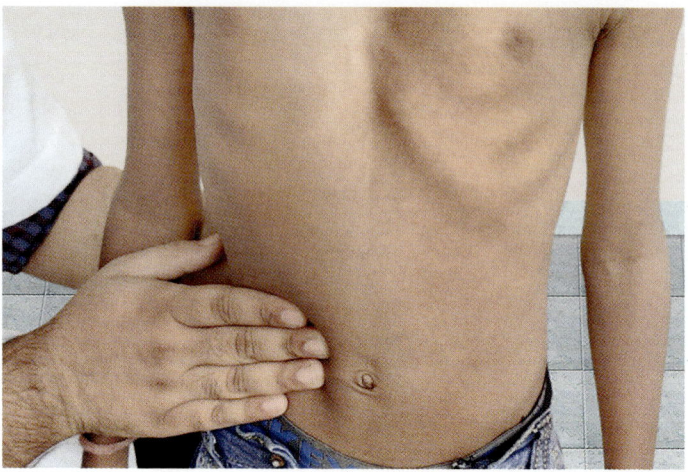

Fig. 3: Examination of abdomen in standing position in older children.

- While exposing abdomen and genitalia of the child, care for his privacy should be taken. When a male examiner is examining a female child, he should have another female attendant or nurse in the room.
- The child should ideally be in lying supine on a firm couch with arms by the side and the lower limbs should be flexed at the hip joint to relax abdominal muscles.
- The room should be warm and well illuminated. The examiner should stand on the right side of the patient. The child should be adequately undressed to expose the chest, the abdomen, and the genitalia. The hands of the examiner should be warm before touching the child.

Inspection

The important points for inspection of abdomen are shown in **Box 9**.

Shape of Abdomen

- Abdomen should be inspected while you are standing at the foot end of the patient with your eyes at the level of abdomen of the child. Normally, abdomen is at the level of chest or slightly below it with concave flanks.

> **Box 9:** Points for inspection of abdomen.
> - Shape of abdomen
> - Movements of abdomen
> - Umbilicus
> - Superficial veins
> - Skin striae
> - Visible peristalsis
> - Visible pulsations
> - Groin and scrotum
> - Anal opening

- *Fullness:* The abdomen may be protuberant in infants normally due to lack of tone of abdominal wall muscles. It can also be due to rickets, PEM or hypothyroidism. Upper part of abdomen may be full due to hepatosplenomegaly. Uniform fullness of abdomen along with fullness of flanks indicates ascites. In a case of intestinal obstruction, central distention indicates small bowel obstruction while peripheral distention due to large bowel obstruction.
- *Localized distention:* It may be due to organomegaly, small bowel obstruction or an abdominal lump like Wilms tumor, neuroblastoma, mesenteric cyst, ovarian cyst, etc. A full urinary bladder appears as a globular suprapubic lump which disappears when the child passes urine. Appearance of transient swelling or lump in epigastrium after feeds in an infant suggests congenital hypertrophic pyloric stenosis.
- *Scaphoid abdomen:* In a newborn, scaphoid abdomen indicates congenital diaphragmatic hernia or intrauterine growth retarded. A newborn with scaphoid abdomen and respiratory distress indicates congenital diaphragmatic hernia, while scaphoid abdomen with bilious vomiting, it indicates duodenal obstruction. It may be due to malnutrition in older children.

Abdominal Movements

Normally, there is gentle rise of the abdomen with each inspiration. In diaphragmatic paralysis, the rise is seen with expiration rather than inspiration (paradoxical), sluggish or no respiratory movements of the abdominal wall indicate peritonitis.

Umbilicus

Normally, umbilicus is located at the midpoint of the line joining the tip of xiphoid process and symphysis pubis. It is retracted and inverted.

- Everted umbilicus may be due to gross distention of abdomen like ascites or organomegaly.
- Transverse umbilicus (smiling umbilicus) **(Fig. 4)** is due to gross distention of abdomen like ascites.
- Umbilical hernia **(Fig. 5)** is very common in children less than 2 years of age. It becomes ballooned when the child cries. In most of babies, umbilical hernia decreases in size and disappears in due course of time. Very few children with umbilical hernia may require surgery if it persists or gets obstructed.
- Umbilical hernia may be pathological signs in cases of hypothyroidism, mucopolysaccharidosis, etc.
- In neonates, look for umbilical sepsis and umbilical granuloma.

Skin Scars

Look for any scar or incision mark of prior surgery. The skin may be stretched, tense, and shining in the presence of gross ascites.

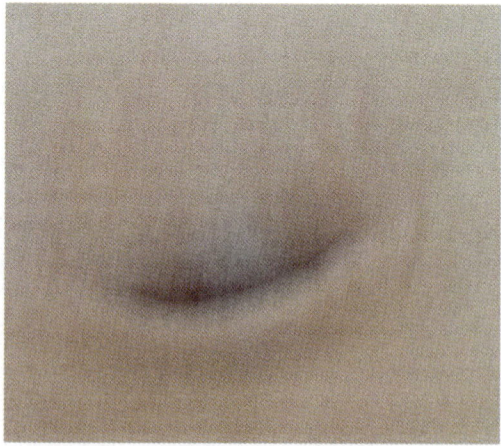

Fig. 4: A smiling umbilicus due to gross ascites.

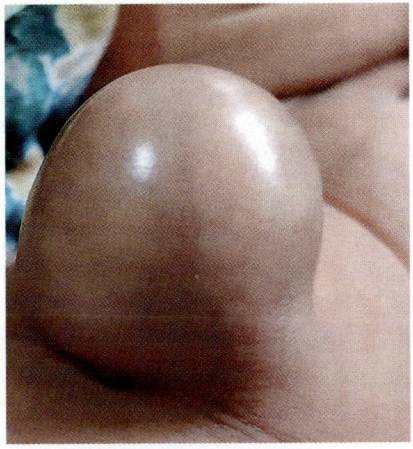

Fig. 5: Umbilical hernia.

Visible Pulsations

- Look for pulsations in epigastrium (right ventricular hypertrophy or aortic pulsations in thin person).
- Look for pulsations over liver.
- Peristalsis may be visible in a case of intestinal obstruction.

Inguinal Regions and External Genitalia

- Look for inguinal hernia.
- Check the presence of testes in scrotum. If testis is absent in scrotum, decide whether it is retractile or undescended.
- Look for hydrocele or any other testicular mass or swelling.
- Look for phimosis, hypospadias, epispadias or any other anomaly.
- Check for ambiguous genitals and synechiae in a female child.

Direction of Blood Flow in Superficial Abdominal Wall Veins (Figs. 6 and 7)

- Small superficial veins may be visible normally over the abdomen. If the veins are distended, prominent, check the direction of blood flow.
- The normal flow of blood in the superficial veins of the abdomen is from the umbilicus upward to the thorax and from the umbilicus downward to the groin.

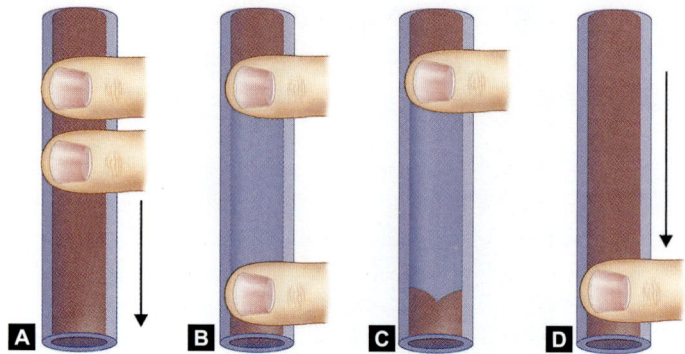

Figs. 6A to D: Method of detecting the direction of blood flow.

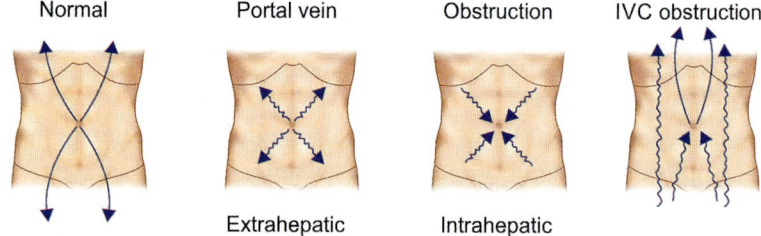

Fig. 7: Diagram of venous return from over chest and abdomen.

- Empty the vein of blood by placing two fingers side by side over the vein.
- Move one finger away while keeping the other fixed.
- Now, release the finger one by one to see the direction through which the blood fills the vein.
- Direction of flow of blood is away from the umbilicus in portal hypertension. There are periumbilical engorged veins with exaggerated flow. It is also called caput medusa.
- In inferior vena caval obstruction, the engorged veins are at the flanks with flow of blood from below upward.
- In superior vena caval obstruction, the engorged veins are above the umbilicus with flow of blood from above downward.

Palpation

It is of prime importance that the infant or child is relaxed while examiner is palpating the abdomen. It is an art and it needs skill,

patience, and distraction techniques. Some of the practical tips are:
- The child should lie supine with the hips flexed and arms by the side.
- Ask the child to relax, if he understands.
- Place your hand and fingers flat on the abdominal wall.
- Press your hand inward during expiration and allow passive outward movement during inspiration.
  The points for palpation of abdomen are shown in **Table 4**.
- Gentle palpation of the abdomen should be done to see how it feels like. A normal abdomen is soft and nontender.
- *Tenderness:* You can see the facial expression of child for pain while examining abdomen, one should not ask the child whether he feels pain. If tenderness is present, it indicates inflammation of underlying organ, then that area should be examined in details in the last.
- *Guarding:* The overlying abdominal wall muscles of the inflamed organ become tense and it is called guarding. It is the protective mechanism to prevent the spread of infection.
- *Rigidity:* The whole abdomen is felt very hard, just like board. It indicates peritonitis or perforation. It should be considered as an ominous sign.
- *Tense abdomen:* It is voluntary contraction of abdominal muscles, commonly seen with older children or adolescents. One cannot appreciate exact findings. Tense abdomen and huge distention can also be due to gas or fluid.
- *Rebound tenderness:* The hand is pressed down gradually on the abdomen and then hand is withdrawn suddenly and completely.

Table 4: Points for palpation of abdomen.

Light palpation	Deep palpation
• Soft • Tender/nontender • Rigidity • Guarding • Tense abdomen • Abdominal wall edema • Abdominal circumference (Girth)	• Liver • Spleen • Kidneys • Urinary bladder • Lump or mass • Fecolith

The patient immediately winces in pain. This is due to inflamed parietal peritoneum springing back along with the abdominal muscles. It is the sign of an inflamed organ.

Abdominal Wall Edema

Look for abdominal wall edema by pinching the skin over the abdomen for 10 seconds **(Fig. 8)**. Presence of indentation or pits on releasing the pinch is suggestive of fluid in the abdominal wall. Alternatively, press the diaphragm of the stethoscope against the lateral abdominal wall and pitting can be seen along the rim of the diaphragm of the stethoscope on releasing the pressure. It is also evident when the tight cloth around the waist like pant is removed as there is indentation on the abdominal wall. For pedal edema, press over shin of tibia or above the malleolus for 30 seconds and see for pitting impression. The presence of pitting impression suggests pitting edema **(Figs. 9A and B)**.

Abdominal Circumference (Girth)

It is measured with the measure tape at the level of umbilicus. Monitoring of abdominal girth is important to assess the progression or reduction in abdominal distention due to ascites or any other cause.

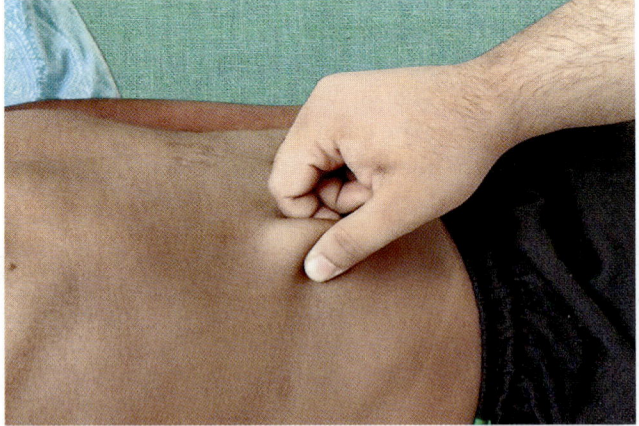

Fig. 8: To look for edema of abdominal wall, the skin of abdominal wall is pinched for 10 seconds and released.

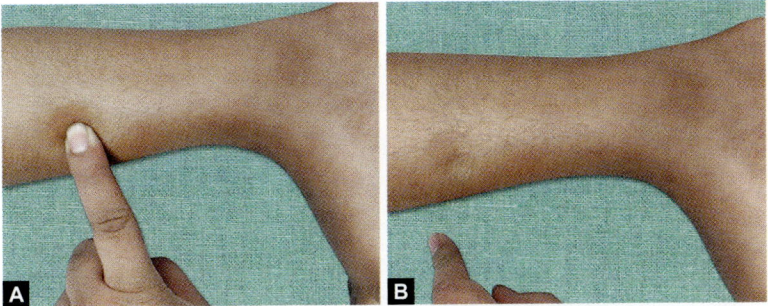

Figs. 9A and B: Demonstration of pedal edema.

Deep Palpation

In an obese child, palpate by dipping the hands deep into the abdomen.

Palpation of liver **(Figs. 10 and 11)**: There are two methods of palpating the liver:
1. Place the right hand over the right iliac fossa such that your fingers are parallel to the ribs and ask the child to take deep breaths. Wait for the liver edge to come and strike the lateral border of the index finger with the inspiration. The fingers should be placed gently over the abdomen and not dug deep which may lead to missing soft liver.
2. Another method of palpation is by keeping your hand parallel to lateral rectus muscle so that the tip of the fingers is pointing toward the ribs. With each inspiration, press the fingers firmly inward and upward to feel the liver edge. If the liver edge is not felt, keep moving up toward the subcostal margin till liver is felt.

Define the lower border of liver:
- Place the right hand over the right iliac fossa such that your fingers are parallel to the ribs, ask the patient to take deep breath, wait for the liver edge to come, and strike the lateral border of the index finger with inspiration. The fingers should be placed gently over the abdomen and not dug deep.
- Measure the size of liver below the right costal margin at midclavicular line (in centimeter and not in number of fingers). It will be for right lobe of the liver.

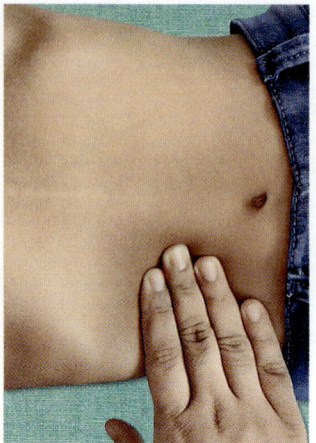 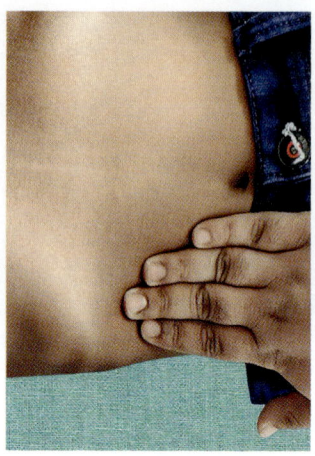

Fig. 10: Palpation of liver. Fingers parallel to subcostal margin.
Fig. 11: Palpation of liver. Fingers perpendicular to the subcostal margin.

Define the upper border of liver:
- Locate the sternal angle. The intercostal space at the level of sternal angle is second space.
- Start the percussion from right second intercostal space to downward. It will be resonant till the upper border of liver is reached, when the note will become dull. The upper border of liver usually lies in the 4th intercostal space.
- In a case of intestinal perforation, free gas in the peritoneal cavity may obliterate upper border of liver on percussion as it becomes resonant instead of dull note.

Span of liver:
- The upper border of liver is defined by percussion and lower border by palpation. The distance between these two borders is span of liver.
- Span of liver gives the actual size of liver. In a case of emphysema or pneumothorax, the pushed liver downward will give the false impression of hepatomegaly, if it is simply measured below the costal margin.

Liver span in normal children at different age is as shown in **Box 10**.

> **Box 10:** Liver span in normal children.
> - Infants → 5–6.5 cm
> - 1–5 years → 6–7 cm
> - 5–10 years → 7–9 cm
> - 10–15 years → 8–10 cm

The left lobe of liver is palpable in the epigastrium, indicates chronic hepatomegaly.

- *Surface:*
  - Gently rolling the fingers over the surface of liver
  - Smooth (Normal), nodular (Cirrhosis).
- *Consistency:*
  - Soft [Viral hepatitis, congestive heart failure (CHF)]
  - Firm (Chronic conditions like tuberculosis, cirrhosis)
  - Hard (Malignancy).
- *Margin:*
  - Rounded (Normal)
  - Sharp and leafy (Cirrhosis).
- *Tenderness:*
  - Viral hepatitis, congested liver (CHF, DF), liver abscess.

Common causes of hepatomegaly are shown in **Box 11**.

Palpation of spleen: Spleen must enlarge at least twice the normal size to become clinically palpable. However, in newborns and infants up to age of 3 months, a just palpable spleen can be normal. The enlarging spleen is traversing from left hypochondrium, to midline and toward right iliac fossa.

There are four methods of palpation of spleen, they are classical method, bimanual method, dipping method, and hooking method.

1. *Classical method:*
   i. The palpation of spleen should begin from right iliac fossa; otherwise one can miss a massively enlarged spleen.
   ii. Palpate the spleen with the right hand over abdomen with fingers pointing toward the left hypochondrium and slowly press the fingers a little into abdomen with each breath.
   iii. Try and feel for the lower end of the spleen as it comes and strikes your fingers at the peak of inspiration.

> **Box 11:** Common causes of hepatomegaly.
>
> *Infants*
> - Intrauterine infections (TORCH)
> - Septicemia
> - Neonatal hepatitis
> - Extrahepatic biliary atresia
> - Galactosemia
> - Glycogen storage disease
> - Congestive cardiac failure
>
> *Older children*
> - Malaria
> - Enteric fever
> - Tuberculosis
> - Hemolytic anemia (Thalassemia)
> - Extrahepatic obstruction
> - Liver abscess
> - Brucellosis
> - Congestive cardiac failure
> - Hepatitis (Viral/Acute or chronic)
> - Malignancies (Leukemia, hepatoblastoma)
> - Wilson disease
> - Mucopolysaccharidosis
> - Glycogen storage diseases
> - Lipid storage diseases (Gaucher disease, Niemann–Pick disease)
> - Budd–Chiari syndrome

    iv. The spleen moves with respiration and has a palpable notch and one cannot get above it. These findings confirm that it is spleen.

2. *Bimanual method (Fig. 12):* If the spleen is not palpable by classical method, not to miss a small palpable spleen (tip of spleen), one should try to palpate it by bimanual method, before one decides spleen is not palpable.
    i. The child should be turn on his right side.
    ii. Try to insinuate the fingers of your right hand beneath the thoracic cage in left hypochondrium.
    iii. Try to push the spleen forward and downward by putting your left palm over left rib cage.
    iv. *Ask the child to take deep breath:* By insinuating fingers beneath the thoracic cage in left hypochondrium, pushing spleen forward and downward and asking the child to take

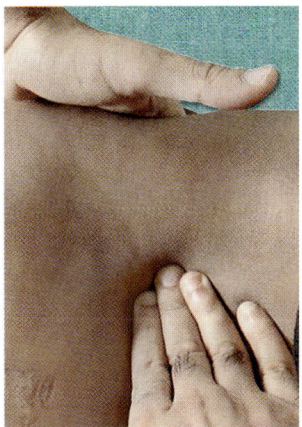

Fig. 12: Bimanual palpation of spleen. The child is turned to the right lateral position. The right hand is placed over the left hypochondrium and spleen tip is searched, the left hand is pushing the spleen downward and forward while child is taking the deep breath.

deep breath, spleen may become palpable if it is enlarged. This method is useful to palpate a just palpable (tip of spleen) spleen.
3. *Dipping method:* In the presence of massive ascites, palpation of spleen may be difficult. Palpate the spleen by exerting sudden thrust by the palpating fingers which will displace the fluid and spleen may become palpable, if it is enlarged.
4. *Hooking method:* Practically, it is not recommended as it is crude method and may cause injury to soft spleen. One should stand on the left side of the patient and try to palpate the spleen by making hook of fingers of your right hand and insinuating it in the left hypochondrium in the thoracic cage. You may get the spleen, if it is palpable.

Differentiation of spleen from other organs:
- The upper border of spleen cannot be reached. You will not be able to insinuate your fingers between the spleen and the left subcostal margin.
- The direction of enlargement of spleen is toward the right iliac fossa.
- The massive splenomegaly can cross the midline.
- A splenic notch is the characteristic of the organ.

Size of spleen:
- The size of the spleen is measured from the left subcostal margin at the midclavicular line to the tip along the direction of enlargement.
- It is also described in centimeter below the left costal margin:
  - *Mild enlargement:* 1–2 cm below left costal margin
  - *Moderate enlargement:* 3–7 cm below left costal margin
  - *Massive enlargement:* >7 cm below the left costal margin
- *Consistency:*
  - *Soft:* Enteric fever, Epstein–Barr virus (EBV) infection
  - *Firm:* Hemolytic anemia, malaria, and kala-azar.
  - *Hard:* Malignancy

Hackett's grading of splenomegaly **(Fig. 13)**:

Grade	Description
0	Normal spleen not palpable even on deep inspiration
1	Spleen palpable below the costal margin, usually on deep inspiration
2	Spleen palpable below the costal margin, but not projected beyond a horizontal line half way between the costal margin and the umbilicus, measured along a line dropped vertically from the left nipple
3	Spleen with lowest palpable point projected more than half way to the umbilicus but not below a line drawn horizontally through it
4	Spleen with lowest palpable point below the umbilical level but not projected beyond a horizontal line situated half way between the umbilicus and the symphysis pubis
5	Spleen with lowest point palpable beyond the lower limit of grade 4.

The common causes of splenomegaly are as shown in **Box 12**.

Palpation of kidneys: The kidneys are palpable by bimanual method **(Fig. 14)**.
- *Right kidney:*
  - Keep the right hand over the right lumbar region and the left hand behind the right loin at the renal angle. The renal angle is formed on the back by the lower border of the 12th rib and outer border of erector spinae muscle.

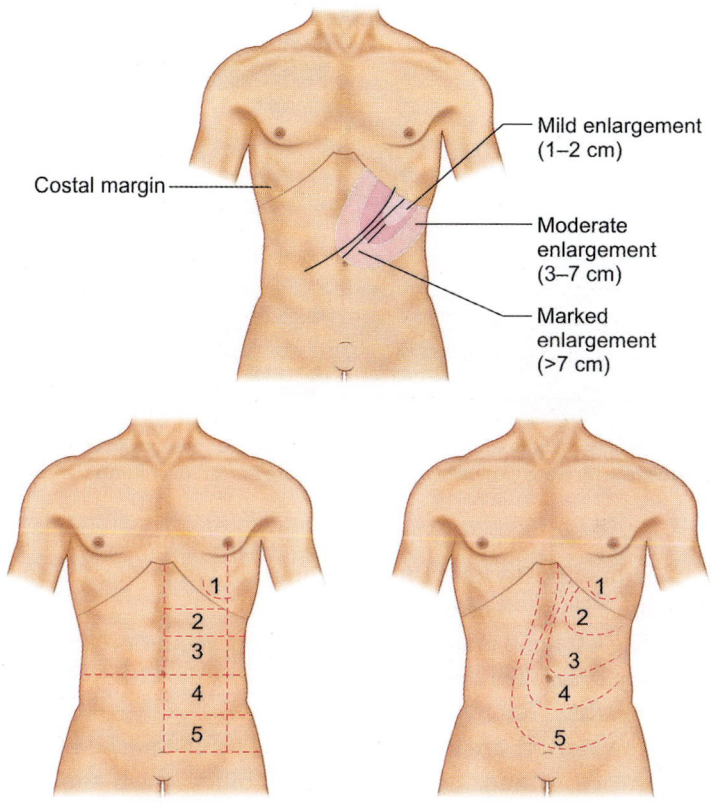

Fig. 13: Hackett's grading of splenomegaly.

Box 12: Common causes of splenomegaly.

- *Infections:*
  - Malaria
  - Typhoid
  - Tuberculosis
  - Kala-azar
  - Bacterial endocarditis (BE)
  - Splenic abscess (Brucellosis, BE)
- *Hematological:*
  - Hemolytic anemia (Thalassemia, sickle cell disease, spherocytosis)
  - Leukemia
  - Lymphoma
- Lipid storage disease (Gaucher, Niemann–Pick)
- Congestion (Portal hypertension)
- Collagen disorders like systemic lupus erythematosus (SLE)

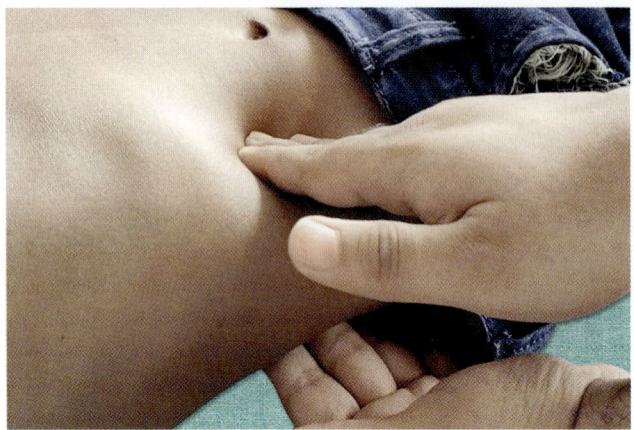

Fig. 14: Bimanual palpation for kidneys. The hand over the loin lifts the kidneys forward which are explored by the other hand placed over lumbar region.

- Press the right hand deep into the abdomen to push the kidney posteriorly during expiration when the abdominal muscles are relaxed.
- The left hand is used to push the kidney anteriorly.
- Try to feel the lower pole of kidney as the child takes deep breaths.
- The kidneys are usually ballotable, can be pushed between the two hands. To elicit ballotability, push the kidney down with the right hand and feel by your left hand kept in the loin when it strikes to the posterior surface of the abdomen.
- The lower pole of the right kidney may be palpable in thin persons.
  - *Left kidney:* Palpate the left kidneys in a similar way by keeping the right hand in the left lumbar region and left hand posteriorly in the left loin. One can stand either on the right or the left side of the patient.

Renal lump: A renal lump may be with Wilms tumor, perinephric abscess, hydronephrosis, renal cyst, etc. Differentiation of renal lump and spleen is practically difficult. It is shown in **Box 13**.

Renal tenderness: To elicit renal tenderness, press your thumb at the renal angle while the patient is sitting and leaning forward.

Urinary bladder: Normally, urinary bladder is not palpate. It becomes palpable as a smooth oval lump in the suprapubic region when it is full. It may be palpable in cases of posterior urethral valve, bladder diverticula, phimosis or voiding dysfunction. The upper border may reach to umbilicus or beyond it. The lump will disappear when the child passes urine and bladder is evacuated completely and it may remain palpable even after micturition due to residual urine in the bladder.

Fecoliths: Fecoliths are hard, dried stool, retained in the rectum and may be palpable in the left iliac fossa in a child with constipation. They are usually multiple and can be indented by pressing a finger into them.

Abdominal lump: Whenever a mass is palpable in the abdomen, confirm that it is not liver, spleen, kidney or urinary bladder. Describe the abdominal lump or mass as shown in **Box 14**.

- *Site or origin:* Confirm whether the lump is intra-abdominal or parietal.

> **Box 13:** Differentiation between renal lump and spleen.
> - A spleen is not palpable bimanually, kidneys are palpable bimanually
> - If you feel splenic notch, it confirms the presence of spleen
> - A direction of enlargement of spleen is toward the right iliac fossa
> - A massive spleen can cross midline but a renal lump does not
> - One cannot reach the upper border of spleen, one cannot insinuate the fingers between the spleen and left thoracic cage, whereas the upper border of a renal lump can be felt

> **Box 14:** Description of an abdominal mass.
> - Site (May indicate organ of its origin)
> - Origin (Intra-abdominal or parietal)
> - Size
> - Shape (Round, elongated, irregular)
> - Margins (Well-defined or ill-defined)
> - Surface (Smooth or nodular)
> - Consistency (Cystic, soft, firm, hard)
> - Mobility (With respiration)
> - Ballotability
> - Presence of signs of inflammation

- Ask the child to lift his shoulder off the couch while you are pressing firmly against the forehead. You can ask him to raise both the extended legs from the couch. If the swelling becomes less prominent or disappears, it indicates intra-abdominal mass. If it becomes more prominent, it is parietal (in the abdominal wall) mass. It can also be examined by straight leg raising test. The child is asked to raise his extended legs in supine lying down position and see whether the mass disappears (intra-abdominal) or becomes prominent (parietal).

Note the site of mass, giving idea of its origin. Also note its size, shape, margins, surface, consistency, etc. The swelling moving with respiration may be arising from liver, spleen, kidneys or stomach. But they do not freely move with palpation.

A swelling, such as mesenteric cyst, may not move with respiration, but moves by palpation.

A swelling which is firmly adherent to the surroundings structure and is not mobile at all may be a retroperitoneal mass, malignancy or chronic inflammation. Presence of impulse on coughing indicates hernia. A renal mass is ballotable. Signs of inflammation like redness, induration, warmness, etc. should be noted. A strangulated hernia may present as an inflammatory inguinal swelling with severe abdominal pain.

Percussion

Percussion of abdomen helps in confirming some of the findings on palpation and tells regarding presence of free fluid in the peritoneal cavity. It is done with the child in supine position and the lower limbs flexed at the hip joints.

Percussion over abdomen helps to differentiate whether the abdominal distention is due to gas or fluid. In the presence of gas in the abdomen, the percussion note will be resonant and if fluid and gas both are present, it will be tympanic.

In a case of intestinal perforation, gas will be present under the diaphragm and liver dullness is obliterated (masking of liver dullness).

Signs of Ascites (Figs. 4 and 15)

In the presence of free fluid in the peritoneal cavity (ascites), different signs will be present depending upon amount of the fluid present.

- *Puddle sign **(Fig. 16)**:* If the fluid in the peritoneal cavity is minimal, it can be detected only by making the patient prone so that he bears weight over his knees and elbows and the

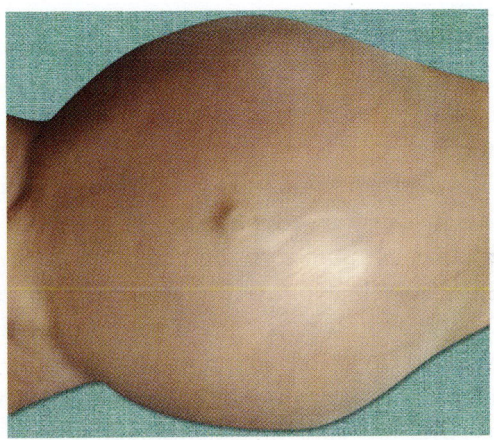

Fig. 15: Abdominal distention due to ascites. Note the fullness of flanks and prominent abdominal superficial veins.

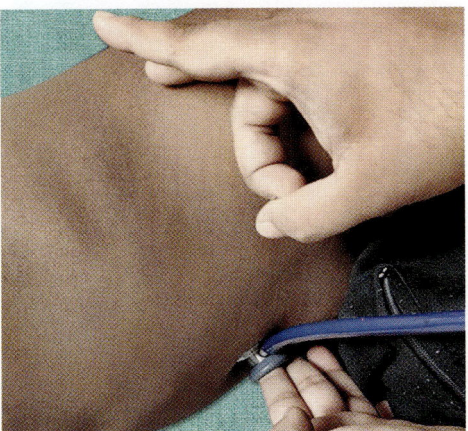

Fig. 16: Puddle sign to assess minimal ascites.

abdomen is off the couch. When the patient assumes this posture, the fluid gravitates down around the center and percussion over the umbilicus will give a dull note.

- *Shifting dullness (Fig. 17):*
  - Child should be lying in supine position. Expose the abdomen and stand on the right side of the patient.
  - Normally, there is resonant note on percussion at the umbilicus.
  - Start percussion from the umbilicus and go laterally toward right or left flank. If it remains resonant throughout up to the flank, this indicates absence of free fluid in the peritoneal cavity.
  - A dull note in the dependent flank suggests presence of fluid because of gravitation.
  - If the flanks are dull, turn the patient to the opposite side without displacing your pleximeter finger. In this position, the umbilicus becomes dependent and the flank is now on top, wait for some time and let the fluid shift toward umbilicus and opposite flank because of gravity. Again, percuss over the same area. A resonant note now confirms that the fluid has shifted to the dependent area.

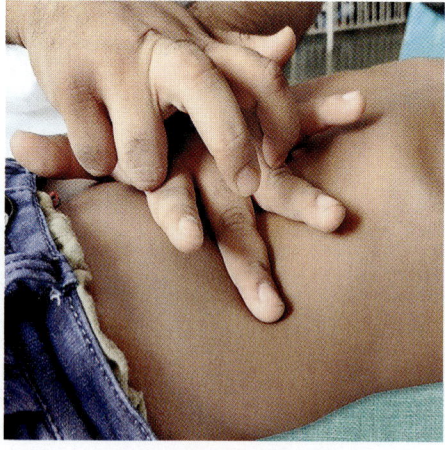

Fig. 17: Shifting dullness.

- The dullness shifts to the umbilicus and flank becomes resonant.
- The shifting can be confirmed by making the child supine again, the dullness will shift back to the flanks and the umbilicus will become resonant.

The shifting dullness may not be present in spite of fluid in the peritoneal cavity either due to encysted fluid or adhesions.

Horseshoe Shape Dull Note

In moderate to massive ascites, the whole peritoneal cavity is full except some area between and around xiphisternum and umbilicus.

- Start percussion from epigastric region, which would be resonant to umbilicus till you get dull note. Mark it.
- From epigastrium to this point, percuss laterally and define dull note at various points both the sides.
- If you join these points, it will give the shape of horseshoe shape.

Fluid Thrill (Fig. 18)

In case of massive ascites, it is not possible to elicit shifting dullness because shift of the fluid by gravity is not possible. In such patients, the whole abdomen is dull, but fluid thrill can be elicited.

- Ask an assistant or a nurse to keep her hand longitudinally in the midline in such a way that ulnar border of her hand touches the abdomen and press it firmly.
- Keep your left palm over the right flank and with right hand give a flick over the left flank. You will feel a thrill that gets transmitted through the fluid under left hand.

To prevent transmission of tapping impulse to travel through the abdominal wall, an assistant or nurse is asked to keep her hand firmly over the middle of the abdomen.

Auscultation

Auscultation over the abdomen is performed to listen the bowel sounds.

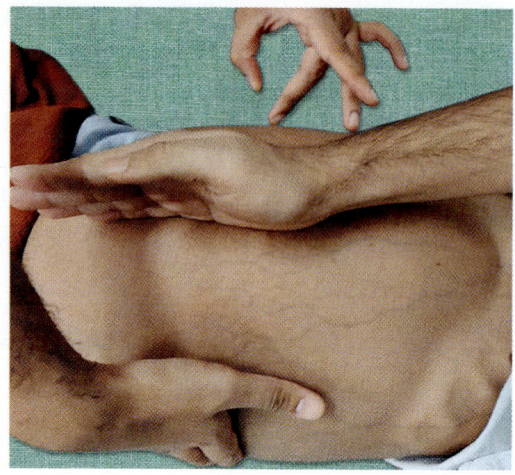

Fig. 18: Demonstration of fluid thrill in a case massive ascites.

Bowel Sounds

- Bowel sounds are normally best heard near the umbilicus.
- The frequency of sound is 10–15/min in small intestine whereas 3–5/min in large intestine.
- Increased bowel sounds are heard in intestinal obstruction, diarrhea, hyperthyroidism, etc.
- Absence or decreased bowel sounds are heard in paralytic ileus, peritonitis, hypokalemia, etc.
- *Borborygmi:* Increased frequency and intensity of sounds (gurgling sounds) often audible to the unaided ears are called borborygmi. It is caused by the movement of fluid and gas in the intestine.

Renal Bruit

Renal bruit should be heard for, in children in whom renal artery stenosis is suspected. Press the bell of stethoscope deep into abdomen over both lumbar regions and try to hear for a bruit.

A venous hum may be audible over liver and spleen in cases of vascular tumors.

Per Rectal Examination

- Per rectal examination is missed in our daily practice. It should be performed in all children presenting with constipation, bleeding per rectum, and any pelvic mass.
- The child and the parents should be explained regarding the examination.
- Ask the child to lie in lateral position with knees flexed toward abdomen.
- Inspect the anus and perianal region for any local infection, an abscess, perianal excoriation, something protruding from rectum, anal fissure, etc.
- Note the site of anal orifice—normal or ectopic.
- The examiner should wear glove, apply lubricant agent (Petroleum jelly) or xylocaine jelly on your little finger.
- Try to insert your little finger in the rectum gently. Note the size of anal orifice (normal or stenosed), tone of anal sphincter, and contents of rectum.
- Empty rectum may be in a case of Hirschsprung's disease. Rectum may be found loaded with hard fecal matter due to functional constipation. Presence of any mass, polyp, etc. should be noted. Try to feel intussceptum in an infant presented with pain in abdomen, mass on right side of abdomen, and bleeding per rectum.
- While removing the figure, the gush of air and fluid indicates Hirschsprung's disease.
- Any blood stain on your finger may be a case of intussusceptions or mucosal bleeding.
- Remove the glove and dispose it properly.
- Note your findings in case paper.

CHAPTER 8

The Respiratory System

Baldev Prajapati, Rajal Prajapati

INTRODUCTION

The history in details and relevant general physical examination are essential components before examination of the respiratory system. The examination of the respiratory system requires considerable skill on the part of the examiner, proper exposure of the child, and quiet, warm, and comfortable room. One should spare some time to observe the child. The sequence of examination should be from least distressing to most distressing.

HISTORY

The history of present illness should be in details with special emphasis on onset (sudden, acute, subacute or insidious), evolution of disease, and response to therapy. List all the symptoms in chronological order. Each symptom should be elaborated in details with certain laid down questions **(Box 1)**. It will provide some clues which will help the clinician for further building up the story of illness. The common symptoms of respiratory system disorders include fever, cough, coryza, sore throat, difficulty in breathing, chest pain, hemoptysis, etc. The presence of fever favors some infection,

Box 1: Laid down questions to elaborate each symptom.
- Onset
- Duration
- Nature and type
- Diurnal variations
- Progress (increasing or decreasing)
- Associated symptoms
- Aggravating and relieving factors
- Response to drug therapy

may be viral, bacterial or tuberculosis. For each symptom, always ask its onset, duration, nature, type, associated symptoms, and aggravating and relieving factors. This information tells us how the disease started, whether it is acute, subacute, chronic, persistent, recurrent, its nature and type may be important clue for some specific condition, associated symptoms and aggravating as well as relieving factors will lead to some system and narrow down the possible conditions. One should go in details of the medicines received by the patient and their effect on course of the symptoms.

Cough

Cough is an explosive expiration. It is a protective reflex that results from stimulation of receptors by some irritant. It begins with deep inspiration, building expiratory pressure over closed glottis followed by explosive expiration. Sudden onset of choking of cough in an otherwise healthy toddler may be due to foreign body aspiration or viral croup syndrome. Intractable cough may be due to viral infection or irritation of tracheobronchial tree due to bronchial asthma, bronchitis, bronchiolitis, etc. Nocturnal cough is common in a case of bronchial asthma, postnasal drip, gastroesophageal reflux disease, etc. Infants and toddlers (<3 years of age) cannot expectorate sputum and they often swallow it and may bring out by vomiting. Barking cough is the characteristic of laryngitis as it occurs in acute laryngotracheobronchitis. Paroxysmal, spasmodic cough occurs in pertussis and foreign body aspiration. Cough with expectorations indicates chronic suppurative lung disease like bronchiectasis, cystic fibrosis, lung abscess, etc. Cough is uncommon in neonates. Its presence in neonates indicates aspiration syndromes or chlamydial and pertussis like infections. Inspiratory whoop is the hallmark of pertussis, but may occur in *Bordetella parapertussis*, adenoviruses, and *Chlamydiae*. The important points to be noted regarding cough are listed in **Table 1**.

Difficulty in Breathing

Children with difficulty in breathing should be evaluated in details. Sudden onset of difficulty in breathing may be due to foreign body, bronchial asthma or viral infections like croup syndrome.

Table 1: Cough.	
Onset	Sudden (foreign body), gradual, recurrent (bronchial asthma)
Duration	Acute (viral), subacute, chronic (tuberculosis)
Nature	Dry (URTI, bronchial asthma); moist (pneumonia, bronchiectasis)
Type	Hacking (tracheitis); barking (viral croup, laryngitis); spasmodic (allergic, asthma); paroxysmal (pertussis)
Cough in neonates	Aspiration, chlamydia, pertussis
Whoop	Pertussis, adenovirus, chlamydiae
Sputum	Amount, color, odor, blood
Severity	Disrupts activity, feeding, sleep, etc. (asthma)
Associated symptoms	Fever (infection), dyspnea (bronchial asthma, CHF), choking, gagging
Aggravating factors	Activity (exertional dyspnea), posture (postnasal drip in lying down position), diurnal, seasonal (bronchial asthma, allergic), nocturnal (bronchial asthma, postnasal drip, GERD)
Relieving factors	Medication, nebulization (bronchial asthma), spontaneously
Treatment taken	Effect of medicines on cough; ACE inhibitors may aggravate cough

(ACE: angiotensin-converting enzyme; CHF: congestive heart failure; GERD: gastroesophageal reflux disease; URTI: upper respiratory tract infection)

Gradually, increasing breathlessness indicates progressive disease like interstitial lung disease, cor pulmonale or congestive heart failure. Level of intolerance will give the idea of its severity. Associated symptoms with breathlessness, like tightness of chest, indicate bronchial asthma while edema feet, diaphoresis, palpitation, and cyanosis indicate cardiac origin. The points to be elaborated for details of difficulty in breathing are shown in **Table 2**.

Signs of Increased Work of Breathing

Identifying tachypnea, retractions, and audible respiratory sounds indicates site of pathology **(Table 3)**. The respiratory sound is produced by some specific mechanism and its presence indicates

Table 2: Difficulty in breathing.

Onset	Sudden, gradual (foreign body, bronchial asthma)
Duration	Acute, chronic
Severity	Level of intolerance—on exercise/on routine activities, at rest, during sleep, inability to feed or speak in sentences
Associated symptoms	Fever, cough, chest pain, edema feet, urine output, cyanosis, etc.
Aggravating factors	Position, time of day, exercise, allergens, irritants, infections, emotions
Relieving factors	Medicines, inhalers, oxygen
Treatment taken	Response to bronchodilators; drugs received like antibiotics, steroids, etc.

Table 3: Respiratory signs and site of lesion.

	Extrathoracic	Intrathoracic	Pulmonary
Tachypnea	+	++	+++
Retractions	++++	++	++
Stridor	+++	+	-
Wheeze	-	++	+++
Grunt	-	-	+

Table 4: Common audible respiratory sounds and their site of origin.

Sound	Site of origin	Phase of respiration when heard
Snuffle	Nasal passages	Inspiration/expiration
Snore	Oronasopharyngeal airway	Inspiration/expiration
Stridor	Extrathoracic airways	Inspiration
Wheeze	Intrathoracic airways	Expiration
Grunt	Lung parenchyma	Expiration

definite pathology **(Table 4)**. The nasal snuffle indicates pathology at nostrils and it is characteristic of congenital syphilis. The nasal snoring is commonly due to adenoiditis. The stridor is produced due to extrathoracic airway obstruction or laryngitis. The wheezing is characteristic of lower airway obstruction. The grunting indicates serious lung parenchymal disease. It is produced by the child by forceful expiration against partial closed epiglottis. It is the effort by the patient to keep the lung inflated in severe respiratory conditions like hyaline membrane disease in the preterm baby or severe pneumonia in older children.

Dysphagia

Acute dysphagia may be due to acute pharyngitis, acute tonsillitis, diphtheria, retropharyngeal abscess, etc. The insidious dysphagia indicates any mediastinal mass and vascular ring.

Hemoptysis

Hemoptysis is uncommon in children. It may be due to bronchiectasis, lung abscess, resolving pneumonia, pulmonary edema, mitral stenosis, pulmonary embolism, tubercular cavity, etc.

Chest Pain

Chest pain is also uncommon in children. The most common causes of chest pain in children are pleurisy, pneumothorax, pneumonia, pericarditis, herpes zoster, coronary insufficiency due to aortic stenosis, Kawasaki disease, gastroesophageal reflux disease causing reflux esophagitis, etc. Some of the features will differentiate cause of chest pain **(Table 5)**.

Table 5: Differentiating features of chest pain.	
Skin pain	History of local rash (herpes zoster) or boil
Musculoskeletal pain	Increased with activity/movement
Pleuritic pain	Localized, catch in breath, aggravating by breathing and cough, sharp pain on deep inspiration, decreases in lateral lying down position on same side; nonpleuritic pain is not related to respiration
Esophagitic pain	Central/retrosternal pain, may be arching and irritability in small children, related with food
Pericardial pain	Central with associated signs of pericardial disease, sharp, stabbing pain, intensifies during lying down, breathing and coughing, sitting up and leaning forward can often ease the pain

Family History
Family history of tuberculosis and bronchial asthma should be routine points to be covered in history taking.

Vaccination History
The vaccination status of the child should be inquired. It provides useful guidelines for exclusion or consideration of certain infections. BCG, DPT, measles, *Haemophilus influenzae* type B, and pneumococcal vaccines offer protection from several respiratory infections.

GENERAL PHYSICAL EXAMINATION
Before starting the examination, spare some time to observe the child to assess its comfort and general appearance. In a dyspneic child, one should note whether accessory muscles of respiration and alae nasi are working or not. Inspiratory dyspnea is due to obstruction of upper airways while expiratory dyspnea is seen in children with obstructive lung diseases. Try to listen the audible respiratory sound, if it is present. The characteristic of sound indicates its site of origin, which becomes important clue to the diagnosis **(Table 4)**. The signs of increased work of breathing **(Box 2)** and signs of acute respiratory failure **(Box 3)** should be noted. It gives clue to severity of disease. State of consciousness and nutrition of the child should be noted. Anemia, cyanosis, and lymphadenopathy should be routinely checked.

Vitals
Vitals (temperature, pulse rate, respiratory rate, BP, and oxygen saturation by pulse oximeter) should be noted.

Box 2: Signs of increased work of breathing.

- Tachypnea
- Retractions (suprasternal/subcostal/intercostal)
- Use of accessory muscles (sternocleidomastoid)
- Flaring of alae nasi
- Head bobbing
- Various sounds (stridor/wheezing/grunting)
- Cyanosis

> **Box 3:** Acute respiratory failure.
> - Apprehension, anxiety, restlessness
> - Tachypnea, dyspnea, chest retractions, cyanosis
> - Air entry to the lungs may be severely compromised due to upper airway obstruction or marked bronchospasms (minimal or absent breath sounds on auscultation)
> - Slow, shallow, gasping or irregular respiration (may be due to CNS depression, neuromuscular disease or terminally exhausted respiratory muscles)
> - *Decreased arterial oxygen saturation:*
>   - <80% by pulse oximetry
>   - PaO_2 <60 mm Hg
>   - FiO_2 >0.6
>   - $PaCO_2$ >50 mm Hg

Respiration

Respiration rate should be counted for full 1 minute with eyes at the level of the chest of the patient. Type of breathing, its character, depth, etc. should be noted. Cheyne-Stokes breathing, Biot's breathing, and apnea occur due to depression of respiratory centers in brain due to various causes like hypoxia, encephalitis, meningitis, raised intracranial pressure, uremia, etc. Cheyne-Stokes breathing is due to involvement of cerebrum, hyperventilation due to midbrain, and apnea as well as apneustic breathing occur due to involvement of medulla oblongata.

ENT Examination

ENT check-up is part of respiratory system examination for upper respiratory tract infections like otitis media and sinusitis. Examination of throat and oral cavity is important.

Clubbing

Clubbing is thickening of the terminal phalanges of fingers and toes. It is due to excessive growth of the connective tissues.

Different Methods of Measuring Digital Clubbing (Fig. 1)

- The ratio of the distal phalangeal diameter (DPO) over the interphalangeal diameter (IPD) or the phalangeal depth ratio is <1 in normal subjects but increases to >1 with digital clubbing.

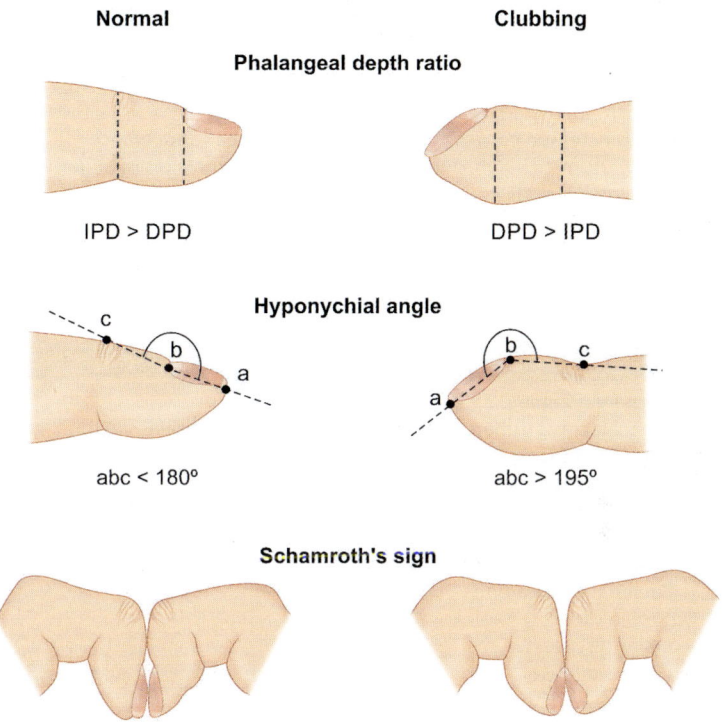

Fig. 1: Different methods of measuring digital clubbing.

- The hyponychial angle is <180° in normal children but >195° in patients with clubbing.
- The dorsal surfaces of terminal phalanges of similar fingers are placed together. In a case of clubbing, the normal diamond-shaped window at the base of nail beds disappears. It is called as Schamroth's sign.

Mechanism of Clubbing

The exact mechanism of clubbing is not known. It is believed that endothelial growth factors released during chronic hypoxia and consequent vasodilatation cause the excessive growth of connective tissues resulting in classical changes of terminal phalanges of fingers and toes, called clubbing.

> **Box 4:** Grades of clubbing.
> - *Grade I:* Fluctuation and softening of the nail bed
> - *Grade II:* Loss of the normal angle between the nail bed and the fold. This is most easily identified by Schamroth's sign
> - *Grade III:* Increased convexity of the nails, parrot beak appearance
> - *Grade IV:* Drumstick sign, due to thickening of the whole distal finger, resembling drum stick
> - *Grade V:* Hypertrophic pulmonary osteoarthropathy (clubbing + thickening of the periosteum); it is less common in children

> **Box 5:** Causes of clubbing.
> - *Respiratory system:*
>   - Bronchiectasis (tuberculosis, cystic fibrosis, ciliary dyskinesia)
>   - Suppurative lung disease (lung abscess, empyema)
>   - Interstitial lung disease
>   - Rarely malignancy of lung or pleura
> - *Cardiac:*
>   - Cyanotic congenital heart disease (most common Fallot's Tetralogy)
>   - Bacterial endocarditis
> - *Gastrointestinal:*
>   - Celiac disease
>   - Crohn's disease
>   - Ulcerative colitis
>   - Cirrhosis of liver
> - *Miscellaneous:*
>   - Familial
>   - Local trauma to digit
>   - Scleroderma
>   - Arteriovenous fistula

Refer **Box 4** for grades of clubbing and **Box 5** for common causes of clubbing.

Chronic Sinusitis

Chronic sinusitis is associated with nasal obstruction with persistent mucopurulent nasal discharge, puffy eyelids, and dark circles under the eyes. The important causes of chronic sinusitis are cleft palate, allergic rhinitis, Kartagener syndrome, immotile cilia syndrome, cystic fibrosis, Hurler's syndrome, immunodeficiency disorders, etc.

EXAMINATION OF CHEST

Anatomical areas for clinical examination of chest are:
- *Front:* Supraclavicular, infraclavicular, mammary, and inframammary areas **(Fig. 2)**
- *Side:* Superior, middle, and inferior axillary areas
- *Back:* Suprascapular, interscapular, infrascapular, and basal areas **(Fig. 3)**

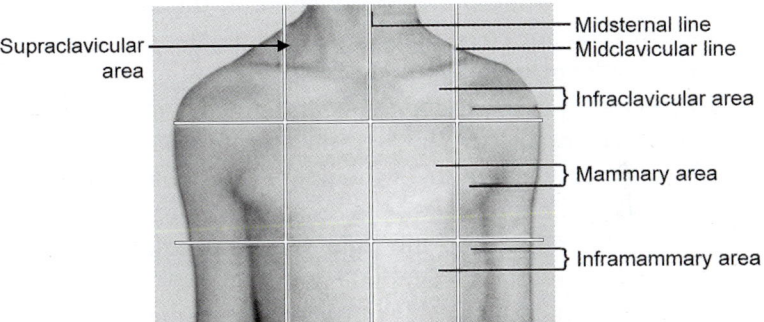

Fig. 2: Anatomical lines and areas in front.

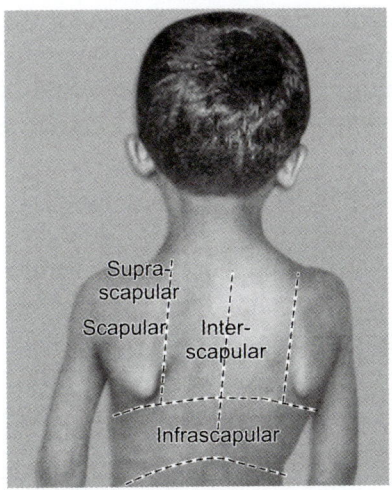

Fig. 3: Anatomical areas in back.

Anatomical Landmarks

- *Angle of Louis (Ludwig's angle, sternal angle):*
    - Transverse bony ridge at the junction of the body of sternum and manubrium sterni
    - Corresponds to 2nd intercostal space (ICS)
    - Corresponds to bifurcation of trachea anteriorly and 4th thoracic spine posteriorly
    - Mediastinum is divided into superior and inferior at this level
    - Corresponds to arch of aorta
- A line drawn from 2nd thoracic spine to the 6th rib in the midclavicular line corresponds to the major interlobar fissure or upper border of lower lobe of the lung.
- The boundary between the upper and middle lobes is marked by a horizontal line drawn from sternum at the level of 4th costal cartilage to meet the major interlobar fissure line on the right side of the chest.
- Upper (also middle on the right side) and lower lobes are accessible to physical examination anteriorly and posteriorly, respectively while all the lobes are accessible in the axillary area.

Inspection

The exposed chest should be inspected from front **(Fig. 4)** by standing at foot end or head end of the patient with eyes at the level of the chest **(Fig. 5)**. The child can be examined in sitting as well as standing with upper extremities by the sides. It should also be viewed from lateral side with eyes at the level of chest **(Fig. 6)**.

Shape of the Chest (Figs. 7A to H)

- Cylindrical or circular in infants
- Normal shape of chest in older children and adults is elliptical (transverse diameter > anteroposterior diameter)
- Barrel-shaped (emphysematous) chest is elongated and shoulders are uplifted (in bronchial asthma)
- Pigeon chest (pectus carinatum)—sternum is prominent (in rickets) **(Fig. 8)**
- Pectus excavatum (funnel-shaped)—depression of sternum (congenital) **(Fig. 9)**

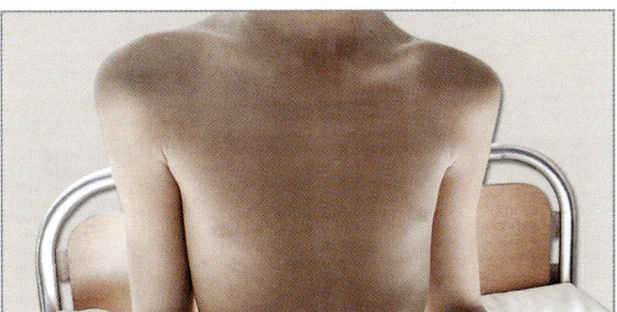

Fig. 4: Inspection of chest from front.

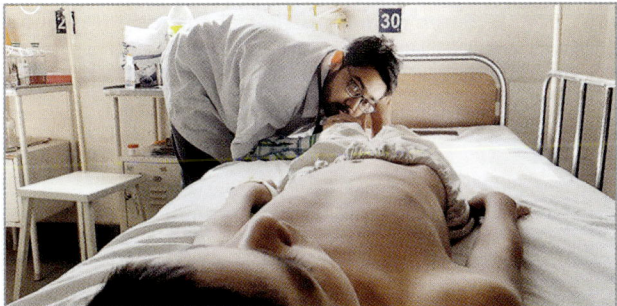

Fig. 5: Inspection of chest from the foot end in the lying position.

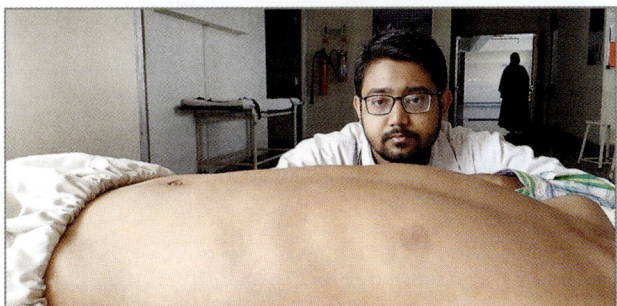

Fig. 6: Inspection of chest from lateral view.

- Harrison's sulcus may be seen in rickets **(Fig. 10)**
- Kyphosis, lordosis, and kyphoscoliosis may give rise to abnormal shape of the chest.

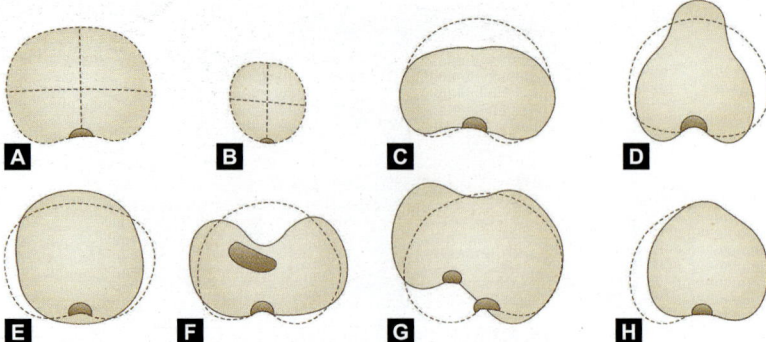

Figs. 7A to H: Cross sections of normal and abnormal forms of chest. (A) Adult chest (elliptical); (B) Infant chest (cylindrical/circular); (C) Flat chest; (D) Pigeon chest (rachitic); (E) Emphysematous (Barrel-shaped); (F) Funnel chest; (G) Kyphoscoliotic chest; (H) Unilateral retraction of chest.

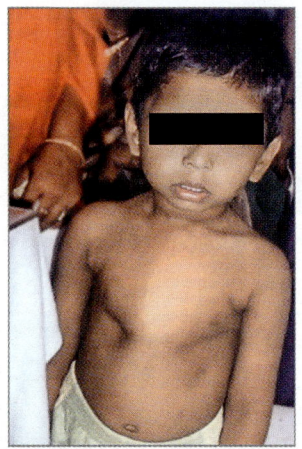

Fig. 8: Pectus carinatum (pigeon chest).

Symmetry

- Note the distance of medial borders of both scapulae from midline on both the sides which is useful to assess any asymmetry of the chest.
- Drooping of one shoulder may occur in patients with fibrocaseous tuberculosis.
- Look for any bulge (intercostal bulging in pleural effusion) or retraction (collapse or fibrosis).

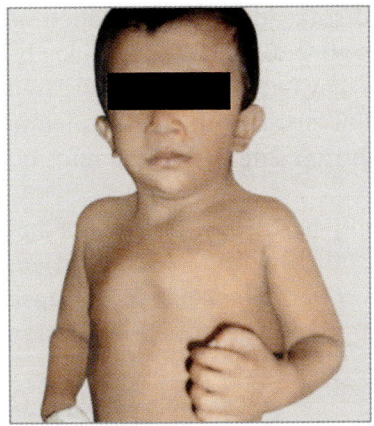

Fig. 9: Pectus excavatum (funnel chest).

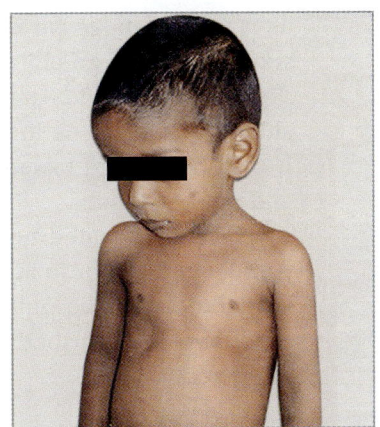

Fig. 10: Harrison's sulcus.

- When empyema points through an ICS as a cystic swelling, it is reducible and cough impulse is present, it is called empyema necessitans.
- Localized bulge of chest may be due to longstanding cardiomegaly (bulging of precordium), intrathoracic mass, and deformities of ribs and spine.

Movements of Chest
- Type of breathing in infants is abdominal or abdominothoracic.
- Indrawing of upper part of abdomen with each inspiration indicates paralysis of diaphragm of that side.
- Chest expansion is minimal or absent with paralysis of intercostal muscles.
- *Look for indrawings:*
  - Suprasternal recession in obstruction of upper airways (laryngeal diphtheria, acute laryngotracheobronchitis, laryngeal or tracheal foreign body)
  - Subcostal indrawing indicates airway disease
  - Intercostal indrawing suggests lung parenchymal disease.
- *Look for position of trachea and apex beat, if visible:*
  - In a child with marked tracheal displacement, clavicular head of sternomastoid muscle would be pushed forward

as a visible bulge on the displaced side. It is called as sternomastoid sign or Trail sign. Normally, trachea may be slightly on right side. Trachea may be pulled toward diseased side due to collapse lung, fibrosis, and thickened pleura. It may be pushed toward normal side by pleural effusion and pneumothorax.
- Apex beat is located normally in 4th ICS (in infants and young children) or in 5th ICS (in children >7 years old) on left side. It may be pulled on pathological side (collapse and fibrosis) or pushed on opposite side (pleural effusion or pneumothorax).

Palpation

- The findings of inspection should be confirmed.
- *Tracheal position:*
  - The position of trachea and apex beat to be confirmed. The trachea is examined in supine position of the child or sitting with slight flexion of neck.
  - Place the index finger into the suprasternal notch, gently push it backward. The finger would touch the trachea in the midline in a normal child. If trachea is deviated, the finger will slide into the tracheosternomastoid space.
  - Place the ring and index fingers on the two sternal attachments of the sternocleidomastoid muscles. Gently, pass the middle finger over the trachea to assess its relationship to the fixed two landmarks, whether trachea is central or on either side **(Fig. 11)**.
  - Look for any tender area, crepitations (subcutaneous emphysema, fracture rib).
- *Chest expansion:* Determine the degree and symmetry of chest expansion by following method:
  - Place the palms on either side of the chest at the level of the nipples, gently opposing the thumbs in the midline **(Figs. 12A and B)**. It can be done at back also by hands placed over the side of the chest and thumbs opposed in the midline over the spine. Ask the child for deep inspiration and observe for the movements of thumbs on both the sides **(Fig. 13)**.

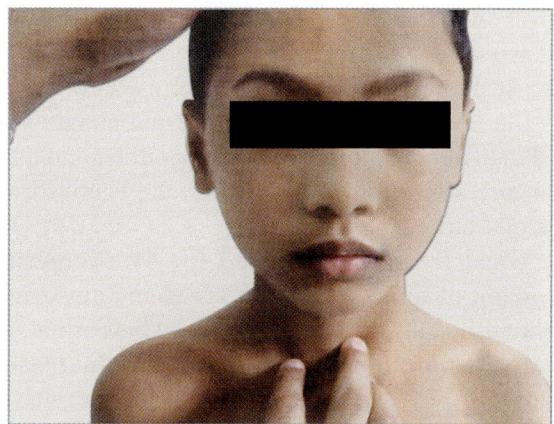

Fig. 11: Technique of palpation for tracheal position.

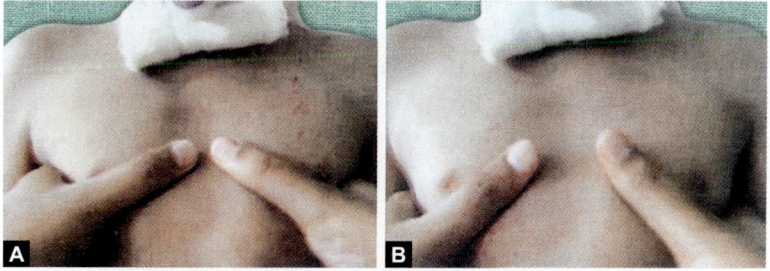

Figs. 12A and B: Assessment of chest expansion at front.

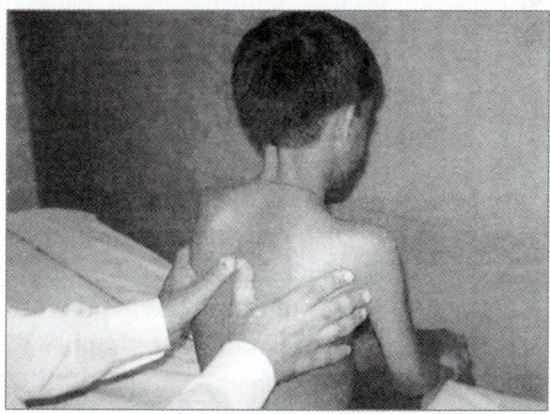

Fig. 13: Assessment of chest expansion at back.

It gives an approximate estimate of degree of chest expansion and assessment of symmetry.
- The use of measure tap will give more accuracy as it quantifies the chest expansion. The normal chest expansion is 3–5 cm in older children and less in toddler and infants.
- Feel for any abnormal sounds (rhonchi, friction rub, coarse crepitations, etc.).
- Tactile vocal fremitus is looked for by comparing tactile transmission of spoken words or cry in infants, over identical areas on both sides of the chest. It may be normal, decreased (pleural effusion, pneumothorax), and increased (lobar pneumonia).

Percussion

Striking the chest wall with the fingers causes underlying tissues to vibrate and the sound is produced. The resultant note (sound) depends on the type of underlying structure whether it is solid, containing air, fluid or both air and fluid. In infants and small children, it may be difficult to derive reliable inference due to small chest.

Method of Percussion

Chest percussion is an art and it can be best learned only by repeated practice and experience.
- Place the hand on the chest of the patient so that middle finger is resting along an ICS. The other fingers should be off the chest.
- Tap the terminal phalanx by the middle finger of the other hand. This action requires movement only at the wrist and not the elbow or shoulder joints **(Fig. 14)**. The tapping finger is called plexor and the finger to be tapped is called pleximeter. The tapping should be sharp and at angle of 90°. Lift the plexor immediately off the pleximeter and listen the note (sound) produced carefully.
- All the areas of the chest should be percussed and compared with contralateral side, immediately.
- Direct percussion of the clavicle (tapping the middle clavicle) is done to percuss the lung apices **(Fig. 15)**.

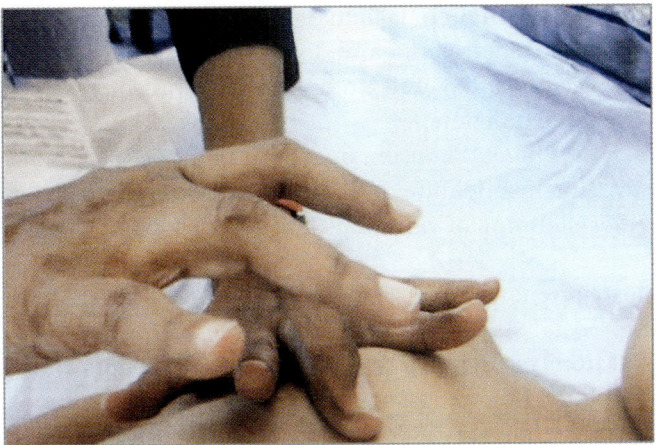

Fig. 14: Method of chest percussion.

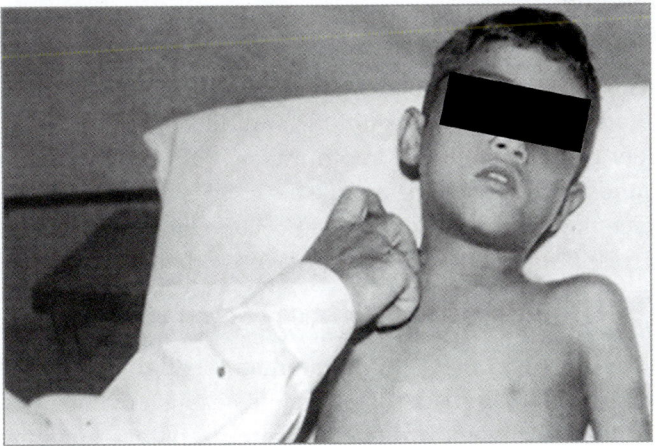

Fig. 15: Direct percussion over the clavicle for assessment of apex of lung.

Types of Percussion Notes

- *Resonant:* The lung tissues contain the air and percussion of lung will give rise to resonant note. The hyperinflated lungs may produce more resonant note.
- *Hyperresonant:* When there is excessive amount of air between the chest wall and underlying lung tissues (pneumothorax), the note perceived is called hyperresonant.

- *Dull note:* When there is fluid or relatively dense or solid structure (pleural effusion and lobar pneumonia), the sound produced is called dull note. The less dull note is referred as impaired dull note.
- *Stony dull note:* When the quality of dull note is compared as between consolidation and pleural effusion, the latter creates greater damping of vibrations and it is described as stony dull note.

Chest percussion on right side, as one comes down from 2nd intercostal space to 5th or 6th intercostal space, the note is changed from resonant to dull note. It indicates upper border of liver. Similarly, percussion of chest on left side, going from lateral to medial, one gets resonant to dull note and it indicates cardiac dull note.

Auscultation

Method of Auscultation

- Deep breathing through the mouth by the patient generates a good airflow. The examiner should demonstrate so that older child can follow it appropriately. In an infant, the breath sounds are evaluated best while the child is crying.
- Place the diaphragm of the stethoscope lightly but firmly over corresponding parts of the chest on both sides. Listen to the breath sounds.
- *All areas should be auscultated in a systematic manner:* Supraclavicular, mammary, inframammary, axillary, infra-axillary, interscapular, suprascapular, and infrascapular of both sides
- The finding should be described in terms of location, intensity, pitch, and timing.

Mechanism of Breath Sounds

Breath sounds are generated in the large airways. As the airflow becomes turbulent during passage through the airways and later transmission through the alveoli, the quality of breath sounds continues changing. Turbulence is created by air that flows within tubes and encounters resistance that alters flow dynamics. For example, air passing through trachea becomes turbulent when it encounters high resistance at the glottis due to the narrow orifice. The resistance causes the velocity of air to increase. When the air is distributed from trachea (single channel) to multiple small airways, considerable sound energy is lost. Besides flow and turbulence, the quality of sound is changed by its frequency. The sounds of varying frequencies take different pathways through the lung.

In general, low frequencies pass through the lung and are directed toward the chest wall, while high frequency sound passes through the airways before being directed through alveoli and then the chest wall. The sounds need not be exactly symmetrical on both the sides even in a normal person.

Types of breathing (Fig. 16):
- *Vesicular breathing:*
  - The normal breath sounds produced in alveoli are called vesicular.
  - The inspiration is loud, high pitched, and long, while expiration is low in intensity and short in duration.
  - Inspiration is immediately followed by expiration.
  - No gap between inspiration and expiration
  - Best heard when the flow is maximal.
- *Bronchial breathing:*
  - Inspiratory and expiratory phases are equal.
  - There is a pause (gap) in between two phases of respiration.

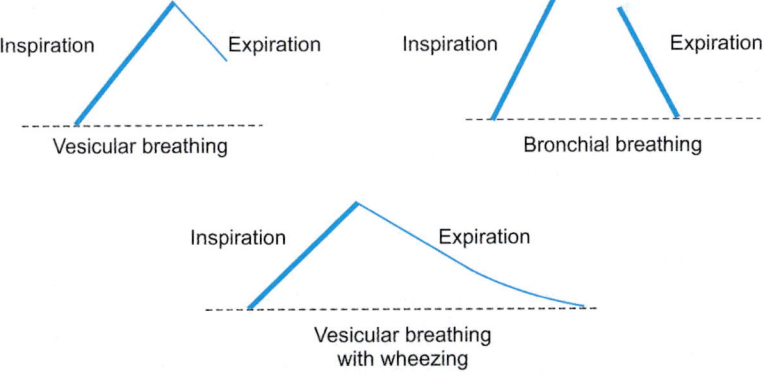

Fig. 16: Diagrammatic pattern of types of breathing.

- Bronchial breathing is heard in consolidation, just above the air–fluid interface in a case of pleural effusion.
- It can be heard over a collapsed portion of the lung, if there is an airway overlying the collapse.
- It may be normally heard over the neck and thoracic spine up to 4th thoracic vertebra.

Types of bronchial breathing:
- High-pitched or tubular (consolidation)
- Medium-pitched (consolidation, small cavity, atelectasis with a patent bronchus)
- Amphoric (bronchopleural fistula)

Intensity of breath sounds may be normal, decreased or absent on one or both sides.

Adventitious Sounds

- *Rattling sounds:* Upper airway sounds transmitted into the chest and heard during auscultation of chest are called rattling sounds. The best example is laryngomalacia.
- *Rhonchus:* It is generated by turbulent air passing through narrowed large airways like trachea and large bronchi (extrathoracic airways). It tends to be low-pitched sound.
- *Wheeze:* Wheeze is produced by oscillations within narrowed airways (bronchiolitis, WALRI). When a large airway is narrowed or obstructed, the wheeze has a single frequency and pitch, and this is described as monophonic. Narrowing of multiple smaller airways over a wide area of the lung creates sounds with varying frequencies and is called as polyphonic wheezing. Wheezing is heard more often during the expiratory phase, since it is produced by limitation of flow. Still, when airway obstruction is severe enough to limit airflow even during active inspiratory phase, wheezing can be heard during inspiration also.
- *Crackles:*
  - Crackles are caused by loss of elastic recoil and premature airway closure. It is produced during inspiration with sudden opening of airways. Crackles are the sounds produced by the explosive opening of airways in territories of lungs deflated to residual volume.

- They are primarily inspiratory, rhythmic, and repetitive, usually not altered by coughing, sensitive to postural changes, and best heard in dependent area of lung.
- There are two types of crackles—coarse crackles and fine crackles. The coarse crackles usually occur in pneumonia while fine crackles in interstitial or restrictive lung diseases. They are also described as Velcro sounds.
- *Rales:* These are bubbling sounds produced by passage of air through the fluid collected in alveoli or bronchioles. It may disappear and again reappear. It may disappear after suctioning of airways. Bronchiolitis is the best example for rales.
- *Crepitations:* These are bubbling, wet sounds produced by passage of air through exudates collected in the alveoli. These are two types of crepitations, fine crepitations, and coarse crepitations. The resolving pneumonia gives rise to fine crepitations while bronchiectasis coarse crepitations.

Vocal Resonance

- The child is asked to repeat some words (one, two, and three) or made to cry. The sound generated from larynx pass through the airways and lungs, the high frequency components get filtered off. However, when there is consolidation, the relatively solid lung does not filter off these frequencies and the sounds are transmitted to the chest wall. These sounds are heard by the examiner with the help of stethoscope kept over the chest wall. It is called as vocal resonance.
- The intensity of vocal resonance may be equal or normal on both the sides.
- It is decreased or absent in pleural effusion, pleural thickening, pneumothorax, emphysema, atelectasis, etc.
- It is increased in consolidation.
- The increased vocal resonance may be so loud that if it appears that sound is produced in the earpieces of stethoscope, is called bronchophony. It is found in lung cavity.
- When the child is asked just to whisper certain words and still there is audible vocal resonance, it is called whispering pectoriloquy. It is found in bronchopleural fistula.

- The nasal twang of vocal resonance is called egophony and is heard at the upper level of pleural effusion due to partially collapsed underlying lung.

Pleural Rub

- It is produced by rubbing of visceral and parietal layers due to inflammation.
- It is well localized, superficial grating, creaking, and leathery sound.
- It is not altered by cough and augmented by snug contact and chest piece of stethoscope to the chest wall.
- It is heard identical in both the phases of inspiration and expiration.
- It increases in intensity when chest piece of stethoscope is pressed against chest wall.
- It disappears when there is collection of fluid in the pleural space and two layers of pleura get separated.
- Pleural rub may be palpable.
- It may be associated with localized chest pain.

Succussion splash: Whenever pleural effusion is suspected, succussion splash should be elicited to rule out hydropneumothorax. The chest piece is affixed at the upper border of dullness and child is suddenly shaken to elicit splash of fluid.

Coin test: A coin is placed in front of chest and tapped with another coin while piece of the stethoscope is placed at an identical spot on the back. A loud bell like sound is heard in the patients of pneumothorax.

CLINICAL FEATURES OF COMMON RESPIRATORY DISEASES (TABLE 6)

Lobar Pneumonia (Consolidation)

- *Symptoms:* Fever, cough, dyspnea, chest pain, and rusty sputum
- *Inspection:*
  - Normal shape and symmetry of chest
  - Chest movements may be diminished on affected side

Table 6: Common respiratory conditions with salient physical signs.

Signs	Consolidation (Lobar pneumonia)	Pleural effusion	Collapse	Pneumothorax	Emphysema
Chest wall	Normal	• Reduced chest movements on affected side • May be bulging of intercostal spaces	Normal or minimal retraction of chest wall	• Hyperinflated (elevated) chest on affected side • Reduced chest movements on affected side	• Barrel-shaped hyperinflated (symmetrical) chest • Chest expansion poor
Mediastinal shift	None	Opposite side	Same side	Opposite side	None
Tactile vocal fremitus	Increased	Diminished or absent	Normal/decreased	Diminished	Diminished
Percussion note	Dull note	Stony dull note	Impaired note	Hyperresonate	• Hyper-resonant • Liver and cardiac dullness might be lost
Breath sounds	Bronchial breathing	• Diminished or absent • Bronchial breathing may be heard at upper border of effusion	Absent/bronchial if bronchus is patent	• Diminished • Amphoric (Bronchopleural fistula)	Diminished with prolonged expiration
Vocal resonance	Increased	Diminished or absent	Diminished	Diminished	Diminished
Adventitious sounds	Fine crepitations	Pleural rub may be heard in early stage of pleurisy	None	Succussion splash if there is hydropneumothorax	Rhonchi

- *Palpation:*
  - Trachea is central
  - Chest expansion may be reduced
  - Tactile vocal fremitus increased
- *Percussion:* Impaired or dull note on percussion
- *Auscultation:*
  - Diminished breath sounds
  - Bronchial breathing
  - Crepitations
  - Vocal resonance increased

Pleural Effusion

- *Symptoms:*
  - Onset may be sudden but is generally insidious
  - Fever, cough, chest pain, and difficulty in breathing
- *Inspection:*
  - Patient prefers to lie on the affected side
  - Respiratory distress (tachypnea, dyspnea)
  - Chest may be bulging (especially intercostal spaces) on the affected side
  - Diminished movements on affected side
- *Palpation:*
  - Trachea and heart are displaced toward the opposite side
  - Less expansion on chest on affected side
  - Tactile vocal fremitus diminished
- *Percussion:* Stony dullness on percussion
- *Auscultation:*
  - Diminished or absent breath sounds on affected side
  - Vocal resonance reduced or absent

Collapse or Atelectasis

Physical examination findings depend on whether an entire lung is involved or a single lobe is collapsed.

- *Symptoms:* History of foreign body inhalation and recurrent chest infections
- *Inspection:*
  - Trachea and heart pulled on the affected side
  - May be narrowing of intercostal spaces on the affected side

- *Palpation:*
  - Shifting of trachea and mediastinum (apex beat) on the affected side
  - Diminished movement and expansion of chest on affected side
  - Tactile vocal fremitus diminished or absent
- *Percussion:* Impaired note on percussion
- *Auscultation:*
  - Breath sounds diminished on affected side
  - Vocal resonance reduced or absent.

Pneumothorax

- *Symptoms:* Sudden dyspnea and chest pain, cyanosis
- *Inspection:*
  - Fullness of neck and upper chest may be due to subcutaneous emphysema
  - Shifting of trachea and apex beat on opposite side may be seen
  - Reduced movements on the affected side
- *Palpation:*
  - Subcutaneous emphysema can be felt, if it is there
  - Shifting of trachea and mediastinum on opposite side
  - Diminished movements and chest expansion on affected side
  - Diminished tactile vocal fremitus on affected side.
- *Percussion:* Hyperresonant on percussion
- *Auscultation:*
  - Breath sounds diminished
  - Vocal resonance reduced
  - Coin test may be positive.

SCHEMATIC PRESENTATION
History and General Physical Examination

- Evaluation of symptoms—fever, cough, difficulty in breathing, noisy breathing, chest pain, hemoptysis, etc.
- Remember to ask for each symptom—onset, duration, nature, type, diurnal variation, associated symptoms, aggravating and relieving factors

- *Points on general physical examination:*
  - Comfortable, dyspneic, tachypneic, alertness, etc.
  - Vitals (temperature, pulse rate, respiration rate, and blood pressure)
  - Signs of increased work of breathing like tachypnea, retractions, various sounds, and cyanosis
  - Nutrition, anemia, lymphadenopathy, ear, nose, throat, and clubbing edema
- *Inspection:*
  - Shape and symmetry of chest
  - Abnormalities like rickets, kyphosis, lordosis, kyphoscoliosis, swelling, scar, etc.
  - Counting respiration rate for full 1 minute
  - Movements of chest
  - Location of trachea and apex beat
- *Palpation:*
  - Confirm location of trachea and apex beat
  - Assess movements and expansion of chest
  - Look for any tenderness or crepitation (subcutaneous emphysema)
  - Tactile vocal fremitus
  - Palpable pleural rub
- *Percussion:* Resonant/impaired note/dull note/stony dull note/hyperresonant
- *Auscultation:*
  - Breath sounds—normal/diminished/absent
  - Type of breathing—vesicular/bronchial
  - Vocal resonance—normal/diminished/increased
  - Adventitious sounds—wheezing/rhonchi/rales/crepitations
  - Pleural rub

The Cardiovascular System

CHAPTER 9

Baldev Prajapati

INTRODUCTION

Many students wonder whether clinical evaluation is relevant in an era of high technology when diagnosis can be easily arrived at by a plethora of sophisticated tests. The discerning clinician, however, knows how to optimally utilize diagnostic tests, cost effectively with maximum safety and benefit for his patient. The pitfalls of misinterpreting diagnostic tests results can be avoided if one is clinically confident of his probable diagnosis. Technology does not absolve the clinician of the need to make a clinical diagnosis but imposes great responsibilities of using technology judiciously and interpreting it wisely. Therefore, the importance of the history and physical examination cannot be over emphasized in the evaluation of infants and children with suspected cardiovascular disorders.

HISTORY

- *Perinatal period:* A comprehensive cardiac history should start with details of perinatal period. Maternal complications during pregnancy, specifically infections in the first trimester should be inquired. Viral infections like rubella and mumps are known for giving rise to congenital rubella syndrome with patent ductus arteriosus (PDA) and endocardial fibroelastosis, respectively to the fetus. *Cytomegalovirus*, herpes simplex virus, and Coxsackie B virus are teratogenic in early pregnancy and may cause myocarditis if infection develops in later pregnancy.
- *Maternal factors:* Advanced maternal age giving rise to chromosomal disorders associated with various congenital heart diseases, gestational diabetes mellitus, and medication exposure are other important factors giving rise to various cardiac malformations **(Box 1)**.

> **Box 1:** Maternal factors giving rise to cardiovascular malformations.
> - *Maternal infections during pregnancy:*
>   – Rubella (PDA)
>   – Mumps (Endocardial fibroelastosis)
> - *Advanced maternal age:*
>   – Trisomy 21 (Down syndrome) with endocardial cushion defect, ASD, VSD, etc.
> - Gestational diabetes mellitus (TGA, VSD, PDA, HOCM, etc.)
> - SLE (Congenital heart block)
> - Mother with CHD (even operated); incidence of CHD increases from 1 to 15%
> - *Medication during pregnancy:*
>   – Phenytoin (Pst, Ast, CoA, PDA)
>   – Alcoholism
>   – Smoking
>   – Progesterone
>   – Estrogen
>
> (ASD: atrial septal defect; CHD: congenital heart defect; HOCM: hypertrophic obstructive cardiomyopathy; PDA: patent ductus arteriosus; SLE: systemic lupus erythematosus; TGA: transposition of the great arteries; VSD: ventricular septal defect; Pst: pulmonary stenosis; Ast: aortic stenosis; CoA: coarctation of the aorta)

- *Maturity and birth weight:* Maturity and birth weight may provide clues. PDA is more common in preterm babies and babies born at high altitude. Small for date babies may be due to intrauterine infections like congenital rubella syndrome with PDA. Large for date infants are often seen in offsprings of diabetic mothers and show a higher incidence of cardiac anomalies. Infants with transposition of the great arteries (TGA) often have birth weight more than average.
- *Recurrent lower respiratory tract infections:* Frequent lower respiratory tract infections, including pneumonia, are common in children with left to right shunts [ventricular septal defect (VSD), atrial septal defect (ASD), PDA] due to pulmonary congestion.
- *Edema:* A child with congestive cardiac failure (CCF) may develop edema. Excessive weight gain in newborns and infants may be a clue to edema. Nonambulatory children may not develop edema over feet, they may have sacral edema. Periorbital puffiness is a more common complaint. Puffiness of eyes and edema are manifestations of systemic venous congestion.
- *Recurrent or persistent wheezing and stridor:* Recurrent or persistent wheezing or stridor may be manifestation of vascular ring causing compression on airways.

- *Symptoms of congestive heart failure (CHF):* In infants, feeding difficulties like prolonged period for each feed, sometimes more than 30 minutes, taking feed with multiple interruptions rather than continuously, excessive perspiration, and becoming dyspneic during taking feed, etc., are symptoms indicating CHF. Eliciting a history of fatigue in an older child during stair climbing, running, bicycle riding or walking short distance is an important information indicating possibility of CHF.
- *Dyspnea:* The onset of difficulty in breathing (dyspnea) in CHF is gradual onset and progressively increasing. The degree of dyspnea can be graded in older children as shown in **Box 2**.
- *Cyanosis:* Cyanosis developing during crying or exercise is an important finding indicating cyanotic heart disease. It is to be differentiated from breath holding spell. Acrocyanosis in full term neonate has no any clinical importance. History of cyanotic spell or squatting indicates possibility of tetralogy of Fallot.
- *Sore throat and joint pain:* History of sore throat and joint pain in the past should be included in the cardiac history routinely, suggesting rheumatic fever.
- *Chest pain:* Chest pain is usually not a manifestation of cardiac disease in the pediatric patient. Pneumonia, pleurisy, pneumothorax, esophagitis due to gastroesophageal reflux, pericarditis, and trauma are common causes for chest pain in children. The cardiac conditions causing chest pain in children are aberrant left coronary artery originating from pulmonary artery (ALCAPA), Kawasaki disease, mitral valve prolapse, pericarditis, aortic stenosis, pulmonary valve obstruction, etc. **(Box 3)**.
- *Palpitation and syncope:* Older children may complain of palpitation (subjective feeling of rapid heartbeats). It may be

---

Box 2: Grades of dyspnea.
- *Grade I:* Dyspnea while climbing stairs or running for a short distance
- *Grade II:* Dyspnea while performing routine activity
- *Grade III:* Dyspnea following light activity like going to bathroom or from one room to the other
- *Grade IV:* Dyspnea even at rest
- *Grade V:* Orthopnea (Breathlessness in recumbent position, relieved by sitting or standing)

> **Box 3:** Cardiac conditions causing chest pain in children.
> - Aberrant left coronary artery originating from pulmonary artery (ALCAPA)
> - Kawasaki disease
> - Mitral valve prolapse
> - Pericarditis
> - Aortic stenosis
> - Pulmonary valve obstruction

> **Box 4:** Neurological manifestations due to cardiac conditions.
> - Cerebrovascular stroke (Embolization or thrombosis secondary to cyanotic CHD with polycythemia, infective endocarditis)
> - Headache (Hypertension, brain abscess in a case of cyanotic CHD)
> - Choreiform movements (Rheumatic chorea)
> - Syncope (Arrhythmias, prolonged Q–T syndrome)
>
> (CHD: congenital heart defect)

due to cardiac arrhythmias and mitral valve prolapse. Syncope may be manifestation of cardiac arrhythmias and prolonged Q–T syndrome. The syncope should be differentiated from epilepsy and functional disorders.
- Some neurological manifestations may be due to cardiac conditions **(Box 4)**.
- Family history should be evaluated in details. History of congenital heart disease (CHD) in mother increases risk of CHD in her offspring from 1 to 15%. In a case of CHD in a sibling, the risk from CHD in next pregnancy is 2.5 times and if two siblings are affected, the risk for the third sibling is 20–30 times. History of essential hypertension and coronary artery disease in family should be routinely sought. History of rheumatic heart diseases and hereditary diseases like Marfan syndrome and Noonan syndrome should also be included.

GENERAL PHYSICAL EXAMINATION

The first and important step is not to miss any life-threatening emergency like cardiogenic shock, cyanotic spell, left ventricular failure, pulmonary edema, and cardiac arrhythmias. These conditions require prompt actions to stabilize the child before proceeding further.

In a stable child, simple observation without disturbing a quiet or sleeping infant is more informative. Look for general appearance, whether the child is ill looking, happy or cranky. Assess whether the child is comfortable or dyspneic, severity of dyspnea, posture, physical growth, nutritional status, etc.

Syndrome with Cardiac Condition

Cardiac disease may be a manifestation of a known congenital malformation syndrome or a generalized disorder affecting the heart and other organ systems **(Table 1)**. Extracardiac malformations may be noted in about 25% of infants with CHD. About 10% of patients have a known chromosomal abnormality.

Sr. No.	Syndrome	Phenotype	Cardiac abnormalities
	Table 1: Common cardiac malformation in association with chromosomal and other syndromes.		
1.	Down syndrome (Trisomy 21)	Brachycephaly, upward slant of eyes, small mouth with protruding fissured tongue, hypotonia, incurved little finger, developmental retardation	Endocardial cushion defect and ventricular septal defect in 50% cases
2.	Trisomy 13 (Patau syndrome)	Microphthalmia, cleft lip/palate, microcephaly, broad flat nose, localized scalp defects, postaxial polydactyly of hands or feet	VSD, ASD, PDA, dextrocardia in 90% cases
3.	Trisomy 18 (Edwards syndrome)	Microcephaly, prominent occiput, small eyes and oral opening, short sternum, clenched hands with overlapping fingers, short dorsiflexed first toe	VSD (90%), PDA (70%), ASD (20%)
4.	Turner syndrome (45, X0)	Lymphedema of dorsa of hands and feet during neonatal period, short stature, broad chest with widely spaced nipples, webbed neck, low hair line, cubitus valgus, amenorrhea	Coarctation of aorta and pulmonary stenosis
5.	Noonan syndrome	Turner-like phenotype, webbed neck, pectus excavatum, cryptorchidism	Pulmonary stenosis
6.	Marfan syndrome	Tall stature, long slender arms and fingers/toes, subluxted lens, lower segment of the body is longer than the upper segment, long span	Dilatation of aortic root with aortic regurgitation, mitral valve prolapse

Contd...

Contd...

Sr. No.	Syndrome	Phenotype	Cardiac abnormalities
7.	Rubella syndrome	Microcephaly, deafness, cataracts, chorioretinitis, metaphysitis	Peripheral pulmonary artery stenosis, patent ductus arteriosus (PDA)
8.	Duchenne muscular dystrophy	Sex-linked disorder with progressive muscular weakness, hypertrophy of calves due to fatty infiltration, positive Gowers' sign, Waddling gait	Cardiomyopathy
9.	Glycogen storage disease (Pompe disease)	Marked hypotonia, macroglossia, hepatomegaly, normal mental development, early death	Cardiomegaly with or without ECG changes (left axis deviation, short PR interval, broad QRS compex)
10.	Hurler syndrome	Coarse features, thick lips and broad nose, cloudy cornea, hepatosplenomegaly, mental retardation	Mitral or aortic regurgitation, coronary artery disease
11.	Ellis–Van Creveld syndrome	Long narrow dysplastic chest (short ribs) and abdomen, notching of upper lip, neonatal teeth, postaxial polydactyly of hands, acromesomelic shortening of limbs, cone shaped epiphyses, small pelvic bones	ASD (50%) or single artrium
12.	Holt–Oram syndrome	Deformities of forearm bones due to absence of radius, absent thumbs	Familial ASD, VSD
13.	William syndrome	Elfin facies, mental retardation, hypercalcemia during infancy	Supravalvular aortic stenosis, pulmonary artery stenosis

(ASD: atrial septal defect; VSD: ventricular septal defect; ECG: electrocardiogram)

Assessment of Growth

Accurate measurement of height, weight, head circumference, arm span, ratio of upper and lower segments, and plotting of serial measurements on standard growth chart are important as both cardiac failure and chronic cyanosis often result in failure to thrive.

Pulse (Heart) Rate

The heart and pulse rates are rapid in children. They are also subject to wide fluctuations especially in newborns and young infants due to crying and excitement. During childhood, the pulse rate may be higher after a meal and in the afternoon, than in the morning. The pulse rate becomes slower as the child grows. The blood pressure varies with age and is related to the height and weight of the child **(Table 2)**.

- *Definition of pulse:* Pulse is defined as expansion of the vessel wall due to propagation of wave produced by movement of blood column ejected from the heart during each systolic contraction which is felt by a palpating finger. **Box 5** outlines the points to be noted during pulse examination.
- *Presence of peripheral pulsations:* The radial pulse is examined using index, middle, and ring fingers with the arm in semipronation and the wrist slightly flexed. If the radial pulse is feeble or

Table 2: Average pulse rate and BP in children at different ages.

	Pulse rate (per min)		BP (in mm Hg)	
	Average	Range	Systolic	Diastolic
Newborn	120	70–170	86	60
1 year	120	80–160	86	60
2 years	120	80–130		
4 years	110	80–120		
6 years	100	76–116	90	60
8 years	90	70–110	96	64
10 years	90	70–110	100	64
12 years	90	65–105	110	70

Box 5: Points to be noted during pulse examination.

- Presence/Absence
- Rate
- Rhythm
- Volume
- Force
- Tension
- Character of pulse
- Radio femoral/Radio radial delay
- Pulse apex deficit
- Condition of vessel wall
- Other arterial pulsations

absent, check the pulsations of bigger arteries like brachial, femoral, and carotid. The radial pulsations may be feeble or absent when the patient is in shock. The femoral pulsations may be diminished in coarctation of the aorta. The upper limb pulsations may be weak or absent in Takayasu arteritis. Radial pulsations may be difficult to palpate or may not be palpable in an obese child and in those with radial artery located behind radius bone or an aberrant pathway of the vessel.

- *Pulse rate:* Pulse rate should be counted when the child is relaxed and comfortable. In an irritable or crying child, pulse rate may be high which should not be mistaken for tachycardia. The pulse should be counted for a complete minute. In an emergency situation, count the pulse for 6 seconds and multiply it by 10 to get the pulse rate per minute. The average pulse rate for different age groups is given in **Table 2**. The tachycardia and bradycardia should be defined as per age of the child **(Table 3)**.

    In conditions like irritable, excessive crying child, fever, and thyrotoxicosis, there may be tachycardia. The pulse rate increases by 10 for each degree of rise in body temperature. If it is not proportionate, it is called as relative bradycardia. The relative bradycardia is seen in enteric fever and brucellosis. Relative bradycardia in enteric fever is not common in young children, it may be seen in older children and adults. The sleeping tachycardia is considered as pathognomic sign of rheumatic fever. Tachycardia may be the early sign of poor perfusion or shock. Common causes of bradycardia are outlined in **Box 6**.

- *Rhythm:* Assess the rhythm of the pulse. The pulse may vary with respiration (sinus tachycardia: heart rate increases with inspiration, sinus bradycardia: heart rate decreases with expiration),

Table 3: Cut off values of resting pulse rate for tachycardia and bradycardia for different age groups.

	Tachycardia	Bradycardia
Newborn	>160	<100
<2 years	>120	<90
In older children	>100	<60

> **Box 6:** Common causes of bradycardia.
> - Physiological (Athlete, Familial)
> - Hypothyroidism (Decreased BMR)
> - Jaundice (Deposition of bile salts and bile pigments at SA node)
> - Raised intracranial pressure (Vagal stimulation)
> - Heart block
> - Drugs (Propranolol, digitalis)
>
> (BMR: basal metabolic rate; SA: sino atrial)

which is called as physiological arrhythmia. If the pulse is irregular, try to define its pattern, atrial fibrillation, atrial flutter, extrasystoles or missed beats.

- *Volume:* The uplifting of middle finger (thrust) measures the pulse volume. Low volume pulse is observed in shock, aortic stenosis, cardiomyopathy, and vasculitis. High volume pulse is present in conditions with hyperdynamic circulation like anemia, thyrotoxicosis, high grade fever, etc. It is also found is aortic regurgitation (AR), mitral regurgitation (MR), PDA, hypertension, arteriovenous fistula, etc.
- *Force:* The pressure required to feel the arterial pulsation is called force. It indicates systolic BP.
- *Tension:* The pressure required to obliterate the pulsations is called tension. It indicates diastolic BP. The proximal finger is pressed to obliterate radial pulsations felt by middle finger. The distal finger is pressed to prevent the pulsations from ulnar artery being conducted into the radial artery through palmar arch.
- *Radiofemoral delay:* Feel the radial and femoral pulsations simultaneously, they are felt together. If not, it is called as radiofemoral delay. It indicates presence of coarctation or aorta.
- *Radio radial delay:* Feel both radial arteries at the same time **(Fig. 1)**, if there is delay in left radial arterial pulsations, it indicates preductal coarctation of aorta.
- *Pulse apex deficit:* Presence of a disparity of 10 or more between auscultated heart rate and the palpated radial arterial pulse rate, both estimated at the same time for a full one minute, is called as pulse apex deficit. Atrial fibrillation, ventricular premature beats like conditions manifest with pulse apex deficit.

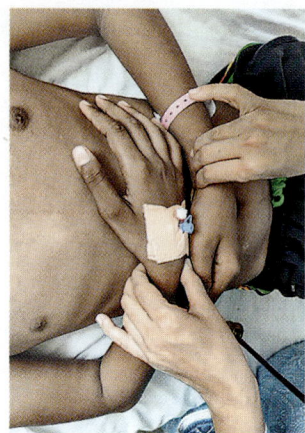

Fig. 1: Method of palpation of radial artery both sides simultaneously for inequality and radio radial delay.

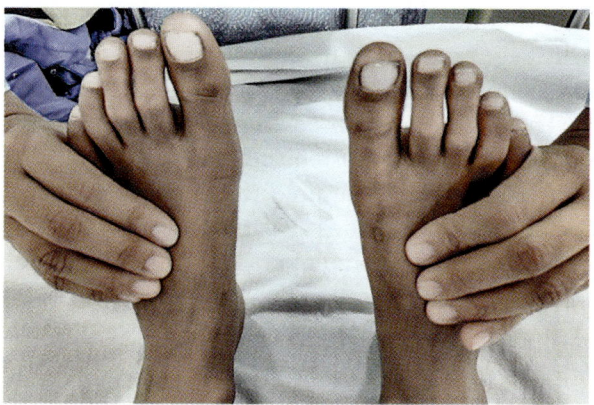

Fig. 2: Method of palpation of dorsalis pedis, both sides simultaneously.

- *Condition of vessel wall:* Vessel wall is normal in children. It is thickened in old age people due to atherosclerosis.
- *Other peripheral pulsations:* Other peripheral pulsations to be examined are carotids, temporal, brachial, axillary, femorals, popliteals, posterior tibials, dorsalis pedis, etc. On examination of dorsalis pedis pulsations both sides simultaneously **(Fig. 2)**, if one side pulsations are delayed, weak or absent, it indicates pathology on that side.

- *Abnormal pulses:*
  - *Pulsus alternans:* Pulsus alternans is defined as the strong (high volume) pulse alternating with weak (low volume) pulse in the presence of normal rhythm. It is found with left ventricular failure and myocarditis.
  - *Pulsus bigeminus:* Pulsus bigeminus refers to regular premature ventricular ectopics occurring alternately after every normal beat. The normal beat is stronger and immediately after ectopic beat which is weaker. This may be misinterpreted as pulsus alternans. But a longer interval (compensatory pause) between them is the characteristic of pulsus bigeminus.
  - *Pulsus trigeminy:* Coupling of three beats due to ectopic ventricular premature beat after two normal beats is called as pulsus trigeminy.
  - *Bisferiens pulse:* This high volume pulse has two palpable impulses in the rapidly rising systolic upstroke, the later second impulse occurs at the peak of the upstroke (tidal wave). It is well appreciated over the carotids. Bisferiens pulse is the characteristic of AR or AR with aortic stenosis (AS) or hypertrophic obstructive cardiomyopathy (HOCM).
  - *Bounding (hyperkinetic) pulse:* Bounding pulse is characterized by high amplitude, large volume pulse with rapidly rising ascending wave. It is present in conditions with high cardiac output with decreased peripheral arterial resistance and wide pulse pressure, e.g., anxiety, exercise, fever, anemia, thyrotoxicosis, beriberi, arteriovenous fistula, AR, VSD, PDA, etc.
  - *Water hammer (collapsing) pulse:* A large volume pulse with abrupt and rapid upstroke followed by equal downstroke due to the rapid and reverse diastolic run off into the left ventricle in AR, PDA, etc., and rapid run off to the peripheral vessels due to decreased systemic peripheral vascular resistance in hyperkinetic states like anemia, fever, pregnancy, thyrotoxicosis, etc.

    Method of elicitation of collapsing pulse **(Fig. 3)**:
    - Feel the radial pulse of the child.

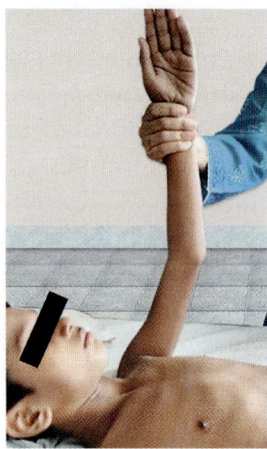

Fig. 3: Examining for water hammer (collapsing) pulse. The arm of the patient is grasped at wrist so that radial pulse is barely palpable. When his arm is uplifted suddenly beyond the plane of the body, radial pulse becomes readily palpable if it is collapsing in character.

- Encircle the arm in right hand just proximal to wrist so that radial pulse is still felt by your palmar surface of gripping hand.
- Encircle the proximal part of the child's forearm with your left hand so as to feel easily transmitted pulsations of brachial artery over the brachioradialis muscle.
- Suddenly elevate the child's arm ventrically above his shoulder.
- You will feel the thump of the water hammer (a famous English toy) collapsing radial pulse on the palmar grip of your right hand and the transmitted impact of the brachial artery pulse across the brachioradialis on your left hand.
- *Hypokinetic pulse:* It is characterized by weak, small volume pulse felt with difficulty. It is found in conditions with low cardiac output, shock, severe cardiac failure, myocarditis, coarctation of aorta, cardiac tamponade, etc.
- *Pulsus tardus:* It is slow rising pulse with a late peak close to the S2, seen in severe cardiac failure.
- *Anacrotic pulse:* It refers to a slow rising, percussion wave with late peaking, small volume radial pulse. It is diagnostic of aortic stenosis and severe mitral stenosis.

> **Box 7:** Causes of pulsus paradoxus.
> - *Cardiac:*
>   - Cardiac tamponade
>   - Pericardial effusion
>   - Constrictive pericarditis
> - *Pulmonary:*
>   - Acute severe bronchial asthma

- *Pulsus paradoxus:* The term pulsus paradoxus is a misnomer as it represents an exaggeration of a normal phenomenon. There is marginal physiologic decrease in systolic BP during inspiration, from 5 to 10 mm Hg. Pulsus paradoxus is defined as difference of BP more than 10 mm Hg taken during expiration and inspiration. Often, this difference is more than 20 mm Hg. The common causes of pulsus paradoxus are listed in **Box 7**.

Arterial Blood Pressure

Blood pressure is defined as the lateral pressure exerted on the vessel wall by the blood, while flowing through it. The systolic BP is chiefly determined by the force of contraction of the left ventricle. The diastolic BP is regulated by the arteriolar resistance. BP should be measured routinely as a part of the physical examination of children. Every child over the age of 3 years should have his BP measured once a year and during every visit to the doctor during adolescence. The BP should be measured in all the four limbs.

Measurement of Blood Pressure

There are four methods by which BP can be measured:
1. Sphygmomanometer method
2. Flush method (mainly for newborns)
3. Oscillometer method
4. Doppler method.

Sphygmomanometer method:
- *Prerequisites:* It is a conventional method. In routine daily practice, the BP is measured in the upper arm (brachial artery).

The child should be lying comfortably in bed or sitting with arm kept at the level of heart. The appropriate size of cuff which should cover two-thirds of upper arm (or width of the cuff should be 40% of the circumference of the arm) should be used. The recommended cuff size in infants below age of 1 year is 2.5 cm, 1–4 years is 5 cm, 5–9 years is 9 cm, and over 10 years is 13 cm. The use of a narrow BP cuff is associated with high systolic BP reading and vice versa. The cuff is applied snugly over the upper arm by keeping its lower edge at least 2 cm above the cubital fossa. The manometer should be kept at the level of heart and should be conveniently placed easy to see it.

- **Method of measuring BP:**
    - Palpatory method: Inflate the pressure cuff while palpating the brachial pulse. The reading at which brachial pulse disappears is suggesting systolic BP.
    - Auscultatory method: Inflate the cuff 20–30 mm Hg above the reading of palpatory method and then listen through the diaphragm of stethoscope placed over the brachial artery. Deflate the cuff slowly by decrements of 2–3 mm Hg and the point when Korotkoff sounds are first heard is indicating systolic BP. When the cuff is further deflated, the Korotkoff sounds become muffled and finally disappear which indicates diastolic BP. Sometimes, the Korotkoff sound does not disappear and in that case muffling of sounds is taken as criterion for diastolic BP.

For recording lower limb BP, the child is asked to lie in prone position. The cuff is applied over the thigh and stethoscope is placed over the popliteal artery in the popliteal fossa. Normally, the lower limb systolic BP is more by 10–30 mm Hg while the diastolic BP is identical in upper and lower limbs. The pulse pressure is the difference between the systolic and diastolic BP and is indicative of pulse volume. Ideally, BP should be measured in all the four limbs, especially when coarctation of aorta or Takayasu disease is suspected.

Flush method: The limb should be raised and squeezed till the hand or foot becomes pale. The cuff should be rapidly inflated so that blanching is noted. The pressure should be gradually and slowly released by 5 mm holding for about 5 seconds at each step.

The point at which the flushing of the hand or foot is seen represents the systolic pressure which is about 5 mm Hg less than that obtained by the auscultatory method. The diastolic pressure cannot be recorded by this technique. Flush pressure is not affected by the cuff size to any great degree. Flush method is mainly used in newborns.

Oscillometer method: When the pressure in the cuff is released, the point at which the oscillometer needle begins to flick regularly is the systolic BP and the point where the oscillations are maximal denotes the diastolic pressure.

Doppler method: This is the most reliable method. The baby is made to lie in supine position and an approximate sized cuff is fitted around the arm. The probe of the ultrasonic Doppler is placed over the radial artery at an angle of 15°. The exact position of the radial artery is located by listening to the hissing sound through the headphone attached to the Doppler cuff which is inflated quickly till the hissing sound ceases. Then the pressure is gradually released and the point at which the hissing sound reappears corresponds to the systolic pressure. Diastolic pressure cannot be recorded by this method.

Normally, standing pressure is higher than supine pressure. The difference between the leg and arm BP is normally 10–15 mm Hg. In children both diastolic and systolic BP increase with emotional tension. Most children have high BP in the late afternoon or evening than in the morning.

Blood pressure varies with the age of the child and is closely related to height and weight **(Table 2)**. Significant increases occur during adolescence. Serial measurements should always be obtained in the evaluation of the patient with hypertension.

Congestive Heart Failure

In younger children rather than obvious edema over dependent parts, there is excessive weight gain. Mother may complain that clothes of the child are no longer fit, their fitting has become very tight within a short time. Older children will present with both periorbital and pedal edema **(Figs. 4A and B)**. Other manifestations of CHF are dyspnea, cough, decreased urine output, tender liver, prominent neck veins, splenomegaly, etc. **(Box 8)**.

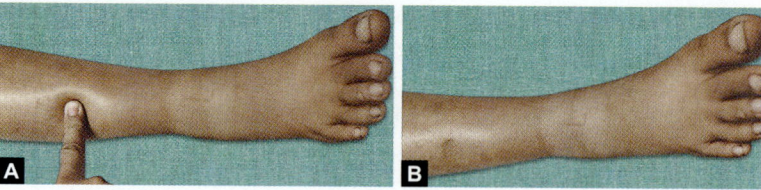

Figs. 4A and B: Demonstration of pedal edema. It should be pressed over shin of tibia or malleolus for 30 seconds and see for pitting impression.

> **Box 8:** Signs and symptoms of congestive heart failure.
> - Sudden or insidious onset of increasing breathlessness, dyspnea, orthopnea
> - Decreased exercise intolerance
> - Easy fatigability
> - Cough, especially in lying down position
> - Wheezing
> - Feeding difficulties (Prolonged time, suck–rest–suck cycle)
> - Excessive sweating
> - Facial puffiness, edema
> - Decreased urine output
> - Cold extremities
> - Right quadrant abdominal pain (Hepatic congestion)
> - Prominent neck veins

Cyanosis

Mild cyanosis may be difficult for early detection and clubbing of the fingers and toes is not usually manifested till late in the first year of life, even in the presence of severe arterial oxygen desaturation. Cyanosis is best observed over the nail beds, lips, tongue, and mucous membranes. Cyanosis can be of two types, peripheral and central. Acrocyanosis common in newborns due to cold which disappears with proper wrapping them or making the room warm. Hypoglycemia can also cause cyanosis. Severe respiratory conditions like bronchial asthma and bronchiolitis can also cause cyanosis which decreases or disappears on correction of hypoxia. Cyanosis due to cardiac cause can be uniform or differential. Uniform cyanosis means that the right to left shunt is taking place at atrial, ventricular or the ascending aorta level. Differential cyanosis indicates that there is right to left shunt through the PDA. The blood flow from the pulmonary artery to the aorta through

PDA goes down in the descending aorta. It is possible only if there is severe pulmonary arterial hypertension (PAH). The majority of patients will have pink fingers with blue toes indicating that great arteries are normally connected to the respective ventricles. If the fingers are blue but the toes are pink or less blue (reversed differential cyanosis), the diagnosis would be complete transposition of great arteries since the pulmonary artery in the complete transposition carries more oxygenated blood than the aorta, connected to the right ventricle. The two components which result in differential cyanosis are PAH causing a right to left shunt and the PDA which results in blood with a lower saturation (normal great vessels) or higher saturation (transposed great vessels) reaching the toes.

Hepatomegaly

Examination of liver is important as part of CVS examination. Enlarged and tender liver is seen in a case of right heart failure.

Jugular Venous Pressure

Jugular venous pressure (JVP) is an indirect measurement of central venous pressure (CVP). It reflects the right atrial pressure. It is measured as the vertical height from the sternal angle to the pulsations in the internal jugular vein. In infants and young children, it is difficult to measure the JVP due to their short necks.
- Methods of measuring JVP (**Fig. 5**):
    - The child should be in supine in a reclining posture on examination cot.
    - Elevate the head and shoulders at an angle of 45° with the help of a backrest.
    - Keep the neck slightly extended and to the left making sure that the neck muscles are not contracted.
    - The sternal angle is located. Identify internal jugular venous pulsations seen in between two heads of the sternocleidomastoid muscle.
    - Measure the vertical height in centimeter by keeping a scale horizontally projected from the topmost point of JVP to a measuring centimeter ruler or scale kept vertically at the level of sternal angle.

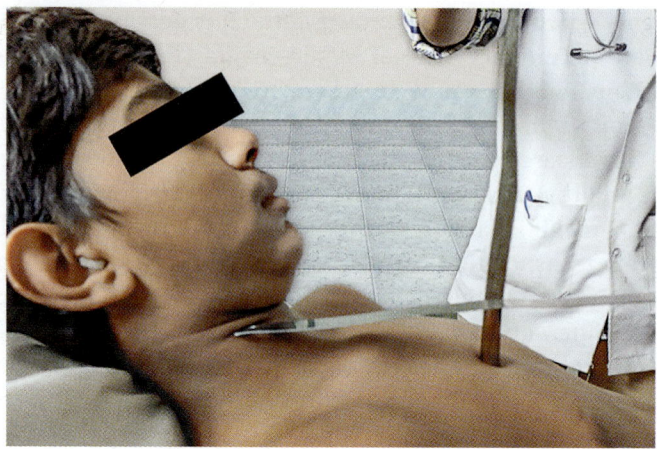

Fig. 5: Method for evaluating jugular venous pressure (JVP). The patient is made to lie in supine position with the head end propped up at 45°, head turned away to the opposite side and neck relaxed. The sternal angle is taken as the zero point and the maximum height of pulsations in the internal jugular is measured with two plastic rulers as shown in photograph. The vertical distance from sternal angle to the imaginary line drawn from the upper end of jugular venous column gives JVP which is measured in centimeters.

> **Box 9:** Causes of raised jugular venous pressure.
> - Right heart failure
> - Pericardial effusion
> - Fluid overload
> - Superior vena cava obstruction
> - Tricuspid stenosis or regurgitation

- JVP more than 3 cm from the sternal angle is considered as abnormal.
- Add 5 cm to this reading to get the CVP, as the center of the right atrium is 5 cm below the sternal angle.
- Raised JVP indicates systemic venous congestion and causes are shown in **Box 9**.

Hepatojugular Reflux

The liver (right hypochondrial area) should be pressed for 30 seconds and simultaneously looked for JVP. There may be transient rise in JVP up to 3 cm normally. If the rise is more than 3 cm or if the rise is more than 15 seconds, the hepatojugular reflux is said to be positive. It is seen in right heart failure and tricuspid regurgitation.

Venous Pulsations

Inspection of the jugular veins may provide considerable information. Still, due to short neck and deposition of fat around the neck, examination of jugular venous pulsations is not practical in infants and young children. It should be carried out in older children.

The patient should be propped up in bed at an angle of about 45° with the neck muscles relaxed. Distension and pulsation of veins situated above the sternal angle are abnormal. Increased venous pressure transmitted to the internal jugular vein may appear as venous pulsations without visible distension. Such pulsations do not occur in normal children reclining at an angle of 45°.

Venous pulsations can be differentiated from those of arteries:
- Venous pulsations vary with the position of the patient and usually have multiple components whereas those of the carotid artery are single, abrupt, and do not vary with the patient's position.
- Abdominal pressure, especially over the right hypochondrium, increases the height of venous pulse, but has no effect on carotid pulsations.
- Mild compression of the external jugular vein in the supraclavicular fossa will abolish venous pulsations, but will not affect carotid pulsation.
- The height of venous pulsation increases with expiration and decreases with inspiration, arterial pulsations are not affected by respiration.

The venous pulse has three positive waves a, c, and v and two negative waves or descents, x and y. The "a" wave is due to atrial contraction (atrial systole). This is followed by the "x" descent, which is interrupted by a small "c" wave. The "c" wave coincidences with the onset of ventricular systole and results from the movement of the tricuspid valve ring into the right atrium as the right ventricular pressure rises. The "v" wave indicates a passive rise in pressure as venous return to the atrium continues during ventricular systole while the tricuspid valve is closed. When the tricuspid valve opens, blood enters the right ventricle rapidly and there is consequently a lowering of the right atrial pressure the "y" descent.

Since the great veins are in direct communication with the right atrium, the changes of pressure and volumes of this chamber are transmitted to the veins, e.g., in CCF, the increased right atrial pressure is transmitted to the neck veins. In tricuspid insufficiency, some of the right ventricular systolic pressure is transmitted to the right atrium and results in large, conspicuous venous pulsations, which correspond to ventricular systole and produce a fusion of the "c" and "v" waves. In complete heart block, if the right atrium contracts when the tricuspid valve is closed, "a" large venous pulsations will occur. In superior vena cava obstruction the JVP is increased, but the veins do not pulsate.

Splenomegaly

Splenomegaly may occur due to bacterial endocarditis.

Skin and Joints

Look for subcutaneous nodules **(Fig. 6)**, erythema marginatum, chorea, and joint swelling suggestive of rheumatic activity.

Clubbing

Apart from noncardiac causes, clubbing is seen in cyanotic CHDs. Presence of cyanosis, conjunctival injection, and clubbing indicates a long duration of the condition. Clubbing is also seen in a case of bacterial endocarditis. Other clinical features of bacterial endocarditis are shown in **Box 10**.

Fundus Examination

Roth spots (flame-shaped hemorrhages with cotton wool pale center) may be seen in children with bacterial endocarditis. Dancing retinal vessels are characteristics of AR and PDA.

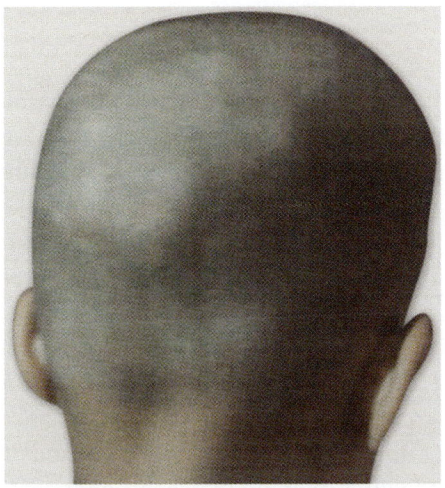

Fig. 6: Subcutaneous nodules over occipital region in a case of rheumatic fever.

> **Box 10:** Signs and symptoms of infective endocarditis.
> - Fever
> - Pallor
> - Clubbing
> - Palmar erythema
> - Hepatosplenomegaly
> - *Janeway lesions:* Nontender nodular lesions over palms and soles
> - *Osler nodes:* Painful, tender, erythematous nodules or swelling at the palmar surface of pads of fingers and toes
> - Splinter hemorrhage in the nails
> - *Roth spots:* Oval, flame-shaped hemorrhage in fundus
> - *Neurological deficits:* Due to embolic phenomenon

EXAMINATION OF CARDIOVASCULAR SYSTEM

It is customary to examine the cardiovascular system in the order of inspection, palpation, percussion, and auscultation, but it is often necessary to auscultate first when the child is calm or sleeping because once the child cries excessively or becomes irritable, it is difficult to decide auscultatory findings. Therefore, the most valuable information must be taken as a priority to be completed but the clinical presentation should always follow sequential pattern.

Inspection

- *Precordium:*
  - Precordium is the area of anterior chest wall overlying the heart. Precordium should be inspected tangentially from the foot end of the bed while the child is in supine position.
  - Look for symmetry and shape of chest wall, pectus carinatum, pectus excavatum, Harrison sulcus, apical impulse, and pulsations in different regions like left parasternal region, epigastric area, suprasternal and neck.
  - In the absence of pleural or pulmonary conditions or skeletal anomalies, precordial bulge indicates chronic cardiac condition.
  - The location of apical impulse is noted if visible. With cardiomegaly, it may be displaced downward and laterally if the left ventricle is enlarged and only laterally if the right ventricle is enlarged. It may not be seen in an obese patient or if the apical impulse is located behind a rib.
  - Increased precordial activity (hyperdynamic cardiac impulse) can be visible in a case of cardiac enlargement due to volume overload like large left to right shunt (VSD, PDA), severe valvular regurgitation (AR, MR), severe anemia, etc. It may be normal in a thin patient.
- Pulsations (of enlarged collateral vessels) may be seen on the back in the region around the scapulae in older children with severe coarctation of aorta.
- Tracheal shift points to mediastinal shift as the cause of displaced cardiac impulse.
- Any scar (post thoracotomy of poststernotomy), swelling or sinus to be looked for.

Palpation

The objectives of palpation over the precordium are to localize, characterize, record, and interpret the characteristics of apical impulse, point of maximal impulse (apex beat), precordial pulsations over different areas, heaves and thrusts, palpable sounds, and thrills.

> **Box 11:** Cardiac palpation.
> - Apex beat
> - Precordial pulsations
> - Heaves and thrusts
> - Palpable heart sounds
> - Thrills

Palpate routinely and symmetrically all the specified areas of palpation over precordium and adjacent areas like apex, mitral area, aortic area, pulmonary area, tricuspid area, left parasternal region, right parasternal region, suprasternal notch, epigastric area, right and left supraclavicular areas, and over carotid arteries **(Box 11)**.

Apex Beat

- *Definition of apex beat:* It is the lowermost and outermost point of cardiac impulse imparting a perpendicular thrust to the palpating finger.
- *Method of palpation of apex beat* **(Figs. 7A to C)**:
    - Put the palm over the precordium and try to locate the position of heart and cardiac impulse.
    - Putting the finger in intercostal spaces with cardiac impulse, try to locate the intercostal space with maximum intensity of cardiac impulse.
    - Put the tip of the finger perpendicularly at the point with maximum thrust. It is the apex beat.
    - Count the intercostal spaces from 2nd intercostal space (corresponding to sterna angle) to downward and decide intercostal space in which apex beat is located.
    - Apex beat is described in relation to midclavicular line or anterior and midaxillary lines (in case of cardiomegaly).
- If apex beat is not found in supine position, it should be sought with left lateral position of the child or in a sitting posture. The nipple is a variable anatomical landmark and therefore, apex beat should not be described in reference to location of nipple.
- The normal position of the apex beat is age-dependent in children. In infancy, it is in the 3rd intercostal space.

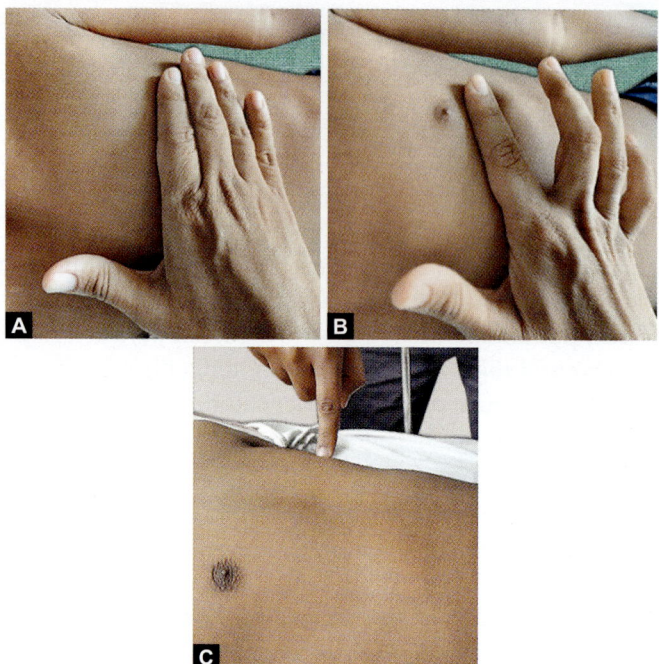

Figs. 7A to C: Method of palpation of apex beat. Note the three steps. (A) First put the palm over precordium and try to locate the position of heart and cardiac impulse; (B) Secondly, try to locate the intercostals space with maximum intensity of cardiac impulse; (C) Finally, put the tip of finger perpendicularly at the point of maximum thrust. It is the apex beat.

In the 3–4 years of age, apex beat is located in the 4th intercostal space just lateral to midclavicular line. Between 4 and 8 years, it is in the 5th intercostal space in the midclavicular line and beyond the age of 8 years, it is palpable in the 5th intercostal space about 1 cm medial to midclavicular line.
- Apex beat is normally well localized.
- If it is not found on the left side, it should be checked for on the right side.
- The right-sided apex beat may signify dextrocardia or left-sided thoracic space occupying conditions like congenital diaphragmatic hernia. The right-sided apex beat may be due to pulmonary conditions, pushing the mediastinum on the opposite side (pleural effusion or pneumothorax on left side) or pulling the mediastinum on same side (collapse of lung on right side).

- The apex beat may be displaced laterally and downward in left ventricular enlargement and only laterally in right ventricular enlargement.
- *Type of apex beat:*
    - Hyperdynamic: The apex beat is forceful, very rapid and normal in duration. Hyperdynamic apex beat is produced by ventricular volume overload conditions like VSD, PDA, AR, and MR. It is also produced by high cardiac output states like anemia, pregnancy, and beriberi.
    - Heaving: It is a forceful, broad, and well-sustained apex beat. In this apex beat, the palpating finger is elevated and remains so for some time. It is the characteristic of left ventricular hypertrophy due to pressure overload lesions like aortic stenosis, coarctation of aorta, systemic hypertension etc.
    - Tapping: It is forceful, sharp, and not sustained. It is the characteristic of right ventricular hypertrophy (e.g., rheumatic mitral stenosis).

Left Parasternal Heaving (Fig. 8)

It is best felt by placing the ulnar border of the examiner's palm vertically on the left sternal border in supine position of the patient. It should be assessed for its force and duration and can be graded as shown in **Box 12**. Left parasternal heaving is felt in a case of right ventricular hypertrophy in conditions like pulmonary stenosis or pulmonary hypertension.

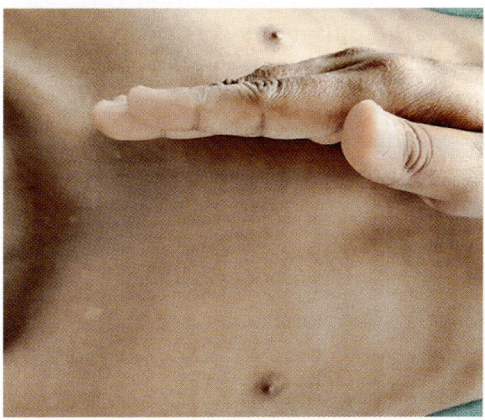

Fig. 8: Palpation for parasternal heave. It is best felt by placing the ulnar border of examiner's palm vertically on the left sternal border in supine position of the patient.

> **Box 12:** Grading of left parasternal heaving.
> - *Grade I:* Just touches hand
> - *Grade II:* Palpable but compressible
> - *Grade III:* Palpable but not compressible

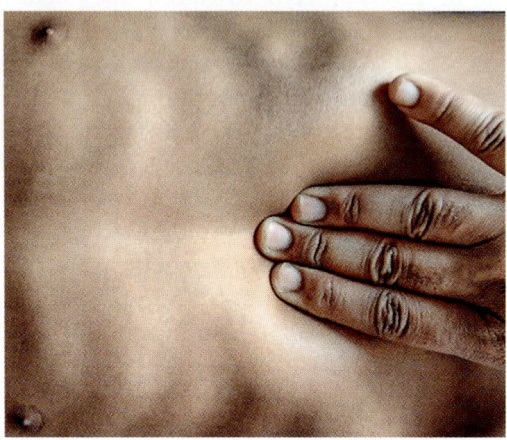

Fig. 9: Palpation for epigastric pulsations, by gentle palpation in subxiphoid region with pad of fingers of right hand.

Epigastric Pulsations

The pulsations in epigastric region can be felt by gentle palpation in subxiphoid region with the pad of fingers of right hand with mild upward slant toward xiphisternum **(Fig. 9)**. Another way to look for epigastric pulsations is to gently press the thumb in the epigastric notch, the pulsations from an enlarged right ventricle are appreciated at the tip, whereas aortic pulsations are felt at the pulp. The presence of epigastric pulsations are suggestive of right ventricular volume overload states such as ASD and tricuspid regurgitation.

Pulsations in 2nd Left Intercostal Space

The second heart sound may become palpable in pulmonary hypertension. This may suggest a dilated pulmonary artery in conditions like ASD, VSD, and PDA. The pulsations are best appreciated by pulp of palpating finger.

Suprasternal Pulsations

Suprasternal pulsations are often seen and are palpable in suprasternal notch. They are commonly palpable in conditions like AR, PDA, and coarctation of aorta **(Fig. 10)**.

Thrills

Thrills are palpable vibrations associated with cardiac murmurs (palpable murmurs):
- The timing and localization of thrills should be attentively noted. The timing can be decided by presence of thrills and simultaneous palpation of apex beat or carotid pulse.
- A thrill is best appreciated by palpating without stretched palm with heads of the metacarpal bones lying directly over the area of interest. The systolic thrill of VSD is best felt at lower sternal border and that of severe MR at apical region.
- A diastolic thrill at the apex is palpable in mitral stenosis.
- A thrill of aortic stenosis is felt in second intercostals space on right side and that of pulmonary stenosis to the left.
- The thrill of aortic stenosis is also palpable in suprasternal notch and over carotid arteries in the neck.
- If a thrill is palpable, then the grade of the murmur would be more than 4/6.

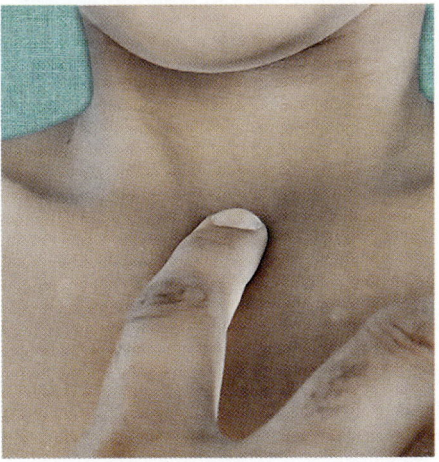

Fig. 10: Palpation of suprasternal pulsations.

Percussion

It has a limited clinical utility and is used to outline cardiac borders and to assess the cardiac size.

- *Define the right cardiac border:*
  - Locate the sternal angle (angle of Louis), a bony prominency (junction of manubrium and body of sternum) in the midline just below the sternal notch **(Figs. 11A to C)**. The corresponding intercostal space to the sternal angle on right side is the 2nd intercostal space.
  - Start percussing from right 2nd intercostal space downward at midclavicular line till you reach the area of dullness (usually felt in the 5th intercostal space). The intercostal space with dullness indicates upper border of liver.

    This step also helps to recognize dextrocardia with or without situs inversus.

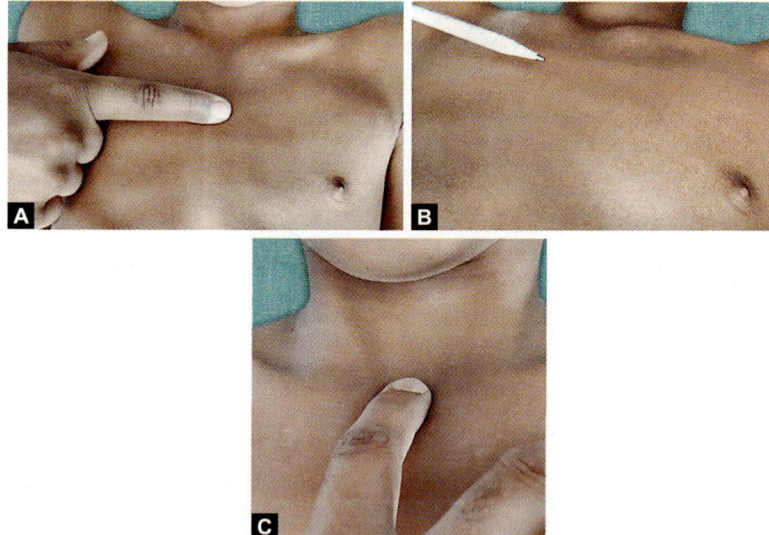

Figs. 11A to C: Identification of sternal angle (angle of Louis) (Ludwig's angle). Transverse bony ridge is felt at the junction of the body of sternum and manubrium sterni, while traversing down from sternal notch. It is sternal angle, very important anatomical landmark.

- After defining upper border of liver, start one space above it, from lateral to medial toward the sternal border, again from resonant to dull note, indicates right cardiac border. Continue to percuss from down to upward and define dull note in all the spaces, defines the right cardiac border.
  The dullness of the right cardiac border does not usually extend beyond the right sternal border, it is behind the sternum. Therefore, dull note of right cardiac border beyond right sternal border indicates cardiac enlargement, usually right atrial enlargement.
- *Define the left cardiac border:*
  - Define the apex beat
  - Start to percuss one space below the apex beat, being lowermost and outermost point of cardiac impulse, no cardiac dullness is expected beyond apex beat, if at all it is, likely due to pericardial effusion. Not to miss pericardial effusion, one space below the apex beat, percussion is started. The art of percussion was devised before era of modern technology, echo study of heart. This an art of clinical examination!
  - From lateral to medial (resonant to dull note), below upward, percussion is performed and point of cardiac border is defined in each intercostal space. Join the points and its left cardiac border.

Interpretations of Percussion Findings

- Extension of dullness beyond the right sternal border indicates right atrial enlargement (ASD, Ebstein anomaly), pericardial effusion, dilated cardiomyopathy, dextrocardia, etc.
- Cardiac dullness beyond the apex beat indicates pericardial effusion.
- Dullness >2.5 cm beyond the left sternal border in the 2nd left intercostal space indicates pulmonary artery dilatation, pulmonary hypertension, pericardial effusion, mediastinal mass, etc.
- Dullness over right 2nd intercostal space may be due to aortic aneurysm, pericardial effusion, mediastinal mass (thymus), etc.

Auscultation

Prerequisites for Good Quality Auscultation

- Stethoscope:
  - Select a good quality stethoscope
  - A two-piece stethoscope with a bell (minimum diameter 2.5 cm) and a diaphragm is desirable
  - Ensure snugly and comfortably fitting ear knobs
  - The angle of ear pieces should be oriented forward and directed toward the external auditory meatus and canals
  - Good quality, thick-walled, weather proof, 25–30 cm (10 to 12 inches) long tubes
  - The diaphragm when tightly applied over the precordium, it filters out the low pitched audible sounds and helps to appreciate selective events of high frequencies, e.g., S2 ejection and midsystolic clicks and soft but high pitched early diastolic murmur of AR, pericardial friction rub, etc.
  - The bell must be applied lightly to listen low frequency heart events like S3 and S4 gallops, mid diastolic rumble of mitral stenosis.
  - The room should be quiet, without noise from fans and air conditioners.
  - The examiner should be unbiased and tension free. His attitude, concentration, focus, practice, training, ready to learn, etc. count a lot for deriving meaningful auscultatory findings.

Steps in Cardiac Auscultation

- Start auscultation from mitral area (apical region) either in sitting position or in supine position. The child may be little turned to the left side.
- From mitral area, move your stethoscope internally inch by inch and at every point auscultate in a same manner.
- Then, proceed to tricuspid area, then upward along the left parasternal margin to pulmonary area.
- Proceed to aortic areas and both carotids in the neck.
- Timing of cardiac events may be decided in relation to carotid artery pulsations or apical impulse by simultaneous palpation.

Areas of Auscultation (Table 4)

- *Apex:* Mitral area
- *Pulmonary area:* 2nd left intercostal space near the left sternal border
- *Aortic area:* 2nd right intercostal space near right sternal border
- *Second aortic area (Erb's area):* 3rd left intercostal space near the left sternal border
- *Tricuspid area:* 4th and 5th intercostal spaces at the lateral end of the left sternal border
- Left and right infraclavicular areas
- Over both carotid arteries in the neck
- Over interscapular regions for collateral murmurs
- Over femorals, brachials, popliteals for pistol shot sounds, Duroziez murmur in AR and peripheral AV malformations
- Cranium, fontanelle, and both lumbar regions.

First heart sound (S1) **(Fig. 12, Table 5)**:
- S1 is louder if diastole is shortened because of tachycardia. It is louder in ASD, mitral stenosis, short PR interval, etc.
- The loud S1 in mitral stenosis indicates that the valve is still pliable.
- A soft S1 may be due to poor conduction through a thick chest wall (obesity), long PR interval or imperfect closure of the valve, as in MR. S1 is soft when the anterior mitral leaflet is immobile because of rigidity and calcification, even in the presence of predominant mitral stenosis.

Table 4: Areas for cardiac auscultation.

Area	Anatomical localization
Mitral area (Apex)	Fourth and fifth left intercostal spaces at midclavicular line
Pulmonary area	Second left intercostal space close to sternum
Aortic area	Second right intercostal space close to sternum
Second aortic area (Erb's area)	Third left intercostal space near left sternal border
Tricuspid area	Fourth and fifth left intercostal spaces just lateral to lower end of sternum

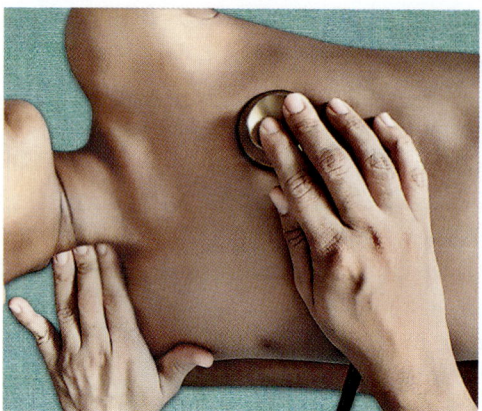

Fig. 12: Auscultation of S1 by timing with carotid pulsations.

Second heart sound (S2) **(Table 5 and Box 13)**:
- Paradoxical or reserved spitting occurs when the aortic valve closes later than the pulmonary valve, like severe aortic stenosis, left bundle branch block, etc.
- The split of S2 is said to be fixed when A-P2 interval does not vary with respiration. Wide and fixed splitting of S2 is characteristic of ASD.
  As the patients with large ASD, receive the blood from left atrium across ASD as well as normal systemic venous return, right atrial inflow remains relatively constant during inspiration and expiration. Therefore, the volume and duration of right ventricular ejection are not significantly increased by inspiration and there is no appreciable inspiratory exaggeration of the splitting of S2. This phenomenon of fixed splitting of the second heart sound is of great clinical value in a case of ASD.
- Loud P2 is characteristic of pulmonary hypertension.

Third heart sound (S3):
- S3 is frequently heard in normal children and patients with high cardiac output.
- In a patient with clinical signs of cardiac failure and tachycardia, presence of S3 is pathological and may be identified as a "gallop". It indicates impairment of ventricular function like myocarditis, cardiomyopathy, AR, MR, etc.

The Cardiovascular System

Table 5: Abnormal heart sounds: mechanism of production and significance.

Sound/Timing	Abnormality	Features and location	Mechanism	Significance
S1	Loud	Best heard mitral area (apex)	Sudden closure of mitral valve	Mitral stenosis
Systole	Ejection click	• Sharp sound, appearing immediately after S1 • Best heard at the base	Delayed opening of semilunar valves	Aortic or pulmonary stenosis with mobile valves
	Mid systolic click	• Late in onset • Best heard at mitral area	Mitral valve prolapsed into atrium	Mitral valve prolapsed
S2	Loud	Best heard at the base	Abrupt closer of semilunar valves	• Systemic hypertension • Pulmonary hypertension
	Split	Best heard at the base	Asynchronous closure of aortic and pulmonary valves	• Wide fixed splitting (ASD, RBBB) • Narrow split (Pulmonary hypertension, AS) • Paradoxically split S2 (AS, LBBB)
Diastole	Opening snap	• Sharp sound appears before first heart sound • Best heard at apex in expiration	Sudden opening of an abnormal mitral valve	Mitral stenosis with mobile valve
	3rd heart sound	• Occurs shortly after S2 • Best heat at left parasternal area or at mitral area	Diastolic distention of diseased myocardium	• May be heard in normal children • Right or left cardiac failure
	4th heart sound	• Occurs before S1 • Best heard in left parasternal area	Forceful atrial contraction against raised ventricular pressure	Left or right ventricular failure

(ASD: atrial septal defect; LBBB: left bundle branch block; RBBB: right bundle branch block)

> **Box 13:** Clinical significance of abnormal S2.
> - Increased intensity (loud) of P2 (Pulmonary hypertension)
> - Decreased intensity of P2 (TOF, severe PS, pulmonary atresia)
> - Widely split and fixed S2 (ASD)
> - Narrow split S2 (Pulmonary hypertension)
> - Single S2 (TOF, severe PS, severe aortic stenosis)
> - Paradoxically split S2 (Severe aortic stenosis, LBBB)
>
> (ASD: atrial septal defect; LBBB: left bundle branch block; PS: pulmonary stenosis; TOF: tetralogy of Fallot)

- S3 in cases of large VSD and severe MR is best heard with the bell of stethoscope at apex during expiration and with the patient in left lateral position.
- S3 in case of large ASD is best heard at left sternal border or just beneath the xiphoid and is usually louder during inspiration.
- S3 usually disappears with treatment of cardiac failure.

Fourth heart sound (S4):
- The fourth heart sound (S4) is a low pitched, presystolic (end diastolic, heard just before S1) sound produced in the ventricle during ventricular filling.
- It is best heard with bell of stethoscope.
- S4 is absent in patients with atrial fibrillation.
- S4 is frequently found in patients with aortic stenosis, hypertrophic cardiomyopathy, and systemic hypertension.
- It is loudest at the apex with left lateral position of the patient.
- With tachycardia, S3 may merge with S4, known as summation gallop.

Opening Snap

Opening snap (OS) is a brief, high pitched, early diastolic sound, which is usually due to stenosis of AV valve, most often mitral stenosis. It is generally best heard at to left lower sternal border and radiates well to the base of the heart. The A2–OS interval is inversely related to severity of mitral stenosis. More severe is mitral stenosis, higher is the left atrial pressure, and therefore earlier the OS of the mitral valve.

Pericardial Friction Rub

- Inflammation of pericardial sac with a friction between its parietal and visceral layers with or without accumulation of fluid may cause a pericardial friction rub.
- They are best audible with the diaphragm of the stethoscope in 2nd and 3rd left intercostal spaces.
- These sounds are high pitched, leathery, and scratchy in character. They seem to be close to ear. They are best appreciated with the patient in leaning forward or in knee-chest position.
- The most common causes of pericardial rub are rheumatic carditis and chronic constrictive pericarditis.
- Pericardial rub is transient and can change within few hours.

Pericardial Knock

It is a sound that occurs earlier in the diastole than usual S3 and is higher pitched. It is found in patients with constrictive pericarditis. Due to restrictive effect of the adherent thickened pericardium, there is abrupt halt in diastolic filling.

Cardiac Murmur

Innocent or functional murmurs are common in children, especially in the newborn period. In older children, they may appear after changes of posture and may disappear in erect posture. In general, the innocent or functional murmurs are systolic in timing. Rarely, they may be diastolic in timing. Any murmur should be described under specific points to derive its meaningful importance **(Boxes 14 and 15)**.

Box 14: Points to describe a murmur.

- Timing in a cardiac cycle (Systolic, diastolic)
- Duration (Early systolic, pansystolic, etc.)
- Loudness (Grade of murmur)
- Frequency (Pitch)
- Quality
- Configuration
- Site of maximum intensity
- Radiation to other areas
- Response to physiological maneuvers

Box 15: Conduction or radiation of murmurs.
- *Well-localized murmurs:* Mitral stenosis, pulmonary valve stenosis, tricuspid valve stenosis
- *Mitral regurgitation:* Left axilla
- *Aortic stenosis:* Carotid arteries and apex
- *Patent ductus arteriosus:* Back
- *Ventricular septal defect:* Right sternal edge

Table 6: Grading of systolic murmur.

Grade	Description
I	Barely audible
II	Medium intensity
III	Loud but no thrill
IV	Loud with a thrill
V	Very loud still requires the stethoscope to be on chest wall
VI	So loud that the murmur can be heard with the stethoscope off the chest

Mechanisms of cardiac murmurs:
- High rate of flow across a normal valve (anemia)
- Forward flow through a stenotic or diseased valve (stenosed valves, narrow vessel)
- Backward flow through a regurgitant valve or septal defect (MR, AR, VSD, PDA, ASD, etc.)
- Forward flow through a normal valve into a dilated distal vessel (Poststenotic pulmonary artery dilatation).

Systolic murmurs: Systolic murmurs are subdivided into pansystolic murmurs and ejection systolic murmurs. The intensity of systolic murmurs is graded from I to VI **(Table 6)**.

Systolic ejection murmurs start a short time after a well heard 1st heart sound, increase in intensity, peak, and then decrease in intensity, they usually end before the 2nd sound. However, in patients with severe aortic or pulmonary stenosis, the murmur may extend beyond the first component of the 2nd sound, thus obscuring it. These murmurs are found clinically in aortic and pulmonary stenosis and in conditions associated with a large left to right shunts.

Pansystolic murmurs: These are caused by the flow of blood from a ventricle or an artery that retains a higher pressure throughout systole than the receiving chamber or vessel. The murmur begins soon after the first heart sound and continues up to the second heart sound. They are heard most frequently in patients with mitral or tricuspid insufficiency and in ventricular septal defect.

Diastolic murmurs: Diastolic murmurs (also graded I–VI) are divided into the following:
- A rumbling, longer diastolic murmurs at the apex, accentuated at the end of diastole (presystolic) usually indicates anatomical mitral valve stenosis.
- A rumbling mid diastolic murmur at the apex is caused by increased transmitral flow in condition with large left to right shunts at ventricular or great vessel level, or with increased flow because of mitral insufficiency.
- A rumbling mid diastolic murmur at left mid and lower sternal border may be due to increased blood flow across the tricuspid valve such as occurs with ASD or less commonly due to tricuspid stenosis.
- A high-pitched blowing diastolic murmur along the left sternal border, beginning with PAH or due to pulmonary valve insufficiency.
- Following surgical repair of Fallot's tetrad, early, low-pitched diastolic murmur along the left mid and upper sternal border is also common.

Continuous murmur: It is a systolic murmur that continues or spills into diastole and indicates continuous flow as in PDA or other aortopulmonary communication. It should be differentiated from a to and fro murmur which indicates that the systolic component of the murmur ends at or before the 2nd sound and the diastolic murmur begins after atrioventricular valve closure, e.g., aortic or pulmonary stenosis combined with insufficiency.

Innocent murmurs: "Functional" "innocent" or "insignificant" are terms used for murmurs not related to any anatomic abnormality of the heart or any demonstrable cardiac disturbance. The term "innocent" is better for conveying meaning. These children have a normal ECG and chest X-ray. It is important to reassure the parents that the cardiac functions are normal and that it is not necessary to limit the child's activities. At a single, random auscultation, approximately 30% of children may be found to have an innocent murmur. The murmur is heard with repeated auscultations over a period of years.

A murmur that has any of the following characteristics should never be labeled as innocent murmur:
- Presence of any clinical cardiac abnormality
- Pansystolic murmur
- Diastolic murmur
- Loud murmurs
- Continuous murmurs except venous hum.

A venous hum is produced by the turbulence of blood in the jugular venous system. It has no pathologic significance and may be heard in the neck and anterior portion of the upper chest. It is heard in both systole and diastole and can be exaggerated or made to disappear by varying the position of the head or by light compression over the jugular venous system in the neck. Supraclavicular bruits are common. In children, innocent cardiac murmurs may also be produced by the straight back syndrome. This consists of loss of concavity of the upper thoracic spine with resultant decrease of the anteroposterior diameter of the chest. This syndrome results in innocent systolic ejection murmurs and at times the murmur is accentuated in late systole. Lateral chest X-ray is diagnostic. This condition is benign and requires no therapy.

The physician should explain that innocent murmur is simple a "noise" and does not indicate the presence of a significant cardiac defect. With growth of the child, innocent murmurs are less well heard and often disappear completely.

At times, additional studies may be indicated to rule out a CHD, but routine electrocardiogram, chest X-ray or echocardiographic examination for well children with innocent murmurs should be avoided.

SCHEME OF PRESENTATION

- *General physical examination:*
  - Comfortable
  - Dyspnea (Grade)

- Growth (with growth chart) and development
- Dysmorphism
- Skeletal deformities
- Vitals (Pulse, RR, BP, SpO$_2$)
- Anemia
- Cyanosis
- Jaundice
- Clubbing
- Edema
- Lymphadenopathy
- Osler nodes
- Subcutaneous nodules
- Erythema marginatum
- Arthritis
- Chorea
- Signs of CHF
- Signs of BE
- Signs of rheumatic activity

- *Inspection:*
  - Precordium (bulge)
  - Precordial pulsations
  - Neck vessels, suprasternal and epigastric pulsations
  - Collateral vessels
  - Apex beat (visible or not)
- *Palpation:*
  - Site and type of apex beat (normal, heaving, tapping)
  - Palpable heart sounds
  - Left parasternal heaving
  - Thrills (palpable murmurs)
- *Percussion:*
  - Outline right and left cardiac borders
  - Dullness beyond apex beat
  - Percussion of aortic area, pulmonary area
  - Check for pericardial effusion
- *Auscultation:*
  - Auscultation of mitral area, pulmonary area, aortic area, tricuspid and left parasternal areas, neck, back

- Heart sounds (intensity, split, 3rd heart sound, 4th heart sounds, gallop rhythm)
- Opening snap and ejection clicks
- Cardiac murmurs (site of maximum intensity, grade of murmur, timing, character, conduction, radiation)
- Extracardiac murmurs
- Pericardial rub.

CLINICAL DIAGNOSTIC SIGNS OF COMMON CARDIAC CONDITIONS

Ventricular Septal Defect

- In spite of congenital defect, the manifestations usually develop around 8–10 weeks of age when pulmonary pressure decreases and there is establishment of left to right shunt.
- Recurrent lower respiratory tract infections are common.
- There may be unsatisfactory weight gain.
- Wide pulse pressure, hyperdynamic precordium, forceful apex beat, systolic thrill over left parasternal region (4th and 5th intercostals space) are usual clinical findings.
- There may be splitting of S2 and loud P2. Third heart sound may be audible at apex. Systolic murmur (may be pansystolic) with more than grade IV at left parasternal region at 4th and 5th intercostals space is common. A diastolic flow murmur in the mitral area may be heard in children with large defect.

Patent Ductus Arteriosus

- Commonly present in newborns, more common in preterm babies.
- Hyperdynamic circulation and collapsing pulse (water hammer pulse) are attention drawing features.
- Heaving apex beat, systolic thrill at 2nd left intercostal space, loud S1, and narrow splitting of S2 are common findings. Machinery, continuous murmur best heard over 2nd left intercostals space, radiating toward left neck is constant finding on auscultation. Diastolic murmur at the mitral area may be heard due to large blood flow across the mitral valve.

Atrial Septal Defect

It may manifest in older children. Recurrent lower respiratory tract infections may be attention drawing.
- Left parasternal heaving is common finding on examination. Wide and flexed splitting is an important clinical feature of ASD. Soft, grade 2 to 3 systolic murmur over 2nd and 3rd intercostal spaces is heard. In the presence of lower respiratory tract infection, this soft murmur may be missed easily. The murmur is due to increased pulmonary blood flow and not due to left to right shunt. Cardiac failure is rare.
- Chest X-ray may not show cardiomegaly, but hilar dancing on fluoroscopy of chest is very common. rSR pattern and right bundle branch block in ECG are very characteristic of ASD. ECG changes are so characteristic that if it is absent, diagnosis of ASD should be reconsidered.
- Associated congenital mitral stenosis (Lutembacher syndrome) with ASD is known.

Tetralogy of Fallot

- Most common cyanotic CHD in children, beyond the neonatal period, 75–80% of total cyanotic CHDs in children.
- Pulmonary outflow tract obstruction (pulmonary valvular stenosis, postvalvular stenosis, pulmonary artery stenosis), over riding of aorta, subaortic VSD, and right ventricular hypertrophy are its components.
- Cyanosis, clubbing, anoxic spells and squatting are common features.
- Prominent "a" waves in the jugular venous pulse, mild right ventricular hypertrophy, single S2 (absent P2), ejection systolic murmur over pulmonary area, and absence of CHF are suggestive of tetralogy of Fallot.

Transposition of Great Vessels

- Most common cyanotic heart disease in neonates and especially infants of diabetic mothers.
- Cyanosis with CHF since early infancy, right ventricular hypertrophy, loud and single S2, short systolic ejection murmur

of pulmonary stenosis or systolic regurgitant murmur of VSD or no murmur are common clinical features of transposition of great vessels.

Tricuspid Atresia

- Nearly 50% of children with tricuspid atresia present with symptoms on their 1st day of life and 80% becomes symptomatic by the end of 1 month.
- Cyanosis, anoxic spells, prominent "a" waves in jugular veins, pulsatile liver, left ventricular type apex beat, and nonsignificant or absent cardiac murmur especially in neonates are specific features of tricuspid atresia.
- Left axis deviation and left ventricular dominancy in ECG are highly suggesting tricuspid atresia.

Pulmonary Stenosis

- Bulging precordium, prominent "a" waves in jugular vein, left parasternal heaving, soft S2, wide and variably split S2, and harsh systolic murmur best heard during expiration in pulmonary area are clinical features of pulmonary stenosis.
- The intensity and duration of murmur and delay in P2 component of S2 are indicators of severity of lesion.

Coarctation of Aorta

- Femorals are feeble or absent and delayed as compared to simultaneously felt radial or brachial pulsations. Palpation of femoral pulsations should be routine in all the newborns, not to miss this condition. Initial for few days after birth, feeble femoral pulsations may be missed due to PDA.
- Blood pressure in the upper limbs is more compared to lower limbs. In a case of preductal coarctation of aorta, raised BP would be recorded only in right upper limb. BP should be measured in all the four limbs routinely.
- Span may be longer than height.
- Palms may appear more pink than soles. Collateral vessels linking the subclavian arteries and intercostal arteries may be seen or felt over interscapular and infrascapular areas.

- Precordial examination shows evidences of left ventricular hypertrophy and aortic ejection systolic murmur. Ejection systolic or continuous murmurs may be audible over the back due to presence of collateral or flow of blood through narrow segment of aorta.
- The child may present with cardiac failure.

Mitral Stenosis
- Feeble pulse, tapping apex beat (right ventricular hypertrophy), palpable S2, and left parasternal heaving (right ventricular hypertrophy) are characteristic findings on palpation.
- Loud S1 in mitral area, OS, mid diastolic rough, and rumbling with presystolic accentuation are classical findings of mitral stenosis on auscultation. A loud first heart sound and OS indicates presence of a relatively pliable noncalcified valve. A short mid diastolic rumble (Carey–Coomb murmur) due to mitral valvulitis may be heard in patients with acute rheumatic carditis without any established mitral stenosis.

Mitral Regurgitation
- Pulse volume is good. Wide pulse pressure is characteristic.
- Hyperkinetic, heaving apex beat, and systolic thrill in mitral area on palpation.
- Muffled or inaudible S1, high-pitched pan systolic murmur (murmur starting immediately after the first heart sound and continuous up to and through second heart sound) which is conducted toward the axilla and back are suggestive of mitral regurgitation.

Aortic Regurgitation
- There are features of "aortic run off" like:
  - Collapsing or water hammer pulse (Corrigan's pulse)
  - Wide pulse pressure
  - Prominent carotid pulsation (Corrigan's sign)
  - Pistol shot sounds
  - de Musset's sign, nodding of head with each systole due to filling of carotid vessels
  - Hill's sign, exaggeration of systolic pressure difference between brachial and femoral arteries.

- Apex beat is forceful and heaving.
- First heart sound is soft and aortic component of second sound is delayed and accentuated.
- High pitched, blowing and early diastolic murmur in the aortic area, best heard with diaphragm of the stethoscope over the left upper parasternal area when the patient sits up, leans forward, and breathes out. The increased flow of blood across the aortic valves may produce an ejection systolic murmur. In severe AR, a low pitched diastolic flow murmur called as Austin–Flint murmur may be audible at mitral area.

Aortic Stenosis

- Feeble pulse, narrow pulse pressure heaving apex beat, and systolic thrill over aortic area on palpation.
- Delayed aortic component of S2, "diamond-shaped" ejection systolic murmur conducted to neck vessels are characteristic findings of aortic stenosis. S2 may be single or paradoxically split.
- Williams syndrome is characterized by peculiar "elfin facies", hypercalcemia, mental retardation, and supravalvular aortic stenosis.

Myocarditis

- Marked tachycardia, low-intensity heart sounds, and gallop rhythm are characteristics.
- Cardiomegaly on clinical examination as well as on chest X-ray.
- Signs and symptoms of CHF are common.
- Regurgitant murmur may be produced by gross enlargement of heart with dilatation of the valves.
- Cardiac arrhythmias in form of ventricular premature beats or conduction disturbances are common.

The Nervous System

CHAPTER 10

Baldev Prajapati

INTRODUCTION

The ever-increasing sophistication and accuracy of neurodiagnostic procedures might cause younger physicians to view the neurologic examination of the pediatric patient as obsolete and, like cardiac auscultation, a nostalgic ceremony engaged in by physicians trained before magnetic resonance (MR) imaging and DNA hybridization. This is not how I view it. Excessive reliance on diagnostic procedures at the expense of an organized plan of approach, the "let's order a CT scan and an EEG and then take a look at the kid" attitude, not only has been responsible for the depersonalization of neurologic care, and the escalation of its cost, but also has made the analysis of neurologic problems unduly complex for the pediatrician or general practitioner.

—John H Menkes

A comprehensive neurological evaluation with detailed history, thorough clinical examination, and use of investigations is the key to reach the correct neurological diagnosis in children. One should try to derive answers to following questions on examination of nervous system to reach the diagnosis:
- Does the child has neurologic disorder?
- Site of lesion (anatomical localization)
- Nature (type) of lesion (pathology)
- Cause of disease (etiology)

COMMON SYMPTOMS RELATED TO CENTRAL NERVOUS SYSTEM (BOX 1)

Seizures

Paroxysmal excessive electric neuronal discharge results in seizures which may be motor, sensory or autonomic. As a first step, it is important to decide whether it is a seizure or seizure mimicking event like breath-holding spell, syncope, benign paroxysmal vertigo, migraine, and shuddering attacks. If clinician had an opportunity to watch the episode, it becomes easy to differentiate seizures from seizure mimics. Whenever possible, it is very valuable to see a video clip of the episode. If the parents have not taken the video clip, they should be asked to do so whenever such an event recurs.

The detailed history should be obtained, keeping in mind following points:
- *Age:* The causes of seizures are different at different ages. Common causes of seizures in neonates are shown in **Box 2**. Febrile seizures are common in the age group of 6 months

Box 1: Common symptoms related to central nervous system.
- Seizures
- Headache
- Vomiting
- Excessive crying
- Irritability, lethargic
- Sensorial changes
- Personality changes
- Giddiness
- Poor school performance
- Delayed development
- Regression of milestones
- Vision disturbances
- Sleep disturbances
- Urinary and/or bowel disturbances
- Gait disturbances

Box 2: Common causes of seizures in neonates.
- Hypoglycemia
- Hypocalcemia
- Hypomagnesemia
- Hypoxic ischemic encephalopathy
- Bacterial meningitis
- Intracranial hemorrhage
- Central nervous system (CNS) malformations
- Inborn error of metabolism (IEM)

to 5 years and very rarely first episode of febrile seizures develops after the age of 3 years.
- Is it first episode or recurrent? Repeated seizures may be due to epilepsy, febrile seizures, metabolic disorders, etc.
- Positive family history for seizures may indicate genetic epilepsy syndromes.
- Presence of an aura and automatism preceding the episode of seizure occurs in complex partial seizures. Aura is usually an unpleasant feeling or a stereotypical visual or auditory hallucination or abdominal discomfort. Automatisms are involuntary motor activities occurring during or after an epileptic seizure and they are usually followed by amnesia. Such automatic behavior can be grimacing, chewing movements, etc.
- *Type of seizures:* It is important to know the type of seizures, whether it is focal or generalized. The focal seizures may be indicating underlying structural lesion which may require neuroimaging for precise diagnosis and treatment.
- *Duration of an episode:* Duration of typical febrile seizures is usually less than 10 minutes. Status epilepticus is defined as 5 or more minutes of either continuous seizure activity or repetitive seizures with no intervening recovery or consciousness.
- *Provoked or unprovoked seizures:*
  - Provoked seizures could be febrile seizures, hypoglycemic seizure, seizures due to dyselectrolytemia, etc.
  - Bacterial meningitis and meningoencephalitis should be differentiated from febrile seizures by looking for other features of meningitis and encephalopathy.
  - Developmental delay, perinatal asphyxia, perinatal or postnatal injury or family history are likely to be associated with unprovoked epileptic seizures.
- Examination should be focused on presence of neurocutaneous markers like café-au-lait spots, shagreen patch, and port-wine stain.
- Look for injury marks over forehead or other body parts which may suggest myoclonic jerks.

The important history taking points for seizures are shown in **Box 3**.

Common causes of seizures in children are listed in **Box 4**.

> **Box 3:** Important history taking points for seizures.
> - *Age:* Neonate/infancy/childhood
> - First episode/recurrent
> - Provoked/unprovoked
> - Focal/generalized
> - *Precipitating factors:* Deprivation of sleep, stress, hunger
> - Presence of aura
> - Postictal period
> - History of perinatal insult
> - History of delayed development
> - History of regression of milestones
> - Family history or febrile convulsions, epilepsy, any central nervous system (CNS) disorder or inborn errors of metabolism

> **Box 4:** Common causes of seizures in children.
> - Febrile seizures
> - Metabolic causes:
>   - Hypoglycemia
>   - Hypocalcemia
>   - Hypomagnesemia
>   - Hyponatremia
>   - Hypernatremia
> - Epilepsy
> - Central nervous system (CNS) infections:
>   - Bacterial meningitis
>   - Tuberculous meningitis
>   - Viral meningoencephalitis
>   - Brain abscess
> - Raised intracranial pressure:
>   - Hydrocephalus
>   - Space occupying lesions—brain tumors, tuberculoma
> - Vascular thrombosis, hemorrhage
> - Neurocutaneous syndromes:
>   - Tuberous sclerosis
>   - Sturge–Weber syndrome
>   - Neurofibromatosis
> - Inborn errors of metabolism
> - Structural anomalies like lissencephaly, absence of corpus callosum, etc.
> - Encephalopathy

Headache

Headache is one of the common neurological symptoms than can be due to variety of causes from nonorganic to serious organic causes such as raised intracranial pressure due to brain tumor.

The common causes of headache in children are shown in **Box 5**. The important history taking points for headache are shown in **Box 6**.

- *Onset:* Ask whether the headache is acute, insidious onset or chronic in nature. Hyperacute headache is seen with subarachnoid hemorrhage. Headache in migraine and cluster headache are usually acute and recurrent. Tension headache and psychogenic headache are usually chronic in nature and insidious in onset. Initially, headache in the morning and then gradually progressive indicates raised intracranial pressure in a case of hydrocephalus, tuberculous meningitis (TBM), space occupying lesion (SOL), etc.
- *Location:*
  - Generalized headache occurs in conditions like central nervous system (CNS) infections, raised intracranial pressure, and hypertension.

Box 5: Common causes of headache in children.

- Migraine
- Cluster headache
- Tension headache
- Headache during fever
- Central nervous system (CNS) infections (bacterial meningitis, tuberculous meningitis, meningoencephalitis)
- Space occupying lesions
- Sinusitis
- Headache secondary to earache or tooth disease
- Trauma
- Postlumbar puncture
- Refractive errors

Box 6: Important history taking points for headache.

- Acute/insidious/chronic/recurrent
- *Nature of headache:* Throbbing/dull aching
- Severity
- Activities are affected or not
- Associated symptoms (nausea, projectile vomiting, fever, etc.)
- Associated photophobia
- Medication required or not; Response to medication
- Whether the headache requires school absenteeism

- Localized headache can be due to various reasons and may indicate etiology. Frontal headache is common with sinusitis and refractive errors. Temporal headache occurs in migraine. Occipital headache may be due to hypertension. Headache occurs around the orbit in cluster headache.
- *Duration and frequency:* Migraine and cluster headaches are episodic and duration of headache ranges from 4 to 72 hours. Chronic daily headache is seen in tension headache. Slowly progressive or worsening headache indicates raised intracranial pressure such as SOLs or hydrocephalus, often associated with projectile vomiting. Any headache which disturbs or interferes with the activity and sleep of the child must be assessed properly.
- *Character:* Headache in migraine is pulsatile or throbbing in character. Dull, boring headache is characteristic of tension headache. Thunder scalp headache, worst headache in one's life is highly indicative of subarachnoid hemorrhage.
- Unilateral headache is seen in classical migraine.
- *Precipitating and aggravating factors:* Episodes of migraine are precipitated by stress, sleep deprivation, hunger, and certain foods. Headache due to raised intracranial pressure gets aggravated by coughing and straining and decreases after an episode of vomiting.
- *Functional impairment:* A patient of migraine likes to take rest and sleep in dark room. In a case of tension headache, the patient continues to work and it does not disturb the sleep.
- *Associated factors*:
  - Nausea, vomiting, photophobia, and visual aura are common with migraine headache.
  - Fever, headache, and vomiting may be due to CNS infection.
  - Projectile vomiting and altered sensorium are common with raised intracranial tension.
  - Nasal discharge, nasal blocks, and upper respiratory tract infection (URTI) indicate sinusitis.

Altered Sensorium

Altered sensorium is described as impairment in arousal and awareness. Arousal or wakefulness is a function of ascending reticular formation, whereas awareness is a function of cerebral cortex and subcortical structures.

Arousal is described in terms of whether the sleep–wake cycle is preserved or not. Absence of sleep–wake cycle indicates coma.

Awareness in older children is expressed as interest in surrounding, recognition of his parents, indicating for bowel or bladder needs, and indicating for hunger. Awareness in infants is understood in terms of interest in their toys, consolability of child, eye contact with mother, and indicating for food.

Common causes of altered sensorium are listed in **Box 7**.

The following points provide more information:
- Onset, duration, and progress of altered sensorium
- History of seizures at present or in past
- History of fever or other symptoms suggesting CNS infection or systemic disorders
- History of headache, vomiting, visual disturbances, and other features suggesting raised intracranial pressure

---

Box 7: Common causes of altered sensorium.

- Metabolic:
  - Hypoglycemia
  - Hyponatremia
  - Hypernatremia
  - Diabetic ketoacidosis
  - Inborn errors of metabolism
- Infections (bacterial meningitis, tuberculous meningitis, meningoencephalitis, etc.)
- Vascular causes:
  - Cerebrovascular stroke
  - Intracranial hemorrhage
  - Hypertensive encephalopathy
- Increased intracranial pressure:
  - Hydrocephalus
  - Space occupying lesions
- Epilepsy (status epilepticus, postictal state, epileptic encephalopathies)
- Systemic diseases:
  - Hepatic encephalopathy
  - Uremic encephalopathy
- Post-traumatic brain injury
- *Toxins:* Lead poisoning, snake bite

- History of diarrhea or fluid loss indicating dehydration and electrolyte disturbances causing seizures or cortical venous thrombosis
- History of head injury
- History of exposure to toxins
- Personal or family history of migraine, epilepsy or encephalopathy

Vision Disturbances

Vision disturbances is often one of the common presenting complaints. It should be defined as follows:
- Onset and progression of visual impairment:
  - *Sudden onset:* Vascular
  - *Insidious and progressive:* Optic neuritis
- *Associated complaints:*
  - Double vision (ophthalmoplegia)
  - Haloes around bright light (glaucoma)
  - Floating spots (retinal detachment)
  - Visual field defects

Regression of Milestones

There is loss of milestones which already child had achieved. It indicates neurodegenerative disorders. It should be differentiated from delayed development. Both the situations require different approaches.

From details of symptomatology, probable clinical conditions can be considered as shown in **Table 1**.

NEUROLOGICAL EVALUATION BASED ON HISTORY

The initial evaluation of the child should determine the child's general condition and the severity of illness, whether he requires immediate treatment or not. In a critically ill child, he should be first stabilized, further evaluation and management can be performed later.

History is fundamental for diagnosis of CNS disease. Ninety percent of information needed for diagnosis in a case of CNS disorder is obtained by history. One should try to decide the category of disorder from the history as discussed next which will help for further evaluation and management.

Table 1: Symptomatology and probable clinical conditions.

Personality and behavior changes, reduced attention span, scholastic backwardness, regression of milestones	• Degenerative diseases • Tuberculous meningitis
Developmental delay	• Cerebral palsy • Intellectual disability
Vomiting, headache, altered sensorium	Raised intracranial pressure
Motor deficits	• Hemiplegia/hemiparesis • Paraplegia/paraparesis • Monoparesis
Abnormal movements, frequent falls	• Movement disorders • Ataxia
Difficulty in getting up from sitting position/climbing stairs	Muscle weakness (myopathy)
Root pain, paresthesia	Spinal cord, nerve roots involvement
Back pain, bladder and bowel involvement	Spinal cord involvement

The history and the evaluation should begin with points as follows:
- *Age of onset of disease:* An early onset of disease may be linked to perinatal events such as birth asphyxia, malformations, congenital infections, etc. Febrile convulsions are common between the age of 6 months and 5 years. Rheumatic chorea is common in prepubertal girls.
- *Types of onset:*
  - Lesions which suddenly affect the nervous system, cause maximal disability within a few hours, and after a static period of days or weeks, then show a tendency to improve, are usually due to vascular disturbances and sometimes due to trauma.
  - Disability of insidious onset and slow but inexorable progression are often due to degenerative disorders or tumors of CNS.
  - Inflammatory lesions such as infections often develop rapidly but less acutely than traumatic or vascular.
  - Characterized by paroxysmal short-lived disorders of function, followed by rapid and complete recovery. This type of history may be due to epilepsy or migraine or to transient ischemic attacks.

- *Sequence of symptoms:* Ask for sequence, duration, and progress of symptoms. A 2-year-old child presenting with high-grade fever for a day and generalized tonic-clonic convulsions associated with fever, convulsions less than 10 minutes, followed by drowsiness for few minutes and regaining normalcy, suggests febrile seizures. Another child of same age group presenting with fever for 5 days, headache and vomiting for 3 days, convulsions for 1 day, and unconscious since 12 hours, suggests acute bacterial meningitis. It started with high-grade fever (bacteremia), headache, and vomiting (raised intracranial pressure), convulsions and unconsciousness (encephalopathy), sequence duration and progress of symptoms explain pathophysiology of acute bacterial meningitis.
- *Evolution of the disease:* The disease being static, improving, progressive, becoming worse or episodic can provide important information about the disease.
    - Cerebral palsy is a static insult to growing brain.
    - Regression of milestones and progressive neurological disorder is the characteristic of degenerative disease.
    - The illustrations of episodic illness are epilepsy and migraine.

Antenatal and Perinatal History

The points to be noted are:
- History of eclampsia
- History of polyhydramnios/oligohydramnios
- History of intrauterine infections (TORCH infections)
- History of birth asphyxia
- History of preterm/low birth weight
- History of neonatal convulsions/hypoglycemia/hyperbilirubinemia
- History of neonatal sepsis/bacterial meningitis

Immunization History

- Encephalopathy following pertussis vaccine
- Demyelinating insults following influenza or rabies vaccines

- If the child has received certain vaccines, specific diseases can be prevented such as measles vaccine (encephalitis), pneumococcal vaccine (pneumococcal meningitis), *Haemophilus influenzae* type b vaccine (HIB meningitis), meningococcal vaccine (meningococcal meningitis), varicella vaccine (encephalitis, cerebellitis), etc.

Family History

Relevant points are:
- Consanguineous marriage (autosomal recessive diseases)
- Draw three generation pedigree chart
- History of migraine, epilepsy, degenerative diseases, etc.
- History of tuberculous contact
- HIV status of parents

GENERAL PHYSICAL EXAMINATION

Relevant important points on general examination should be noted. It may provide a clue to consider the neurological diagnosis.
- *Vitals:*
  - Persistent, high-grade fever, not responding to antipyretics may be of central origin due to hypothalamic lesion.
  - Irregular respiration is known in case of involvement of pons and medulla.
  - Bradycardia may be a sign of raised intracranial pressure.
  - Transient hypertension is known in raised intracranial pressure, Guillain–Barré syndrome, poliomyelitis, etc.
- Dysmorphic facial features may be due to syndromic disorders and other causes.
- Mental status
- *Nutritional status:* Some of the nutritional deficiencies are known to cause CNS manifestations like iron deficiency anemia, protein–energy malnutrition (PEM), vitamin B_{12}, niacin, thiamine, and other deficiencies. Copper metabolic disorders like Wilson disease and Menke's syndrome are known.
- Anthropometry will provide details of his growth and other disorders like hypothyroidism, homocystinuria, PEM, etc.
- Posture of the child like opisthotonus in tetanus, decorticate and decerebrate rigidity, and dystonia.

- Head size and shape may provide information regarding microcephaly, craniosynostosis, etc.
- *Anterior fontanelle (AF):* Open and bulging may be in a case of hydrocephalus, acute bacterial meningitis, TBM, raised intracranial pressure, etc.
- Neurocutaneous markers like café-au-lait spots and shagreen patches.
- Hair changes.
- Eye examination for papilledema, cataract, KF ring, cherry red spot, etc.
- Spinal abnormalities like meningocele, meningomyelocele, pilonidal sinus, tuft of hair, etc., which may be markers for dysraphism of spinal cord.
- Look for features of specific syndrome like Down syndrome, MPS, Turner syndrome, Marfan syndrome, etc.

NEUROLOGICAL EXAMINATION

For methodological and thorough clinical assessment of neurological system, one should have common tools as shown in **Figure 1** and he should follow scheme as shown in **Box 8**.

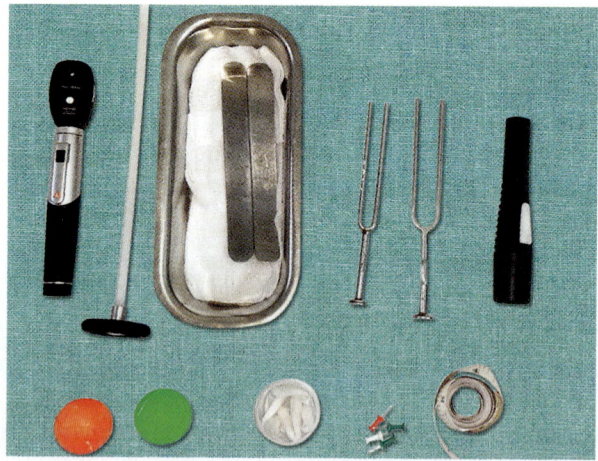

Fig. 1: Common tools for neurological examination: Measuring tapes, cotton wisps, spatula, torch, percussion hammer, tuning forks, ophthalmoscope, red and green colored balls, etc.

> **Box 8:** Scheme of neurological examination.
>
> - Higher functions:
>   - Consciousness (Glasgow Coma Scale)
>   - Orientation of time, place, person
>   - Handedness
>   - Speech
>   - Memory
>   - Developmental quotient/intelligence quotient
> - Cranial nerves
> - Motor system:
>   - Muscle tone
>   - Muscle power
>   - Nutrition/wasting
>   - Coordination
>   - Involuntary movements
> - Sensory system:
>   - Cortical
>   - Superficial
>   - Deep
> - Reflexes
>   - Superficial reflexes
>   - Deep tendon reflexes
> - Signs of meningeal irritation
> - Cerebellar signs
> - Skull and spine
> - Gait
> - Urinary and bowel functions

Consciousness

Consciousness is defined as awareness regarding external as well as internal milieu.

Consciousness has two components, arousability (wakefulness) and awareness. Cognitive functions mean the construction of thought process that includes remembering, problem solving, and decision-making which evolves through childhood to adolescence.

Mental functions are tested in an alert, awake child. If the levels of arousal are reduced, then awareness is also reduced. One cannot evaluate awareness in an unarousable (unconscious) child.

- *Consciousness:* Awareness regarding external as well as internal milieu
- *Drowsy:* Arousable with light stimuli, responding appropriately for sometime

- *Stupor:* Arousable with painful stimuli, remains awake till stimulus is applied, goes to original status as soon as stimulus is removed.
- *Semiconscious:* Nonspecific response to only deep painful stimuli.
- *Unconsciousness:* No response to any stimulus
- *Coma:* Prolonged stage of unconsciousness. Coma may be followed by persistent vegetative state.
- AVPU and Glasgow Coma Scale (GCS) are two commonly used scales for clinical evaluation of unconscious child as shown in **Box 9** and **Table 2**.

Orientation of Time, Place, and Person

Orientation cannot be evaluated properly in children below the age of 5 years. The assessment of orientation should be age sensitive and questions should be tailored for patient's age.

Box 9: AVPU Pediatric Response Scale.
- (A) *Alert:* Awake, active, appropriately responsive
- (V) *Voice:* Voice responsiveness
- (P) *Pain:* Pain responsiveness
- (U) *Unresponsive:* Not responding to any stimulus

Table 2: Glasgow Coma Scale (GCS).

Parameter	Glasgow Coma Scale	Adelaide Coma Scale
Eye opening • Spontaneous • Responds to speech • Responds to pain* • Nil	 4 3 2 1	As in Glasgow scale
Best motor response • Obeys commands • Localizes pain • Withdrawal of limb • Flexion to pain • Extension to pain • Nil	 6 5 4 3 2 1	As in Glasgow scale

Contd...

Contd...

Parameter	Glasgow Coma Scale		Adelaide Coma Scale	
Best verbal response				
• Oriented	5		Oriented	5
• Confused	4		Words	4
• Inappropriate words	3		Vocal sounds	3
• Incomprehensible sounds	2		Cries	2
• Nil	1		Nil	1

*Pain is imparted either by strong pinch, applying pressure on the finger nail with a pencil, squeezing big toe or applying pressure over the supratrochlear notch located on the medical end of upper margin of orbit. Coma score of <12 suggests severe head injury, score of <8 suggests need for intubation and ventilation and a score of <6 suggests need for intracranial pressure monitoring.

A 3–4 years old alert child should be able to tell his name and gender and identify his parents. An older child may be able to answer regarding time, place, and different persons like near relatives and friends.

Memory

Memory has three components, registration, retention, and recall. The immediate, short-term, and long-term memory depends on functioning of these basic components. Immediate memory is tested by naming four to five objects and asking the child to repeat it shortly. Short-term memory can be assessed by asking simple questions regarding daily routine activities such as what he had taken in lunch or dinner, what home work he got previous day, etc. Long-term memory can be tested by asking the child to tell short story, a poem, telephone number of his residence, etc.

Intelligence

Judgment, reasoning, perception, thinking, and vocabulary should be tested by asking age appropriate simple questions. Assessment of intelligence quotient (IQ) is time-consuming and rigorous and done by clinical psychologists.

An IQ between 90 and 110 is considered as average. Intellectual disability is classified as mild (IQ 55–69), moderate (IQ 40–55), severe (IQ 25–40), and profound (IQ <25).

Speech and Language

Speech is defined as the faculty of communicating, expressing or understanding thoughts, and ideas through the medium of symbols, which may take the form of spoken or written words.

Speech should be evaluated for quality of voice, articulation, and langue milestones. Language includes testing speech, reading, and writing.

- Langue is a system of words or signs that people use to express thoughts in the form of speech, gesture, sign language or written symbols.
- *Speech and handedness:* Language is lateralized to the dominant hemisphere, which is generally the left hemisphere for a right-handed child and vice versa. Due to this, left hemispheric lesions frequently cause aphasia in right-handed individuals. Interestingly even among left-handed individuals, majority (70%) are still left hemispheric dominant, only 13% are right hemispheric dominant and the remaining 17% are mixed.
- *Loss of language:* It is called aphasia. It could be receptive (Wernicke's aphasia) or expressive (Broca's aphasia) or global. It should be differentiated from dysarthria (disorder of articulation), dysphonia (disorder of vocal cords), and stammering (functional disorder of speech). Dysarthria may be due to extrapyramidal disorders.
- Abnormality or absence of speech by 18 months of age and inability to make meaningful sentences by age of 3 years is abnormal and indicates possibility of autism or aphasia.

Lobe Functions

- Apraxia is the inability to accomplish previously learned and performed complex motor actions even though motor system, sensory system, understanding, and coordination are relatively intact. The child may not be able to comb the hair, wear the shoes or drink a cup of tea properly, if he is asked to do so. It suggests parietal lobe dysfunction.
- Right and left orientation occurs by age of 4 years. You may ask simple questions like show your left hand, touch your left ear with right hand, show my right hand, touch my right hand with

your left hand, etc., to access it. The disorder indicates involvement of parietal lobe.
- Agnosia is the inability to understand the meaning of symbolic significance of ordinary sensory stimuli even though the sensory pathway and sensorium are intact. If the child is asked to show his thumb or little fingers and not able to do so, is the example of agnosia. With closed eyes, an object (like coin) is put in a hand of the patient and if he is not able to recognize it, it is called astereognosis. With the closed eyes of the child, if you write a number or letter on his hand, he is not able to identify it, it is called as agraphesthesia.

Frontal Lobe Dysfunction
- Vague psychiatric disorders
- Emotional instability
- Lack of concentration
- Dementia, impaired intellectual capacity
- Loss of recent memory
- Becomes careless about his dress and appearance
- Micturition disturbances (may micturate in public or becomes incontinent)
- Anosmia (loss of smell)

Occipital Lobe Dysfunction
- Visual hallucination
- Homonymous hemianopia

Temporal Lobe Dysfunctions
- Visual hallucination
- Altered state of consciousness
- Receptive dysphasia

Hypothalamic Dysfunction
- Obesity
- Sleep disturbances
- Features of diabetes insipidus

Cranial Nerve Examination

There are 12 cranial nerves **(Box 10)** and they can be categorized as sensory, motor, and mixed. All cranial nerves, except first and second, originate in the brainstem. Therefore, cranial nerve examination is an excellent tool to localize a brainstem lesion.

Olfactory Nerve (Cranial Nerve I)

- Neonates, infants, and toddlers can detect olfaction and can express with facial expression but cannot express verbally.
- Olfactory nerve is purely a sensory nerve and it is routinely not tested, unless some specific problem is suspected.
- It can be tested in children above the age of 5 years.
- *Method of examination:*
    - Ensure that nasal passages are patent.
    - Eyes of the child should be closed.
    - Each nostril should be examined separately.
    - Use the familiar and nonirritant substances like peppermint, soap, and chocolate. Avoid irritant substances because that may stimulate trigeminal nerve and give a false interpretation.
    - Anosmia (absence of perception of smell) and hyposmia (reduced perception of smell) can occur due to cribriform plate damage following meningitis and head injury. Perception of smell can also be impaired due to herpes simplex viral encephalitis, corona viral infection etc.

> **Box 10:** Cranial nerves.
> - Olfactory (sensory)
> - Optic (sensory)
> - Oculomotor (motor)
> - Trochlear (motor)
> - Trigeminal (mixed)
> - Abducens (motor)
> - Facial (mixed)
> - Vestibulocochlear (sensory)
> - Glossopharyngeal (mixed)
> - Vagus (mixed)
> - Accessory (motor)
> - Hypoglossal (motor)

Optic Nerve (Cranial Nerve II)

Optic nerve is a sensory nerve. The components of examination of optic nerve are shown in **Box 11**.

Pathway of optic nerve: The optic nerve consists of fibers derived from the ganglionic cells of retina. Optic nerves from both the eyes join to form the optic chiasma in middle cranial fossa. At optic chiasma, fibers from nasal sides cross over to temporal side to form optic tract. Each optic tract passes backward and outward from optic chiasma to reach lateral geniculate body. Fibers from lateral geniculate body carry visual information through optic radiation to visual cortex. Some of the fibers in the optic tract end in pretectal nucleus for pupillary reflexes and superior colliculus for extraocular movements.

Visual acuity:
- At birth, the vision is about 20/400 but matures to 20/20 by 1–2 years of age.
- If a child can follow moving object, it suggests that he has intact cortical vision.
- Infants with poor vision fail to fix and follow the light. They often develop nystagmus by 2 months of age. Menace reflex demonstrates gross vision and is performed in infants, uncooperative, mentally subnormal children, and children with vegetative state. A finger is suddenly brought towards the patient's eye. Blinking of eyes in response to this is suggestive of grossly normal vision.
- Formal testing is done by Snellen chart, which is possible in older and cooperative children.

Field of vision: The visual pathways are organized in such a way that different patterns of visual field abnormality result from different sites. The visual fields are divided vertically through

> **Box 11:** Components of examination of optic nerve.
> - Visual acuity
> - Field of vision
> - Color vision
> - Pupillary reactions
> - Fundus examination

the point of fixation into the temporal and nasal fields. On your right, as you look ahead, is temporal field of your right eye and the nasal field of your left eye. The visual fields are described from the child's point of view.

Field defects are said to be homonymous if the same part of the field is affected by the eyes, e.g., a right homonymous hemianopia means there is a field defect in the temporal field of right eye and nasal field of left eye. Whereas a bitemporal hemianopia would be a heteronymous field defect.

Homonymous field defects are called congruous, if the field defects in both eyes match exactly, or incongruous, if the field defects do not match exactly.

Localization of the lesion can be described as the field defect **(Table 3)**. Visual fields are clinically tested by confrontation test.

Confrontation test (Fig. 2):
- The visual field of the child is compared with the visual field of the examiner.
- The examiner sits at about 50 cm distance and in front of the child (confront).
- Both the eyes are tested separately and in all the four quadrants.
- For testing the child's left eye, his right eye is occluded and the left eye of the examiner is occluded.
- The child is asked to look directly into the examiner's eye.
- The examiner holds his finger outside his visual field in the middle of one quadrant and moves the finger slowly to the central field. The child is instructed to say "yes" when he starts to see the finger.
- If the field of defect is found clinically, the child should undergo a perimetry assessment by an ophthalmologist.

Table 3: Localization of field defects.	
Field defect	Localization
Mono ocular	Lesion anterior to optic chiasma
Bitemporal	Lesion at the optic chiasma
Homonymous field defect	Lesion behind the optic chiasma
Incongruous homonymous	Lesion in the optic tract
Congruous homonymous	Lesion behind lateral geniculate bodies

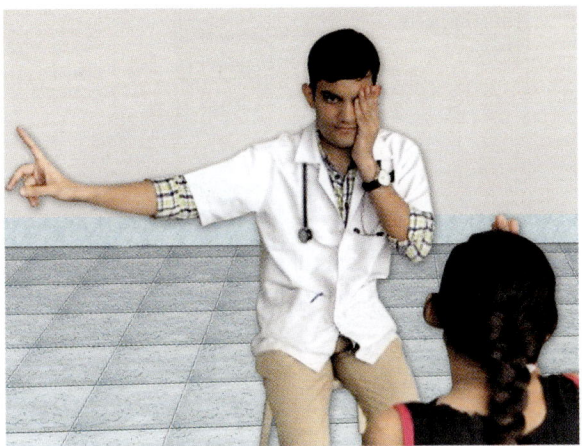

Fig. 2: Testing for field of vision by confrontation test.

Color vision: Color vision can be assessed in children older than 3 years of age by Ishihara chart. The Ishihara test is a diagnostic test of color perception for red and green color. Deficiencies are carried out by using pseudoisochromatic plates. A child develops the ability to recognize different colors by 18 months of age and starts noticing shapes, texture, and sizes. A child can name at least one color by the age of 3 years.

Pupillary reaction:
- Pupillary light reflex (both direct and consensual) should be tested in a dark room by shining the light suddenly with a torch from the side of the eye after asking a child to look at a distance, showing some attractive object or toy. Both the eyes are tested. The test is essential in children with coma, head injuries, stroke, and brain tumors. The reflex consists of optic nerve as afferent, center in pons (Pretectal and Edinger–Westphal nucleus of oculomotor nerves), and the efferent being oculomotor nerve.
- Direct reflex shows constriction of the pupil on the same eye.
- Consensual reflex shows constriction of the pupil in the opposite eye. It is due to bilateral innervations of Edinger–Westphal nucleus of oculomotor nerve.
- *Accommodation reaction:* Ask the child to look at a distant object. Bring your index finger or a pen suddenly in front of

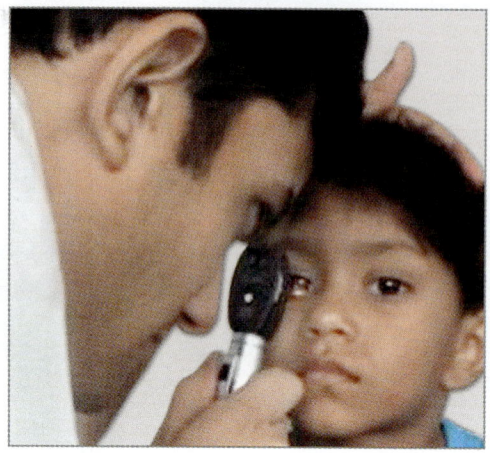

Fig. 3: Fundus examination by ophthalmoscope.

eyes and ask the child to fixate on finger or pen. Observe the movements of eyeballs and pupils. Adduction of both the eyes and constriction of pupils is the normal response.

Fundus examination (Fig. 3): It should be routine as a part of clinical examination of CNS.
- Papilledema is suggestive of raised intracranial pressure. It is a contraindication for lumbar puncture.
- Optic nerve atrophy, retinal infarcts, and retinal hemorrhage are other important findings.
- Cherry red spot in retina is seen with Tay-Sachs disease, Niemann-Pick disease, and gangliosidosis.
- Presence of Roth spot is characteristic of bacterial endocarditis.

Oculomotor (III), Trochlear (IV), and Abducens (VI)

These are pure motor nerves, they control the movements of eyes (eyeballs, upper eyelids, and pupils), and are tested together.
- Look for ptosis, position of the resting eyeballs, squint, spontaneous movements of eyes, nystagmus, and other abnormal movements like opsoclonus.
- Movements of both the eyes when they move in the same direction together are called as conjugate eye movements and are controlled by the centers in frontal lobe, pons, and midbrain. Paralysis of these supranuclear regions gives rise

to the supranuclear gaze palsies. The infranuclear lesions lead to paralysis of muscles of the eye.
- Conjugate eye movements can be elicited by command in conscious, co-operative child or doll's eye phenomenon in an unconscious child.
- *Doll's eye phenomenon (oculocephalic reflex):*
  - The infant is placed supine and head is suddenly turned towards either side. The baby's eyes lag behind like a doll, i.e., there is conjugate deviation of the eyes toward the opposite side.
  - No importance in conscious patient.
  - Present in normal newborn, in patients with coma, impairment of optic fixation.
  - Absence of doll's eye phenomenon in a comatosed child is indicative of damage to brainstem or due to increased intracranial pressure and transtentorial herniation.
  - Presence of doll's eye phenomenon in a comatosed child is indicative of intact brainstem and unconsciousness may be due to cortical lesion.
- All extraocular muscles, except superior oblique (supplied by 4th cranial nerve) and lateral rectus muscle (supplied by 6th cranial nerve), are supplied by 3rd cranial nerve.
- The manifestations of oculomotor motor nerve palsy are shown in **Box 12**.
- The common causes of palsies of these nerves are cerebral palsy, raised intracranial pressure (6th nerve palsy as a false localizing sign), brainstem tumors, meningitis, Guillain–Barré syndrome, etc.

Box 12: Manifestations of oculomotor nerve palsy.

- Diplopia
- Ptosis (drooping of upper eyelid) due to paralysis of levator palpebrae superioris
- Eye is fixed in lateral and downward position, due to unopposed action of lateral rectus and superior oblique muscles
- Pupil is dilated due to unopposed action of dilator pupillae which is supplied by sympathetic fibers accompanying nasociliary branch of ophthalmic nerve
- Exophthalmos
- Enophthalmos

Trochlear (IV) Nerve Palsy

- Isolated 4th nerve palsy is rare.
- There is an upward deviation of the affected eye in the abducted position due to the unopposed action of inferior oblique muscle.
- Diplopia may occur on attempted downward gaze while climbing down the stairs.
- There may be compensatory torticollis.

Abducens (VI) Nerve Palsy

- Paralysis of lateral movement of the eye
- Convergent squint as the affected eye tends to deviate medially.
- Diplopia on looking toward the affected side
- Compensatory torticollis

Trigeminal Nerve (V Cranial Nerve)

Trigeminal nerve is a mixed nerve. It is tested for both components—sensory and motor.

- Sensory component is tested for pain, touch, and temperature sensations over face. It has three divisions—ophthalmic, maxillary, and mandibular.
- *The following general rules are essential to follow while testing sensory component of this nerve:*
    - Eyes should be closed.
    - Light touch should be tested by a cotton wisp. Touch both sides scalp, cheek, and chin.
    - Pain sensations should be tested by toothpick point or a safety pin.
    - Sneeze is elicited on stimulation of nose. Pain solicits withdrawal and crying in newborns and infants.

Corneal reflex:

- The test elicits sensations from the cornea in the ophthalmic division of the trigeminal nerve (afferent part) and the motor part (efferent part) of the reflex is via both facial nerves to cause blinking on both the sides normally.
- Corneal reflex is a brainstem reflex and the center lies in pons.

- *Method of elicitation of corneal reflex (Fig. 4):*
  - Explain the child regarding the testing.
  - Confirm that child is not wearing contact lenses.
  - Ask the child to look at ceiling or opposite side and the cornea is touched on the lateral side with a sterile cotton wisp to avoid visual blink.
  - Do not touch the central part of cornea as it can damage it. Take care to not touch eyelashes or conjunctiva.
  - Test on both the sides.
  - Normal response consists of blinking on both the sides.
  - If the trigeminal nerve is affected, neither eye blinks and if there is unilateral facial nerve involvement, normal eye blinks.
  - Absence of unilateral corneal reflex and loss of pain sensation suggests 5th cranial nerve involvement.

Testing motor division: The motor division of 5th cranial nerve innervates the muscles of mastication. Ask the child to clinch his teeth and feel the bulk of masseter and temporalis muscles. Ask the child to open the mouth and to move lower jaw side to side to check functions of pterygoid muscles. Observe for the deviation of the jaw or asymmetry of muscle contraction. A unilateral lesion results in the deviation of the jaw to the affected side.

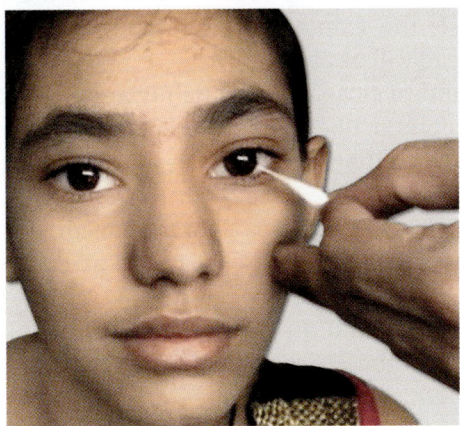

Fig. 4: Testing for corneal reflex.

Jaw jerk: Trigeminal nerve is both afferent and efferent for jaw jerk. To elicit the reflex, ask the child to open the mouth slightly. Place your finger over child's chin. Strike your finger with reflex hammer. Normally, jaw jerk is not elicitable. If it is elicitable, it is interpreted as exaggerated. It indicates supranuclear lesion of trigeminal nerve. In nuclear or infranuclear lesion, the jaw jerk is absent.
- Isolated lesion of this nerve is uncommon. Involvement of trigeminal nerve is seen with other cranial nerves in conditions like tuberculous meningoencephalitis, brainstem glioma, fracture of base of skull, herpes zoster, cavernous sinus thrombosis.

Facial Nerve (VII Cranial Nerve)

The facial nerve is important in clinical medicine as its involvement is common in CNS disorders. It is mainly a motor nerve, but also has a sensory component. The motor division supplies all the muscles of face. The sensory division conveys the taste sensations from the anterior two-thirds of the tongue. The manifestations of facial nerve palsy are as follows **(Figs. 5A to D)**:
- Unilateral facial weakness or palsy manifests by the asymmetry of the face. There is loss of nasolabial fold, dropping of corner of the mouth (orbicularis oris weakness), and drooling of saliva (weakness of buccinators) on the affected side. It should be differentiated from congenital absence of Depressor Angularis Oris **(Fig. 6)**.
- Ask the child to look upwards and see for the wrinkles over forehead. If the frontalis muscle is involved, the wrinkles over forehead will be absent.
- Ask the child to close the eyes tightly and try to open them to test orbicularis oculi. If the muscle is weak, then the child is unable to close the eyes properly, and there is also widened palpebral fissure.
- Ask the child to smile and to clench the teeth, if orbicularis oris and levator angularis oris are weak, the affected side does not move out like the normal side.
- Ask the child to hold the air in mouth, if there is facial nerve paralysis, then the air escapes through ipsilateral side due to weakness of buccinator muscle.
- Asymmetry of face in a crying newborn makes facial nerve palsy obvious.

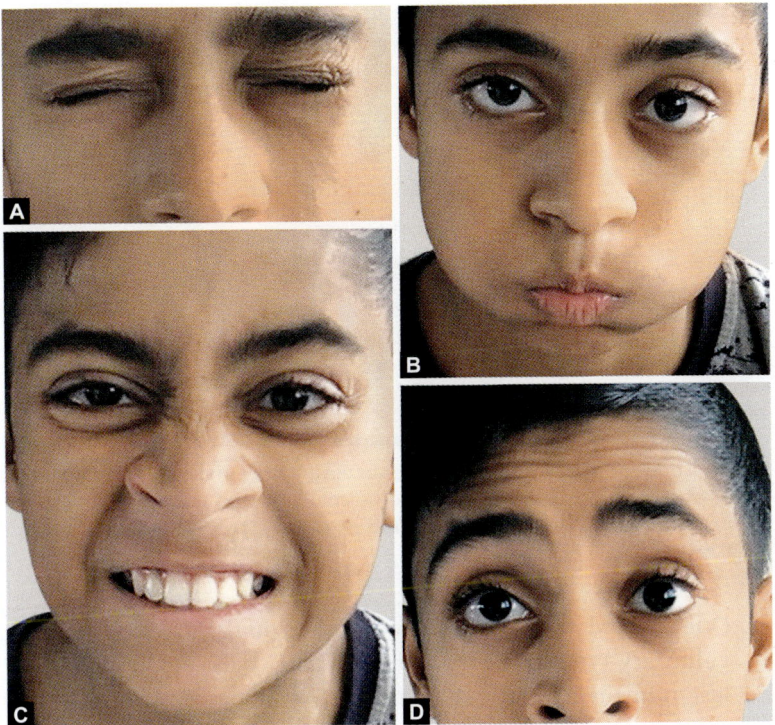

Figs. 5A to D: Testing facial nerve motor function. (A) Close eyes; (B) Holding air in the mouth; (C) Clinching the teeth, look for symmetry of nasolabial folds on both sides and deviation of angle of mouth; (D) Wrinkling the forehead.

Upper motor neuron and lower motor neuron facial palsy:
- In upper motor neuron (UMN) lesion, upper part of the face will be spared as it is bilaterally innervated, therefore wrinkling over forehead, eye closing, and blinking are not affected.
- Lower motor neuron (LMN) lesion (lesion from the facial nerve nucleus in the brainstem to anywhere along its pathway) affects half of the whole face (both upper and lower halves) on the ipsilateral side.
- In LMN lesion, Bell's phenomenon is observed, in which corneal reflex is lost and weakness is accentuated when the child cries or smiles. It develops on the same side of lesion.
- Reduction of tears on the affected side is due to lacrimal gland involvement following involvement of parasympathetic fibers.

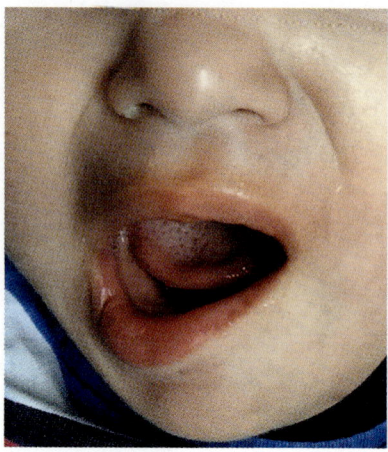

Fig. 6: Congenital absence of Depressor Angularis Oris. Note the corner of angle of mouth is moved toward the normal side and the lower lip moves downward and outward, nasolabial fold is not affected, differentiating from facial nerve palsy.

- One should try to distinguish emotional movements from voluntary type in a supranuclear facial palsy lesion. In UMN lesion involving corticobulbar fibers, weakness is seen more on volitional movements but is seen less on emotional movements such as crying and smiling, which is called volitional facial palsy.
- The sensory component supplies the taste sensation to the anterior two-thirds of the tongue. Practically, it is hardly tested.

Common causes of unilateral facial palsy:
- *Unilateral UMN facial palsy:* The common causes are stroke, demyelination, and lesions involving cerebrum, cerebral peduncle or upper pons at the level of facial nerve nuclei along with hemiplegia on same side.
- *Bilateral UMN facial palsy:* It is very rare, can be seen in affection of corticobulbar involvement, due to bilateral stroke, severe head injury and some neurodegenerative disorders.
- *Lower motor nerve palsy:* It is commonly seen in practice due to various reasons like Bell's palsy, meningitis, Kawasaki disease, middle ear infection, trauma in parotid region, following surgery in middle ear, and parotid gland or lower face. Guillain–Barré syndrome, myasthenia gravis, etc., can present

with LMN facial palsy. It can occur in newborns following birth injury due to forceps delivery or prolonged labor.
- Facial nerve palsy and congenital absence of depressor angularis oris should be differentiated. In congenital absence of depressor angularis oris, the corner of mouth is moved toward the normal side and the lower lip moves downward and outward, nasolabial fold is not affected.

Vestibulocochlear (VIII) Nerve

Vestibulocochlear is purely sensory nerve. It has two components—vestibular and cochlear. The cochlear division is tested for hearing and vestibular for equilibrium (labyrinthine function).

Vestibular function: It is not tested routinely, but in cases of vertigo, nystagmus, dizziness, and coma. To check for brain death and brainstem functions, caloric test is performed. Before performing caloric test, one should confirm that tympanic membrane is intact.
- A rotational test is performed by keeping the child sitting erect, head tilted forward by 30° and turning him several times, 10 rounds in 20 seconds in a full circle on a revolving chair. One should observe deviation of the eyes and nystagmus. Each ear separately cannot be tested.
  Normally, on rotation, the fast component of nystagmus is on the side of rotation and the slow phase of nystagmus is in the opposite direction. On stopping the rotation, direction of fast and slow phases of nystagmus is reversed.

Hearing assessment:
- Newborns respond to a loud sound by startle response, crying or showing a change in behavior.
- An infant aged >3 months turns to sounds produced by objects such as bell or rattle. For an older child, observe the response to a ticking watch, finger rub, snapping the fingers with thumb or whispers used from behind the back of the child. The child should be asked to repeat the whispered words or numbers. Start snapping the fingers at 10 cm away from the child's ear and ask him on which side the sound is heard. The sound stimulus should not be visible to the child. If the child does not respond, the tuning fork tests should be performed.

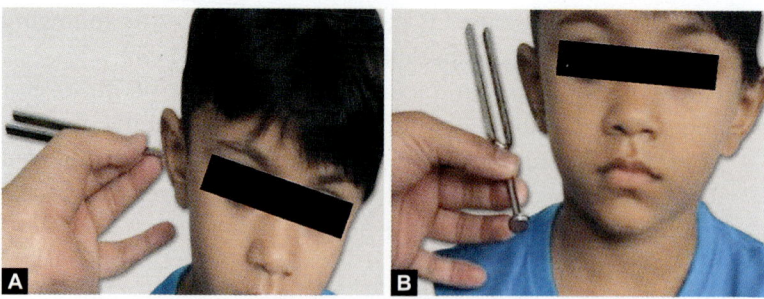

Figs. 7A and B: Rinne's test.

- Rinne test and Weber test can be performed by using a tuning fork of 256 Hz. Hearing should be compared on both sides.
- *Rinne test (Figs. 7A and B):* The tuning fork is held against the mastoid bone for testing bone conduction till the sound is not heard, then the vibrating end is held near the external ear of the same side for the testing air conduction.
  Normally, the air conduction is better than bone conduction. If a reverse of that is found, it suggests conduction abnormalities in the middle ear. In sensorineural defect, both air and bone conduction are affected.
  - Normally, air conduction is better than bone conduction, Rinne test positive.
  - In conductive hearing loss, bone conduction is better than air conduction, Rinne test negative.
  - In sensorineural hearing loss, both air conduction and bone conduction are impaired, retaining their normal relationship of air conduction is better than bone conduction.
- *Weber test (Fig. 8):* The vibrating tuning fork is placed at vertex, glabella or nasal bridge on forehead and the child is asked, in which ear is it better heard?
  - Normally, the sound is equally heard in both the ears.
  - In conducting hearing loss, sound is better heard in the involved ear, lateralized to affected side.
  - In sensorineural hearing loss, sound is heard better in the normal ear, lateralized to normal side.
- *Schwabach test:* The child's hearing by bone conduction is compared with the examiner's hearing by placing the vibrating tuning fork against the child's mastoid process and then

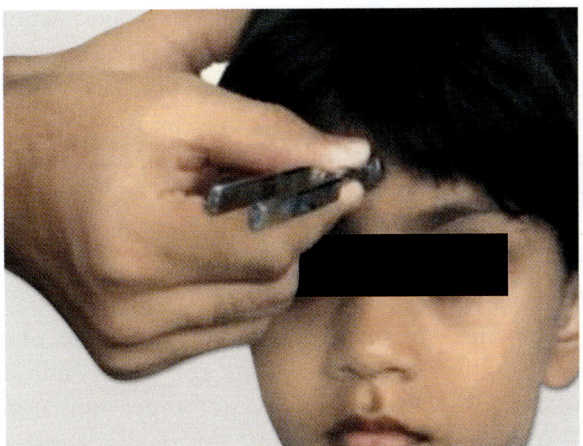

Fig. 8: Weber's test.

> **Box 13:** High risk conditions for hearing deficit.
> - Preterm/low birth weight
> - Neonatal hyperbilirubinemia
> - Craniofacial anomalies
> - Perinatal asphyxia
> - Congenital rubella
> - Cytomegaloviral infection
> - Down syndrome
> - Bacterial meningitis
> - Ototoxic drugs
> - Genetic and familial causes

against examiner's mastoid process. If the examiner can hear the sound after the child has stopped hearing, then it indicates hearing loss is present.
- If hearing impairment is suspected from history and testing, more detailed testing of hearing should be performed by audiometry, brainstem auditory evoked potentials, etc.
- High risk conditions for hearing deficit are listed in **Box 13**.

Glossopharyngeal and Vagus Nerve (IX and X Cranial Nerves)
- Glossopharyngeal nerve carries sensations from the pharynx, tonsils, soft palate, and posterior one-third of the tongue. The motor part of the nerve supplies the stylopharyngeus muscle for the swallowing.

- Vagus nerve controls the pharyngeal constrictor action, palate elevation, and vocal cord action and carries a sensation from the external ear canal, pinna, and behind the ear.
- Both the nerves are tested together by inducing gag reflex and observing the symmetrical retraction of soft palate.
- Ask the child to open the mouth. By throwing light with a torch and depressing the tongue, examine the movements of soft palate and uvula while saying "Ah". Palate should move upward and backward equally on both the sides.
- The gag reflex consists of contraction of the pharyngeal musculature, brief elevation of the soft palate, and elevation of the tongue. The child may get sensation of retching. The response is consensual, the soft palate is elevated and movement is symmetrical regardless of the side touched. Absent reflex suggests peripheral nerve involvement. The afferent fibers of gag reflex are mediated through IX cranial nerve and efferent fibers through IX and X cranial nerves.
- Weak cough reflex indicates involvement of vocal cords.
- Hoarseness of voice, stridor, nasal regurgitation, nasal quality of voice, drooling, and difficulty in swallowing and whispering are manifestations of involvement of IX and X cranial nerves.
- In unilateral IX cranial nerve involvement, there will be no response on touching the affected side. In unilateral vagus nerve involvement, regardless of which side of the pharynx is touched, the palate fails to rise and the uvula deviates toward normal side during palatal movements.
- Isolated involvement of IX cranial nerve is rare, but unilateral X cranial nerve involvement produces weakness of soft palate on the same side and hoarseness of voice due to vocal cord palsy.
- Common conditions involving these two nerves are listed in **Box 14**.
- *Bulbar palsy:* Involvement of bulbar nerves (IX to XII cranial nerves from medulla).
- *Pseudobulbar palsy:* Bilateral involvement of corticobulbar fibers to bulbar nuclei presenting as exaggerated gag reflex seen with spastic quadriplegic cerebral palsy, brainstem tumors, encephalitis, head injury, Gaucher disease, and neurodegenerative diseases.

> **Box 14:** Common conditions involving IX and X cranial nerves.
> - Diphtheria
> - Botulism
> - Bulbar palsy
> - Guillain–Barré syndrome
> - Poliomyelitis
> - Posterior fossa tumor
> - Trauma
> - Encephalitis
> - Demyelinating diseases
> - Tuberculous meningitis

Spinal Accessory Nerve (XI Cranial Nerve)

- It is a pure motor nerve and supplies to trapezins and sternocleidomastoid muscle.
- The nerve is tested by asking the child to shrug the shoulders and feeling for the strength of the trapezius. If the muscle is affected, the child cannot uplift the shoulders.
- Another test is there to place one hand against the right side of child's face and then ask him to turn the head against the hand, the left contracting muscle becomes prominent and can be palpated. Compare both the sides. Another method for testing this muscle, from both sides simultaneously, is by placing hand on the child's forehead, asking him to bend forward, and observing the prominence of muscle on both the sides. The function of this muscle is to rotate the head to opposite side.
- In the newborn, sternocleidomastoid muscle's strength can be indirectly assessed by observing head flexion on the traction response, by observing the resting head posture and by spontaneous head rotation.
- Involvement is seen in dystrophies, spinal muscular atrophy, poliomyelitis, myasthenia gravis, etc.

Hypoglossal Nerve (XII Cranial Nerve)

- Hypoglossal nerve supplies to the muscles of tongue. It is a pure motor nerve.
- It can be examined by observing the tongue in resting position on the floor of the mouth followed by asking the child to protrude the tongue.

- Look for fasciculations (muscular twitching involving the simultaneous contraction of contiguous groups of muscle fibers), atrophy, asymmetry, and deviation.
- Look for movement by asking the child to move the tongue in and out, push tongue side to side against the cheek, and produce lingual speech sounds.
- If hypoglossal nerve is affected on one side, the protruded tongue will deviate on the same side of weakness. It is due to unopposed action of normal genioglossus muscle to push the tongue to the opposite side.
- In bilateral involvement, protrusion of tongue is weak or absent. UMN lesions of the XII cranial nerve are rare and may be seen in cerebral palsy.
- Fasciculation of tongue is characteristic of spinomuscular atrophy (SMA).

Normal cranial nerve examination can be summarized as shown in **Box 15**.

Motor System Examination

The components of motor system are shown in **Box 16**.

Box 15: Summary of normal nerves examination.

- Child is able to identify things by seeing (II), smell (I) and taste (VII and IX)
- Movements of eyeballs normal (III, IV, VI)
- No deviation of angle of mouth, facial asymmetry or drooling of saliva (VII)
- Hearing normal (VIII)
- No difficulty in chewing (V) and swallowing (IX and X)
- No regurgitation of feeds (IX and X)
- Able to turn face side to side (XI)
- Movements of tongue normal (XII)

Box 16: Components of motor system examination.

- Muscle tone
- Muscle bulk (nutrition, wasting)
- Muscle power
- Coordination
- Involuntary movements

Muscle Tone

Muscle tone is defined as continuous and passive partial contraction of the muscles due to minimal continuous motor electrical discharge. It helps to maintain the posture.

On clinical examination, muscle tone is the resistance to passive stretching and movement when the muscle is at rest. Muscle tone can be normal, decreased or increased. Reduced muscle tone is called hypotonia and increased muscle tone is called hypertonia. Hypotonia and increased mobility due to neurological causes should be differentiated from hyperextensibility of joints due to other causes.

Muscle tone can be assessed on inspection, palpation, and measuring range of movements.

- *Inspection:* Abnormal posture may be due to hypertonia, as example, adduction of upper limb against trunk and flexion at elbow is seen in a patient with spastic hemiplegia. Hypertonia of lower limb may be manifested by circumduction at hip and adduction of thigh. Opisthotonus is the best example of increased trunkal extensor tone resulting in arching of the body **(Fig. 9)**.

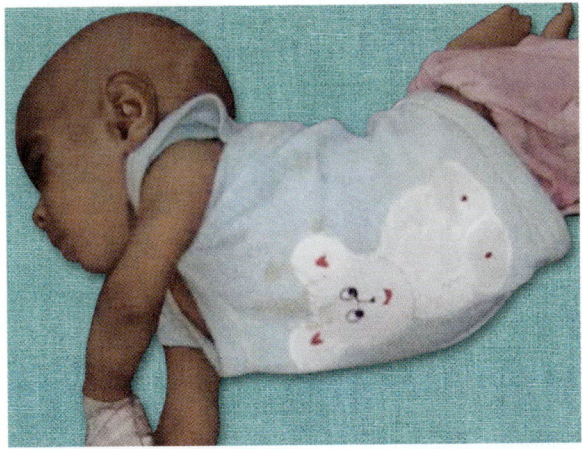

Fig. 9: Opisthotonus: a spasm wherein the head and the heels are bent back making the body like a bow in extreme cases of tetanus and tuberculous meningitis.

Decorticate rigidity **(Fig. 10 and Box 17)** and decerebrate rigidity **(Fig. 11 and Box 18)** should be differentiated. It indicates site of lesion as well as possible prognosis. A frog-like position of lower limbs (abduction at hip and flexion at knee) indicates hypotonia.

- *Palpation:* Palpation of muscle gives the feeling regarding tone of muscle, firm (normal), flabby and soft (hypotonia), and stiff (hypertonia).
- *Resistance to passive stretching (range of movements):*
    - The testing of muscle tone is done by putting the major joints through their full range of movements and noting up to what degree range of movement is possible.
    - When the child resists voluntarily, his attention can be diverted by talking or asking the questions.
    - Passive movements of the major joints in the upper limb (elbow and wrist) and the lower limbs (knee and ankle) are conventional and reliable methods for assessing muscle tone. The difference in the tone is noted at each joint and compared with normal.

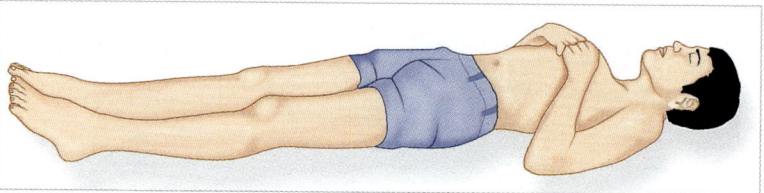

Fig. 10: Decorticate rigidity.

Box 17: Decorticate rigidity.

- Abnormal flexor response
- Consisting of rigid extension of the lower limbs and flexion and supination of arms and fisting of hands
- Maintenance of this body posture is by midbrain of red nucleus without inhibition of diencephalon, basal ganglia and cortical structures
- Lack of cerebral and diencephalic control over brainstem
- Prognosis is favorable

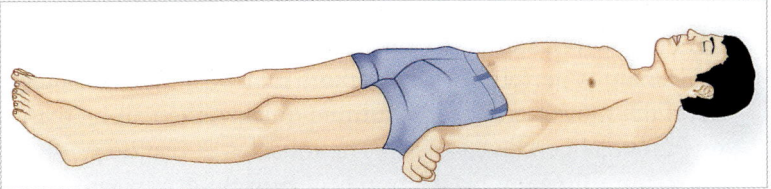

Fig. 11: Decerebrate rigidity.

> **Box 18:** Decerebrate rigidity.
> - Abnormal extensor response
> - Consisting of rigid extension of legs, arms, trunk and head with hyperpronation of arms
> - Lesion is in diencephalon, midbrain or pons
> - Prognosis is not favorable

Flappability: Shake the limb to and fro and observe the movements of distal joint. For example, shake the forearm and observe the movements of wrist. If there is hypotonia, the movements of wrist (flappibility) will be increased. If there is hypertonia, the movements of wrist will be decreased.

- Muscle tone can be decreased by certain drugs like diazepam, severe malnutrition, hypokalemia, renal tubular acidosis, etc. It may also be increased due to anxiety or pain.
- Other causes of hypotonia are LMN lesions like poliomyelitis, Guillain–Barré syndrome and spinal shock, cerebellar lesions, and basal ganglia diseases like rheumatic chorea, etc.
- In the presence of contractures, assessment of muscle tone is difficult.
- Involuntary movements interfere in eliciting muscle tone and may be variable.

Types of hypertonia: Two types of hypertonia are seen in the practice, clasp knife spasticity which results from pyramidal tract lesions and lead pipe or cog wheel rigidity which results from extrapyramidal lesions.

- *Clasp knife spasticity:* There is initial resistance to a fairly rapid passive movement with sudden giving way toward the end

of the movement, flexion or extension. This is a velocity-dependent resistance to the muscle stretch, if the passive movement is performed slowly, there may be a little resistance, but if the movements are performed quickly, then an increased resistance is perceived easily. The muscles at rest do not have more tone but any brisk stretch of muscle group will result in a "catch" at about mid-length of the muscle followed by release of the catch and relaxation of the muscle. The catch and the release have been linked to a closing pen knife, which is the origin of the term clasp knife spasticity. The spasticity is easily felt in the flexon group of muscles of the upper limb and extensors of the lower limb.
- *Rigidity:* There is same resistance in agonist and antagonist muscle group at any point giving rise to same degrees of hypertonia on passive movements. It is not velocity dependent. Rigidity is described as cogwheel if the resistance is stepwise or as a lead pipe if the resistance is uniform to passive movement.

Other methods of assessment of muscle tone:
- *Range of angles in infancy (Amiel-Tison):*
  - It is by visual assessment. The infant should be calm and not crying. Note the angle and compare with the age norms **(Table 4)**. Do not do movement forcibly. If the child starts crying, stop it. The head should be in midline.
  - *Adductor angle:* Place a finger on femoral diaphysis and abduct both lower limbs as fast as possible **(Fig. 12)**.

Table 4: Normal ranges of angles in infancy (Amiel–Tison).

	0–3 months	4–6 months	7–9 months	10–12 months
Adductor angle	40–80	70–110	100–140	140–170
Popliteal angle	80–100	90–120	110–160	150–170
Dorsiflexion angle	60–70	60–70	60–70	60–70
Scarf sign	Does not reach midline	Reaches midline	Crosses midline	Reaches opposite shoulder

- *Popliteal angle:* Flex both the thighs by the side of the abdomen and extend both the knees simultaneously. The popliteal angle, which is formed by the calf and the thigh, is estimated in both legs simultaneously **(Fig. 13)**. Compare the angles on both the sides. Significant asymmetry is indicated by a difference of 10–20° between both the sides.
- *Dorsiflexion angle of the foot:* Hold the infant's leg straight and flex the foot towards the leg. The dorsiflexion angle is formed between the dorsum of the foot and the anterior aspect of the leg **(Fig. 14)**. It is performed in two phases. First, a slow moderate pressure is applied to measure

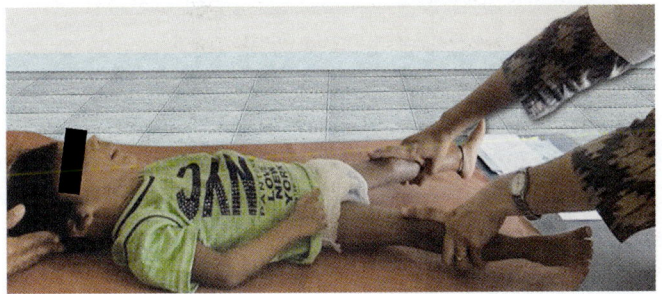

Fig. 12: Assessing the adductor angle.

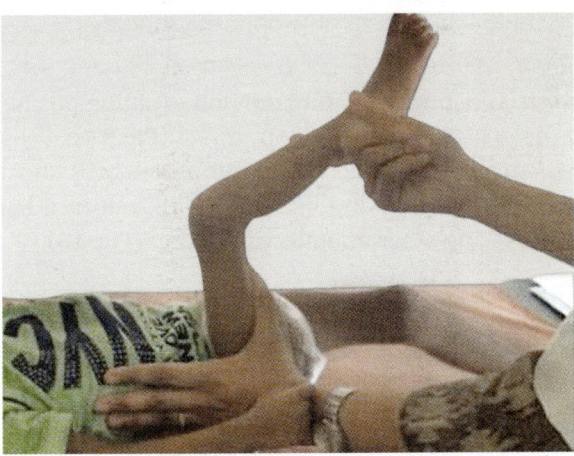

Fig. 13: Assessing popliteal angle.

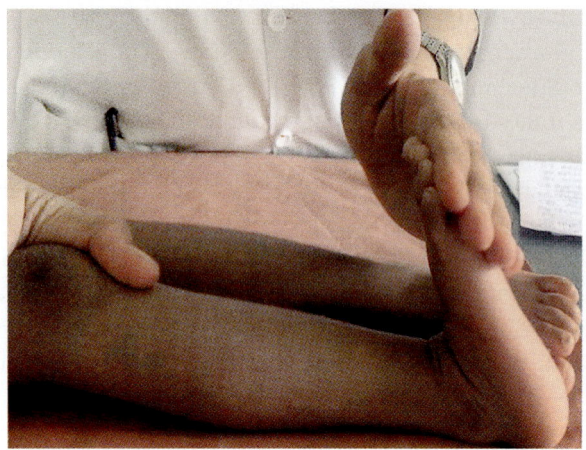

Fig. 14: Assessing dorsiflexion angle.

smallest dorsiflexion angle (slow angle). Then, sudden quick flexion is performed and the angle is measured (rapid angle). Normally, both the angles are equal. A difference between the rapid and slow angles of >10° indicates exaggerated stretch reflex.
- *Scarf sign:* Hold the infant in semi-reclining position. Pull the infant's arm as far as possible across the chest toward opposite shoulder. Note whether the elbow does not reach midline, crosses midline or reaches the opposite shoulder.

Tests for floppy infant:
- *Pull to sit:* Grasp with thumb and pull to sitting position. There will be head lag in a case of floppy infant **(Fig. 15)**.
- *Vertical suspension:* The hypotonic infant will slip through. A floppy infant will hang like a rag doll, but in a hypertonic infant scissoring of lower limbs will exhibit **(Fig. 16)**.

Muscle Bulk (Muscle Nutrition, Muscle Wasting)

Before examining for muscle bulk, one should consider the child's age, built, constitution, obesity, etc.
- Put the limbs in the symmetrical position and look for wasting of the muscles by inspection and palpation, if it is, decide which muscle is wasted and flabby on palpation.

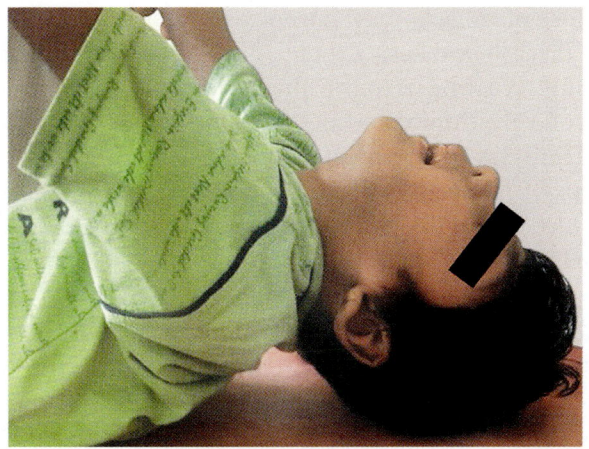

Fig. 15: Pull to sit in a floppy infant. Note the complete head lag.

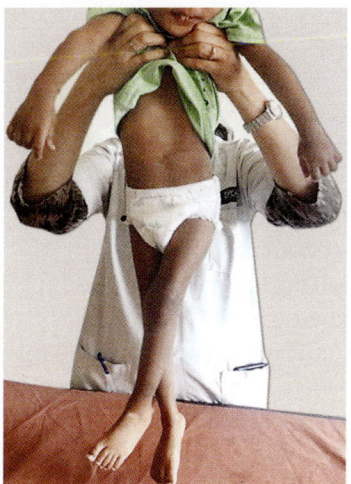

Fig. 16: Scissoring of the lower limbs in a hypertonic child on vertical suspense.

- Measure the circumference of the muscles with maximum bulk, not crossing the joints and at defined distance with reference to bony landmark, e.g., 15 cm above the medial malleolus of lower end of tibia and compare on both sides.
- Difference of 1 cm in muscle girth is significant.

- The loss of muscle bulk (atrophy or wasting) may be due to LMN disease or disuse atrophy. It may be a part of generalized wasting. Wasting is more marked in proximal muscles in muscular dystrophy and poliomyelitis, while it is more so in distal muscles in peripheral neuropathy.
- Localized muscle wasting is suggesting neurological condition like old poliomyelitis, old spastic hemiplegia, injuries, spina bifida, etc.
- Hypertrophy of the muscles can be either localized or generalized and may be due to pseudohypertrophy as seen in Duchenne muscular dystrophy and Becker muscular dystrophy involving mainly calf muscles. Generalized hypertrophy is seen in myotonia congenita and Kocher–Debre–Semelaigne syndrome (hypothyroidism and pseudohypertrophy of calf muscles).

Muscle Power

Muscle power (strength) is defined as the force of contraction that can be generated by an active contraction of each muscle or muscle group. It is graded as 0 to 5 as described in **Table 5**.

- Ideally, individual muscle should be tested, but practically it is difficult. In clinical practice, muscle groups are tested and it provides fairly good information.
- Informal testing of muscle power can be done by simply observing the child. See whether child is ambulatory, playing, transferring an object from one hand to another, walking, running, jumping,

Table 5: Grades of muscle power.

Grade	Movement
0	No movement at all
1	Flickering present
2	Active movement with gravity elimination (side to side movement)
3	Active movement against gravity
4	Active movement against gravity + some resistance
5	Active movements against gravity + full resistance (normal power)

getting up from supine to sitting position, and from sitting to standing or climbing steps.
- The muscle power can be tested by active or passive movements. Start distally, move proximally. Compare both sides.
- The child is asked to perform flexion, extension, supination, pronation, etc. by contracting a group of muscles at a specific joint using maximum power while the examiner tries to prevent it by using a greater force. For example, the child is asked to flex the elbow and the examiner will try to prevent the movement.

  In another method, the group of muscles is put in the final position by completing the movement and he is asked to maintain the same position while the examiner tries to oppose this motion. For example, the child keeps the elbow flexed and tries to keep it flexed while the examiner tries to extend it. Each movement should be tested against resistance.
- Muscle power is tested at all major and small joints, testing all movements occurring at the joint.
- *Some of the tests for declining muscle power are given as follows:*
  - The test for biceps in upper limb is done by asking the child to flex the elbow with his palm facing upward, while triceps can be tested by asking the child to extend the arm **(Fig. 17)**.

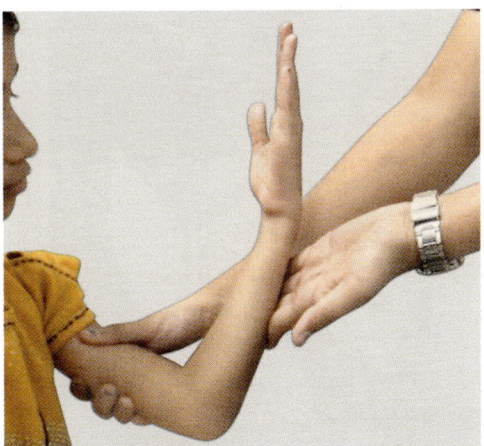

Fig. 17: Testing the power of triceps muscles. Note that the patient is asking to extend the elbow against resistance offered.

- The deltoid muscles can be tested by asking the child to raise his arms above the head.
- The hamstrings (knee flexors) can be tested by knee flexion **(Fig. 18)**.
- The quadriceps can be tested by asking the child to extend the knee while he is sitting on edge of the cot **(Fig. 19)**.
- When the child pushes down the examiner's palm with soles of foot, the power of gastrocnemius and soleus muscles is assessed.

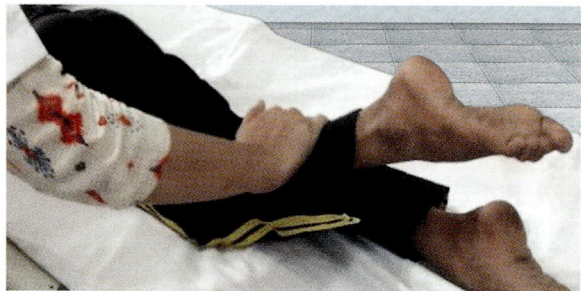

Fig. 18: Knee flexion, testing the power of knee flexors, hamstrings. Ask the child to lie prone. Ask him to flex the knee joint and offer the resistance.

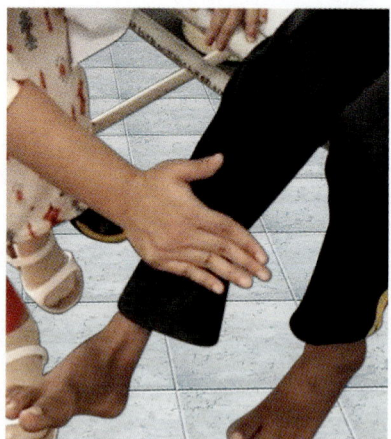

Fig. 19: Knee extension, testing the power of knee extensors. Child should sit with the legs dangling. Ask the child to extend the knee and offer the resistance.

- The ability to stand up from the lying down position requires good muscle power in both pelvic girdle and leg muscles.
- In unconscious child, raise both arms and let them fall back, followed by checking the legs by flexing the knees with soles of feet touching the bed together and then letting them fall back. Observe the difference, weak limb will fall rapidly than the normal one.
- Gower sign is solicited by asking the child to get up from a prone position or squatting position. The child uses his hands as support, and climbs on himself to get into an upright position. It indicates the proximal weakness of pelvic girdle muscles and muscles of lower limbs. It is typically seen in patients suffering from Duchenne muscular dystrophy.
- Testing the hand muscle is shown in **Figures 20A to N**.

Coordination

Coordination is a complex function of muscles. It is the result of intact motor and sensory systems, cerebellar function, and proprioception. Therefore, incoordination is seen in pyramidal and extrapyramidal disorders of motor control, sensory system involvement, and cerebellar disorders.

- To test coordination, one should assess the speed, rhythm, and accuracy of repetitive movements.
- Coordination can be informally assessed in the limbs and trunk by observing the gait during walking, playing, buttoning, unbuttoning, wearing shoes, writing, drinking water with a glass or eating with a spoon.
- It is tested formally in the children aged beyond 6 years.
- Besides cerebellar disorders, coordination can also be affected by visual acuity and sensory losses.
- Ataxia is the most common manifestation of incoordination which results due to affection of cerebellum and proprioceptive sensations.

Tests for coordination in upper limbs:
- *Finger to finger and finger to nose test* **(Figs. 21A and B)**: Ask the child to fully extend and abduct the arm and then to touch

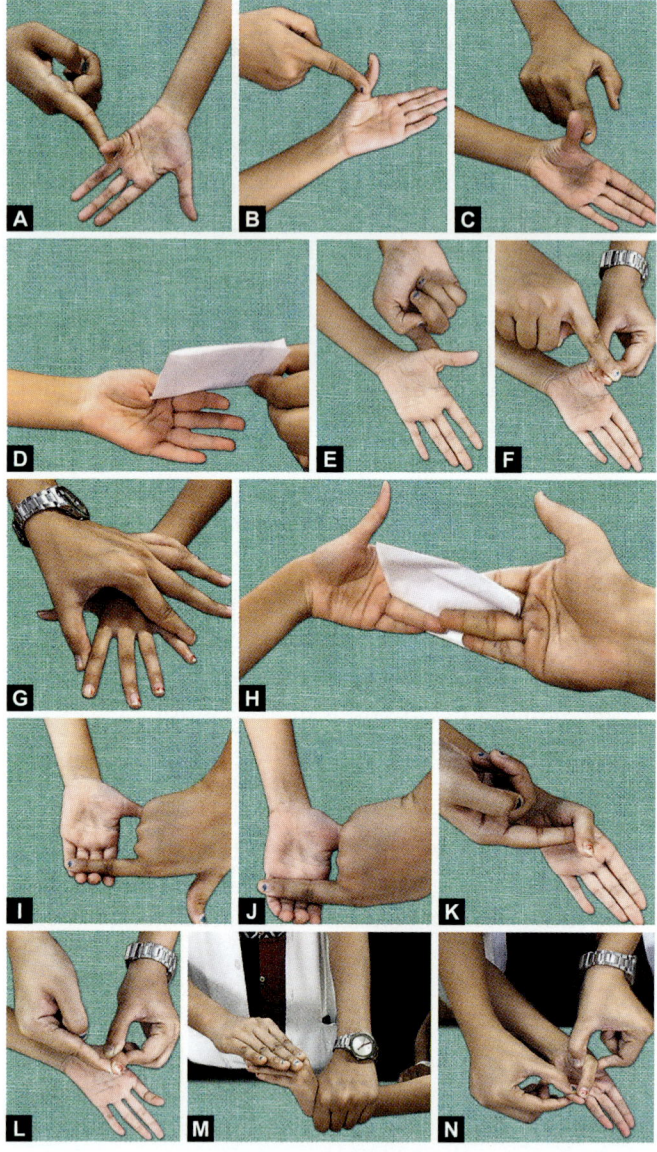

Figs. 20A to N: Testing hand muscles. (A) Abductor digiti minimi; (B) Abductor pollicis brevis; (C) Abductor pollicis; (D) Abductor pollicis card test; (E) Extensor pollicis brevis; (F) Extensor pollicis longus; (G) Finger abductors; (H) Finger adductors; (I) Flexor digitorum profundus; (J) Flexor digitorum sublimus; (K) Flexor pollicis brevis; (L) Flexor pollicis longus; (M) Lumbricals; (N) Opponens pollicis.

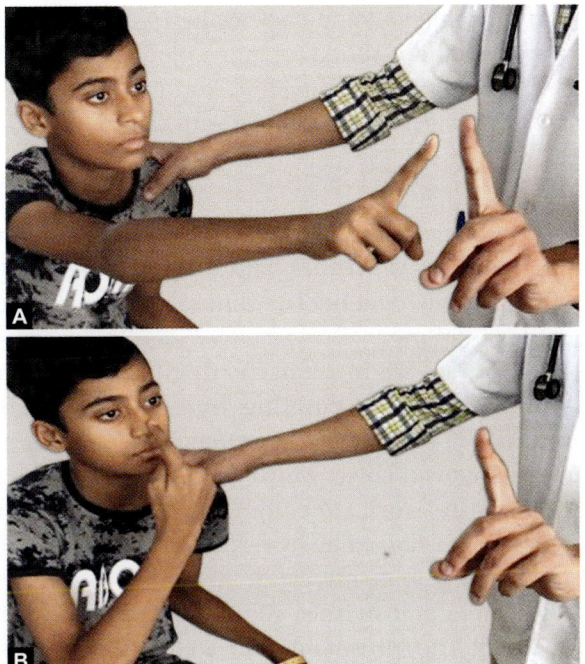

Figs. 21A and B: Finger–finger and finger–nose test to assess coordination. It results in overshooting or undershooting in a case of cerebellar disorder. It is called as dysmetria.

the tip of his nose rapidly with the index finger with hand in mid prone position. The accuracy of touching the tip of nose should be observed. This test should be performed from both sides with eyes open and closed. It is followed by nose-finger-nose test, in which the second target is the tip of examiner's finger. By this test, tremors can also be seen. In cerebellar disorders, the child overshoots the tip of nose.

- *Dysdiadochokinesia:* It is the inability of the child to perform rapid alternative movements such as pronation and supination of the forearm rapidly. It is indicating cerebellar lesion.

Tests for coordination in lower limbs: It is performed when the child is lying in supine position. The child is asked to raise one leg and bring the heel of the foot of that leg down accurately onto the knee of the resting leg and after touching it, move the heel smoothly down the shin of tibia to the foot and back again. In cerebellar disorders, the heel may overshoot the knee, movements may be slow and zigzag, the heel may fall off the shin. For assessment of sensory ataxia, ask the child to perform this test with closed eyes.

Involuntary Movements

Observe the child at rest as well as when he is doing some activities like holding the objects, writing, and playing to see whether he has any abnormal movement. The different types of involuntary movements are as follows:

- *Tremors:* Tremors are involuntary, rhythmic, to and fro alternating movements, resembling trembling or oscillations. Tremors may be present at rest or may develop when the child is reaching out to an object which is called as intention tremors. The intention tremors are common with cerebellar disease. They can also be caused by hyperthyroidism, anxiety or drugs like salbutamol, terbutaline, etc.
- *Tics:* These are habit spasms, commonly seen over face, neck, and shoulders. They do not interfere with voluntary movements. They are stereotype, repetitive, rapid, and transient at the same location or restricted to a muscle group. Tics increase during the period of stress. Head nodding, eye blinking, and shoulder movements are examples of various tics.
- *Chorea:* These are rapid, sudden, and jerky movements. These are nonrepetitive and quasi purposive which may be generalized or localized. Involvement of proximal joints is more common than the distal joints. They increase with stress and anxiety but disappear during sleep. The causes include rheumatic chorea (Sydenham chorea), adverse effects of anticonvulsant drugs, Wilson disease, Huntington chorea, etc. Chorea is due to lesions in the caudate nucleus.
- *Athetosis:* Athetosis is characterized by slow, involuntary, nonrhythmic movements of axial rotation with hyperextension of the limbs. These are due to basal ganglia involvement. Athetosis is known to occur in rheumatic fever and Wilson disease. The lesion is in putamen nucleus.
- *Ballismus:* These are rapid, violent, repetitive, and irregular movements affecting proximal joints and have a constant location,

commonly shoulders and hips. Hemiballismus is common with the lesions in contralateral subthalamic nuclei.
- *Dystonia:* These are spontaneous, involuntary movements. There are sustained muscle contractions that force the affected part of the body into abnormal twisted movements and posture. There may be contractions of agonist and antagonist muscles simultaneously. These are rapid with slow relaxation. It is due to involvement of extrapyramidal system.
- *Myoclonus:* It is a sudden, rapid, and jerk-like movement. There is repetitive contraction of a single muscle or a group of muscles. It may be generalized or localized. It may be flexion spasm of myoclonus epilepsy.
- *Fasciculations:* These are rapid involuntary contractions of one or more units of muscles and are visible just like a flicker on the skin. It is due to inflammation or degeneration of anterior horn cells.

Sensory Systems

Sensory system examination is a difficult task in CNS examination. It requires cooperation from the child and tests are subjective and therefore wide variations may be observed in its interpretation by different examiners. Practically, detailed sensory system testing may not be needed in each child and may not be possible. It will be definitely indicated in a patient with suspected spinal cord disorder, syringomyelia, peripheral nerve disease, etc.

Sensations can be superficial (touch, pain, temperature), deep (vibration, joint position), and cortical (stereognosis, point location, two-point discrimination, graphesthesia, etc.).
- Older child may complain of some points indicating involvement of sensory like loss of sensations (anesthesia), exaggerated sensation (hyperesthesia), tingling, numbness, and burning sensations.
- Peripheral neuropathy is the most common cause of sensory loss in children.
- Lateral spinothalamic tracts carry pain and temperature sensations while ventral spinothalamic tracts carry crude touch sensation and firm pressure to thalamus and then to parietal

cortex sensory area. Dorsal column including tracts of fasciculus gracilis carries the sensations of the touch, vibration, and sense of position.
- Before testing for sensory system, the child should be explained in detail and the test to be demonstrated to him with eyes open. While actual testing, his eyes should be closed.
- Sensory system examination includes test for touch, pain, temperature, vibration, and joint position.
- Light touch testing is done by using a cotton wisp and asking the child to say yes when he feels the touch. Pain can be tested with the sharp and the blunt end of a ball pen and it should be tested after testing for touch sensation. Do not use a needle to test the pain.
- Start with the area that is impaired and go proximal and distal to define the boundaries.
- Compare the sensations on both the sides, distally and proximally and see whether it is symmetrical or asymmetrical.
- If superficial touch and pain sensations are impaired, then check for the temperature by using cold and hot test tubes.
- Deep pain is tested by squeezing the calf muscles and Achilles tendons.
- Pressure is tested in a similar way to testing touch with firm pressure with examiner's finger or thumb.
- Sensory deficit of pain, touch, and temperature suggests peripheral neuropathy. **Table 6** shows the areas affected and their dermatomes.

Table 6: Areas of sensory loss and their dermatomes.

Surface	Dermatome
Lateral surface of upper arm	C5
Tip of the thumb	C6
Medial surface of upper arm	T2
Medial surface of lower arm	T1
Middle of anterior thigh	L2
Medial side of calf	L4
Lateral side of calf	L5
Sole of the foot	S1

Vibration Sensation (Proprioceptive Sensation)

- It is tested by putting a vibrating low frequency tuning fork (128 Hz) on the bony prominence starting from distal parts like big toe, medial malleolus of tibia, radial, and ulnar tuberosities, etc. Other parts are patella, iliac crest, spinous processes, sternum, skull, etc. The child should be explained the difference between touch and vibration sensation.
- Ask the child whether he perceives vibrations. If yes, then ask him to inform you the point when he feels cessation of vibrations. Compare with yourself. If you still perceive and the patient does not, then it indicates vibration sensation is impaired.
- Sensations of vibration and position are lost in subacute combined degeneration of spinal cord and Friedreich ataxia.

Sense of Joint Position (Proprioceptive Sensation)

- Hold the joint to be tested. For example, hold the great toe by thumb and index finger, then move from side to side while the proximal part is held fixed.
- Explain the different joint positions like neutral, up or down by demonstration.
- Ask the child to close the eyes and repeat the test by moving the joint in one position. Ask the child regarding position of joint.
- Return the digit to the neutral position before moving it in some other direction randomly. The child should tell the examiner the correct position. Test both the sides.
- Romberg sign is also the test for proprioception. It can be tested in children more than 5 years of age. It is described with cerebellar signs.

Cortical Sensations

Cortical sensations are as shown in **Box 19**. These tests assess contralateral parietal lobe functions. Before testing, explain the child in details and ask him to close the eyes.

- *Stereognosis:* It can be tested in children more than 5 years of age. The coins, keys or small balls like common objects are used for testing stereognosis. Ask the child to close the eyes and to identify the object given in his hands.

> **Box 19:** Cortical sensations.
> - Stereognosis
> - Graphesthesia
> - Two-point discrimination
> - Point location
> - Extinction phenomenon
> - Barognosis

- *Graphesthesia:* This test can be tested conclusively in children more than 8 years of age. Before testing, explain him in detail and then ask him to close the eyes. Write some number on his palm and ask him to answer which number was written on his palm. It is an ability to identify written numbers or letters on child's skin. If he is not able to do, it is called as graphesthesia. It indicates loss of cortical sensation.
- *Two-point discrimination:* This test is inconclusive for children up to 6 years of age. The special caliper manufactured for this purpose is used for this test. Distal fingers and lips are very sensitive and can discriminate 3–4 mm of separation.
- *Point location (topognosis):* It is the ability to localize the stimuli given at different parts of body with closed eyes.
- *Sensory extinction:* Two stimuli are applied at two identical points on each side. Ask the child to describe how many spots are being touched. Normally, both sides are felt but with sensory lesion, the person will sense only one.
- *Barognosis:* It is the ability to appreciate the difference of the weight on both sides by putting two similar objects with same size and shape but different weight. The objects are given to the child and asked if they weigh different or same.

Examination of Reflexes

The reflex is an involuntary motor response to a sensory stimulus or muscle stretch. For elicitation of a reflex, a spinal reflex arc should be intact. Spinal reflex arc is formed by receptors, afferent nerve fibers carrying signals from sensory limb, an integrating center, efferent nerve fibers carrying signals from the anterior horn cells to the muscle, and the effector muscle which is innervated by efferent nerve fibers that carries out the response.

The reflexes are classified as superficial and deep reflexes. Primitive reflexes are described in the chapter on neonate. These reflexes are also called as developmental reflexes as they appear at birth and disappear in due course of time and are replaced by voluntary movements as the cortical control develops with neurological maturity. Absence of these reflexes or incomplete development at the time of birth is considered as abnormal and signifies neurological developmental disorder or some other reason. Persistence of these reflexes beyond their time to disappear is of great importance, may be an early marker of cerebral palsy or cortical dysfunction. Reappearing of primitive reflexes in some unconscious patient is of great concern.

Superficial Reflexes

Superficial reflexes include corneal reflex, conjunctival reflex, abdominal reflexes **(Fig. 22)**, cremasteric reflex, anal reflex, and plantar reflex **(Figs. 23A and B)**. Corneal and conjunctival reflexes are described with cranial nerve examination and rest are shown in **Table 7**.

- Superficial reflexes are diminished or lost in UMN lesions and plantar response is extensor.

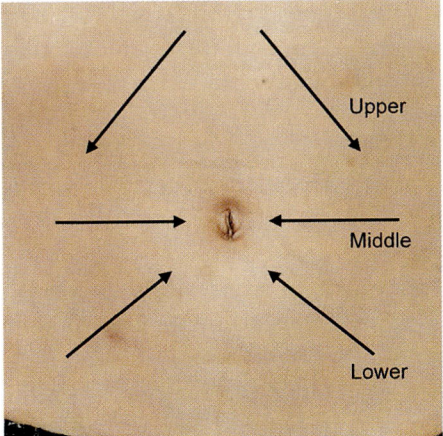

Fig. 22: Eliciting the abdominal reflexes: The abdominal wall is stroked (sharp and gentle) below the costal margins from medial to lateral side. The skin of the lower quadrant is stroked from the lateral to the medial side. This elicits contraction of the muscles of the abdominal wall.

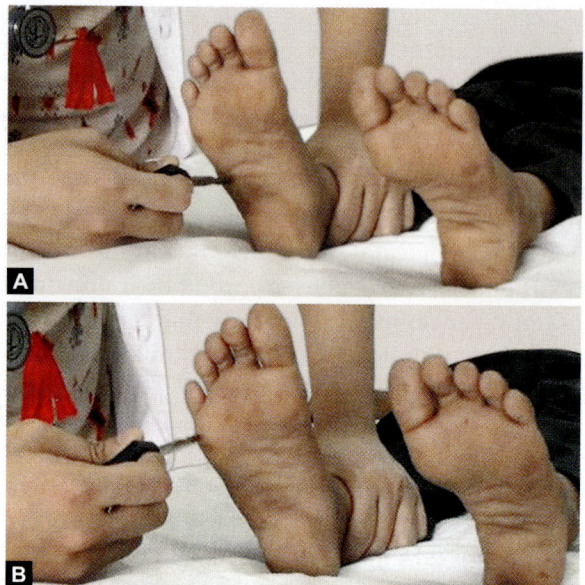

Figs. 23A and B: Elicitation of planter reflex.

- In superficial reflexes, the sensory signal has to not only reach the spinal cord, but also the brain. The motor limb then has to descend the spinal cord to reach the motor neurons. Therefore, these reflexes are lost in conditions that interrupt the pathway between brain and spinal cord.

Deep Tendon Reflexes

These are also known as stretch reflexes. The successful elicitation of deep tendon reflexes (DTRs) requires skill and certain points to be observed as follows:
- The child should be comfortable, relaxed, and properly positioned. Proper exposure of the area to be examined is an important point.
- The examiner should hold the hammer by his thumb and index finger, his movements should be free and at the wrist, not at elbow. The force of the stroke should be sufficient to elicit the reflex. The stroke should be quick, sudden, sharp at the targeted point, and forceful as necessary. The targeted point should be decided by palpation of the tendon.

Table 7: Superficial reflexes and their responses.

Name of the reflex	Spinal nerve roots	Method of elicitation	Interpretation of response
Abdominal reflexes	T6 to T12	Stroke the skin lightly over the abdomen from lateral to medial side with a key or blunt end of hammer in upper (medial to lateral), middle and lower quadrants	• Underlying muscle contracts and umbilicus moves in that direction • Absent abdominal reflexes and brisk deep tendon reflexes indicate pyramidal tract lesions • Upper abdominal reflexes present, but lower abdominal reflexes absent indicating level of spinal lesion
Plantar reflex	L5–S1	Stroking the lateral aspect of the sole from heel to little toe, and then medially from the base of the toes to a great toe with the blunt object like a key	• *Flexor plantar response*: Plantar flexion of the great toe, along with flexion and adduction of other toes • *Extensor plantar response*: Extension (dorsiflexion) of the great toe and fanning of other toes. It is also called as Babinski response. In infants (<1 year), Babinski sign may be positive (extensor response) normally
Cremasteric reflex (in males)	L1–L2	Stroke a line along the medial aspect of upper thigh, watching the movement of testis in scrotum	Elevation of the testis on the same side
Anal reflex	S3–S4	Stroking the perianal area	Contraction of the anal sphincter

- After eliciting the reflex, watch its response, normal, diminished, absent or exaggerated. Look for contraction of muscle and not merely movement of joint.
- Deep tendon reflex should be tested on both sides and compared simultaneously.
- If the reflex (knee jerk) is not elicitable in an alert child, reinforcement methods should be used to distract his attention. He is asked to hook his hands together with flexed fingers and pull them apart as hard as possible and then DTR is tested.

- The methods of eliciting DTR are shown in **Figures 24 to 26**.
- The grading of DTR is shown in **Table 8**.
- The methods of eliciting DTR, their spinal nerve roots, and responses are shown in **Table 9**.
- Ankle clonus can be elicited by bending a knee in a partly flexed position. Take the foot of the patient in your hand at the distal end and quickly dorsiflex with fingers and maintain in same position **(Fig. 27)**. Look for rhythmic oscillations at the ankle joint.

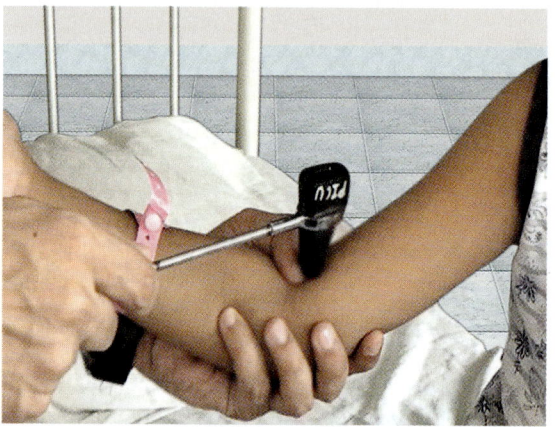

Fig. 24: Elicitation of biceps jerk.

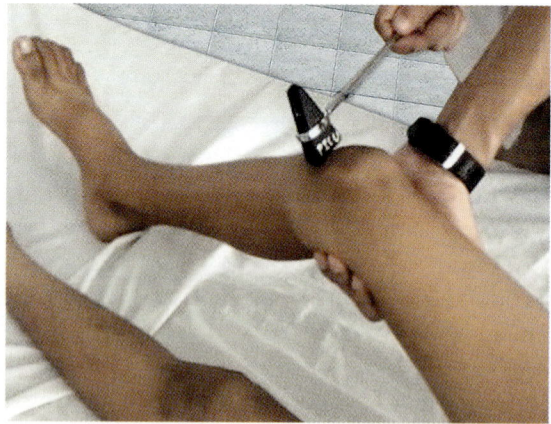

Fig. 25: Elicitation of knee jerk.

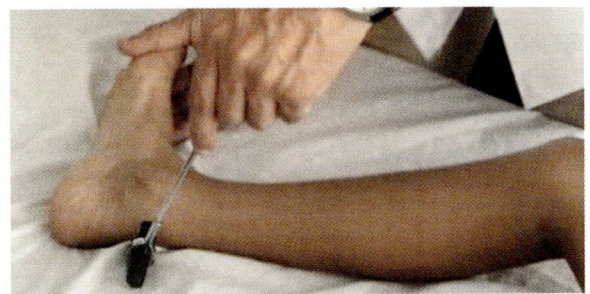

Fig. 26: Elicitation of ankle jerk.

Table 8: Grading of deep tendon reflex.	
Grade	Reflex
O	Absent
+	Present but diminished
++	Normal response
+++	Brisk/exaggerated/hyperactive
++++	Marked hyperactive with clonus

Table 9: Deep tendon reflexes, their spinal nerve roots, method of elicitation, and responses.			
Name of the reflex	Spinal nerve roots	Method of elicitation	Response
Biceps	C5–C6	The child's arm should be partially flexed at elbow. Percuss with hammer on a finger placed over biceps tendon in the antecubital fossa	Visible contraction of biceps muscle and flexion of the elbow
Triceps	C7–C8	In lying down position, flex arm at the elbow at 90° and hold it close to the chest. Percuss the triceps tendon directly above the elbow	Visible contraction of triceps muscle and extension of elbow

Contd...

Contd…

Name of the reflex	Spinal nerve roots	Method of elicitation	Response
Brachioradialis (Supinator)	C5–C6	Flex the child's arm and rest his slightly pronated forearm on examiner's forearm. Strike 1–2 inches above the wrist	Supination and flexion of the forearm and contractions of brachioradialis muscle
Knee jerk (Patellar jerk)	L3–L4	If the child is lying down, flex his knee. The knee should be at angle of about 130°. Keep your one hand below both the knee, supported by forearm and percuss the quadriceps tendon (not patella) directly with the hammer	Note the contraction of the quadriceps and extension of knees
Ankle jerk (Achilles jerk)	S1–S2	Externally rotated legs of the child, with knee and hip slightly flexed. Dorsiflex foot at the ankle. Percuss the Achilles tendon	Look for plantar flexion at the ankle and contraction of the calf muscles

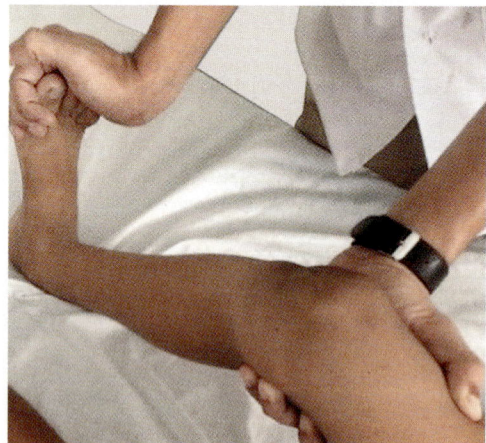

Fig. 27: Elicitation of ankle clonus.

More than six oscillations are considered as sustained clonus. It indicates UMN lesion. Ill-sustained clonus may be seen in the newborns and young infants normally.
- Patellar clonus is elicited in a supine child with extended lower limbs. The upper end of patella should be grasped with one end while the other hand should steady and fix the leg below the knee joint. A brisk downward thrust to the upper end of patella can lead to rapid patellar movements if it is positive **(Fig. 28)**.
- The interpretation of DTR should be done with reference to other features of UMN lesions like spasticity and plantar extensor response.
- Deep tendon reflex may be transiently absent in spinal shock due to UMN lesion, but the plantar reflex remains extensor.
- *Hoffman sign:* It is one of the latent reflexes that appears in spasticity as in case of pyramidal tract lesions. Hold the child's hand at the wrist with the palm facing downward and hanging loosely. The tip of the middle finger is grasped with the examiner's thumb and index finger and the nail of the middle finger is given a snap with examiner's thumb. The normal response is the absence of any thumb movement but in pyramidal tract lesion, there is flexion of thumb.
- The exaggerated DTRs are seen with UMN lesions like cerebral palsy, cerebrovascular stroke, CNS trauma, spinal cord lesions, etc. In hypotonic cerebral palsy, the DTRs are exaggerated even in the presence of hypotonia. In Down's syndrome there is hypotonia and diminished DTRs. Hypotonia with exaggerated

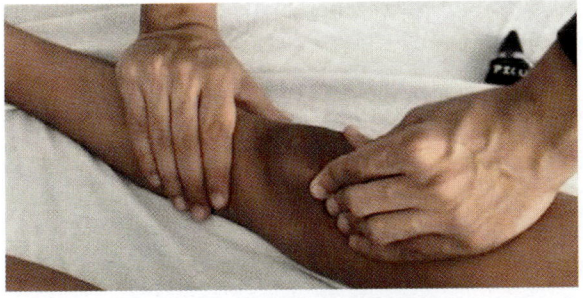

Fig. 28: Elicitation of patellar clonus.

DTRs in Down syndrome indicates atlantoaxial dislocation. Exaggerated DTR may be normally seen in an anxious child. Pendular knee jerk is observed in cerebellar disorders. Diminished or absent DTRs are seen in LMN lesions like Guillain-Barré syndrome, poliomyelitis, spinal shock, etc.

Signs of Meningeal Irritation

The signs of meningeal irritation are present when the meninges are irritated due to inflammation or otherwise.
- *Meningitis:* The inflammation is due to infection. The common infections causing meningitis are bacterial meningitis and TBM.
- *Meningism:* There is presence of meningeal signs (mainly neck stiffness) and is a reflex spasm of muscles to avoid painful flexion of neck, resulting in neck stiffness. It is commonly seen in cases of subarachnoid hemorrhage.
- *Meningismus:* Meningismus is a terminology used to describe signs of meningeal irritation (neck stiffness) present due to other reasons like right upper lobe pneumonia.
- The different tests used to assess signs of meningeal irritation produce tension in the inflamed and hypersensitive spinal nerve roots and resulting signs are protective muscle contractions and postures that minimize the stretching of meninges and the nerve roots.
- Neck rigidity, positive Kernig sign, and positive Brudzinski sign are signs of meningeal irritation. They are commonly present in bacterial meningitis and tuberculous meningitis. They are also caused by subarachnoid hemorrhage, brain abscess, and raised intracranial pressure.

Neck Rigidity (Nuchal Rigidity, Neck Stiffness)
- If the child has altered sensorium, he is placed in supine position. One hand is placed behind the head of the child and the neck is gently flexed. If there is resistance to flexion of neck, the sign is considered positive **(Fig. 29)**.
- If the child is conscious, he is asked to sit and flex his head voluntarily and touch his chin to his chest. The sign is

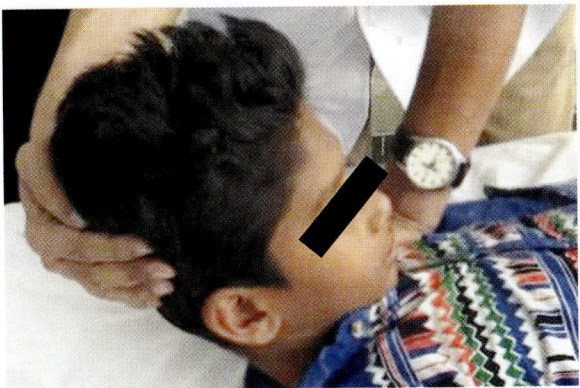

Fig. 29: Eliciting nuchal rigidity.

considered positive if flexion of neck is associated with pain and resistance.
- In an uncooperative young child, neck stiffness is elicited by bringing the head beyond the edge of the table and supporting his head with examiner's hand while trying to flex the head.

Kernig Sign

The patient should be in supine position. His hip and knee joints are flexed to a 90° and then knee is slowly extended by the examiner. The appearance of resistance or pain during extension of the patient's knee beyond 135° constitutes a positive Kernig sign **(Fig. 30)**. The inflamed and hypersensitive nerve roots are stretched which leads to a reflex spasm of the hamstring muscles.

Brudzinski Sign

- It is performed with patient in supine position. The examiner keeps one hand behind the patient's head and other hand on the chest to prevent the patient rising. With passive flexion of the neck, there is reflex flexion of patient's hips and knees in a positive Brudzinski sign **(Fig. 31)**.
- *Brudzinski leg sign*: When one leg is passively flexed, there is reflex flexion of the opposite leg.

Brudzinski sign should not be confused with straight leg raising test which is performed in a case of abdominal lump to differentiate whether it is in abdominal wall or intra-abdominal.

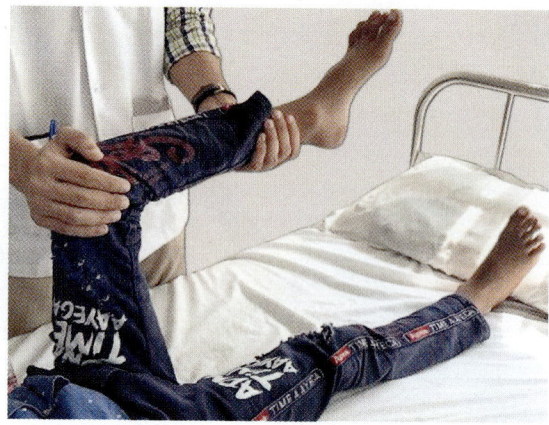

Fig. 30: Eliciting Kernig's sign.

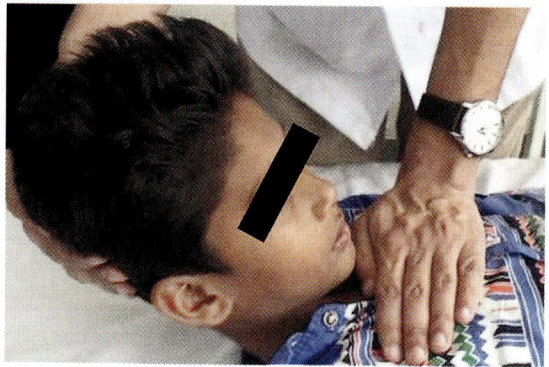

Fig. 31: Eliciting Brudzinski sign.

Cerebellar Signs

The cerebellum is playing the role for maintenance of muscle tone, balance, and coordination. Therefore, any child with incoordination or imbalance should be examined in detail for cerebellar signs. The cerebellar signs are shown in **Box 20**.

Ataxia

Ataxia refers to impaired control of posture or movements of limbs and trunk.
- *Truncal ataxia:* The child is not able to maintain his balance while sitting upright. It is manifested in the form of swaying or

> **Box 20:** Cerebellar signs.
> - Dysarthria
> - Ataxia
> - Nystagmus
> - Dysmetria (past pointing)
> - Intention tremor
> - Dysdiadochokinesia
> - Rebound phenomenon (over shooting)
> - Incoordination
> - Hypotonia
> - Pendular knee jerk

falling while trying to sit upright. It is due to lesions in vermis of the cerebellum.

- *Gait ataxia:* The child is not able to maintain balance while standing and walking. It can be tested as follows:
  - *Romberg sign* **(Figs. 32A and B)**:
    - This is actually a test of proprioception and maintenance of balance is based on vision, vestibular function, and proprioception.
    - The child is asked to stand with his feet close together. The child will sway and tend to fall toward the side of lesion in a case of unilateral cerebellar lesion. In case of bilateral cerebellar lesions, the child will tend to sway backward.
    - If the child can maintain his posture with open eyes but falls or sways with closed eyes, it is called as positive Romberg sign. It indicates lesion of the proprioception (sensory ataxia).
  - *Tandem walking:* This test may not be conclusive till the child is 7 years old. The child is asked to walk in a line in such a way that one foot is placed exactly in front of the other. In cerebellar lesions, the child tends to sway and fall toward the side of lesion.
- *Hypotonia:* It is defined as decreased resistance to passive movements of the muscle. It is different from hypotonia of LMN origin as there is no associated weakness.
- *Rebound phenomenon*: The examiner suddenly releases the resistance when the child is attempting to flex the elbow

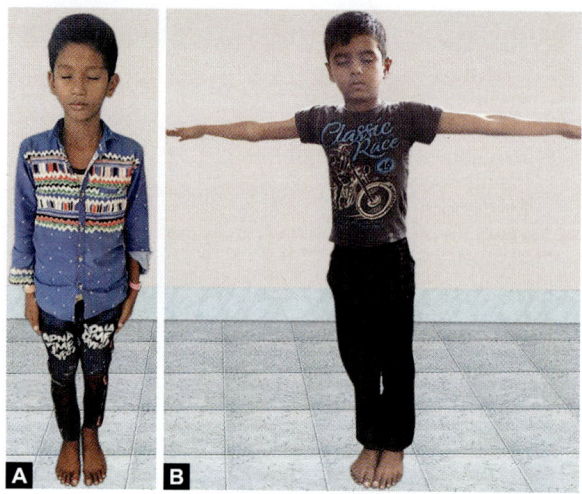

Figs. 32A and B: Romberg sign.

and pulling his forearm against the resistance offered by the examiner. The child's hand inadvertently strikes the face.
- *Dysdiadochokinesia (rapid alternating movements):* It may not be possible to test in younger children, less than 10 years.
- *Tremors*: Intention tremors are present in the child with cerebellar disorders. When the child tries to reach an object, coarse, slow, side-to-side oscillations of the hands appear that increase in intensity as he reaches nearer to the object. Sometimes, the tremors of head, hands, and fingers may be present at even the rest.
- *Dysmetria (past pointing):* The child is not able to decide the exact distance for a particular action and it results in over shooting or past pointing.
- *Pendular knee jerk:* The child is asked to sit at the edge of the table with his legs dangling. On eliciting the knee jerk, there will be 2–3 oscillations of legs at knee joint moving like a pendulum.
- *Nystagmus:* It is defined as periodic, rhythmic oscillations of eyeballs. The oscillations may be approximately of equal amplitude and velocity (pendular nystagmus) or more commonly with a slow initiating phase and fast corrective phase (jerky nystagmus). Besides cerebellar lesions, nystagmus may be due to vestibular lesions, ocular lesions, and brainstem dysfunction.

> **Box 21:** Common conditions causing cerebellar signs.
> - Post viral cerebellitis (most common chickenpox)
> - Drugs (phenytoin, benzodiazepine)
> - Neuroblastoma
> - Cerebellar tumors
> - Congenital malformations like Arnold Chiari malformation
> - Hydrocephalus
> - Lead encephalopathy

- *Dysarthria:* It may be scanning speech or staccato speech. In scanning speech, each syllabus of a sentence is carefully enunciated and separated, staccato speech is jerky and explosive.

The common conditions causing cerebellar signs are shown in **Box 21**.

Gait Examination

Gait examination is very important in neurological assessment of a child as it reveals involvement of various parts of the nervous system like cerebral hemispheres, extrapyramidal system, cerebellum, LMN lesions like Guillain–Barré syndrome, myopathies, muscular dystrophy, and neuropathies.

- It is important to observe the child walking and sometimes running for a distance of a few feet in the examination room. Also, watch how he is getting up from floor and climbing the stairs.
- Toe walking may be normal in young children, however it may be an early clue of spastic diplegia.
- *Hemiplegic gait (Circumduction gait):* With paralysis on one side of the body, the person stands with unilateral weakness on the affected side, arm flexed, adducted, and internally rotated. Leg on the same side is the in extension with plantar flexion of the foot and toes. While walking, the child holds his arm to one side and drags his affected leg in a semicircle (circumduction) due to weakness of distal muscles (foot drop) and extensor hypertonia in the lower limb. This develops following cerebrovascular stroke. With mild hemiparesis, there may be loss of normal arm swing and slight circumduction only.

- *High stepping gait:* It is seen in patients with foot drop, weakness of foot dorsiflexion. There is an attempt to lift the leg high enough during walking so that the foot does not drag on the floor. On bringing the foot to the ground, toes touch first and then heel. It results in high stepping gait with sudden sound, also called as slapping gait. It is seen in peripheral neuropathies, spina bifida, etc.
- *Waddling gait (lurching gait):* When there is affection of the hip girdle, the normal movement of the pelvis does not occur. In order to clear the opposite limb from the ground, the patient bends on the normal side and there is exaggerated lumbar lordosis. The opposite side of the pelvis drops when the lesion is unilateral and it produces a lurching gait. Affection of hip girdle on both sides leads to waddling gait. It is seen in muscular dystrophies like Duchenne muscular dystrophy, spinomuscular atrophy (SMA), etc.
- *Scissoring gait (spastic gait):* The children with scissoring gait have tightness of adductor muscles of the lower limbs, which leads to scissoring of the limbs. They also have stiffness and contractures of the Achilles tendon because of which instead of their entire foot, only their toes touch the ground while walking. It is commonly seen in children with spastic cerebral palsy (preterm born babies).
- *Broad based gait:* In this type of gait, the child tends to walk with the feet separated so that his base becomes broad. He sways from side to side on standing. He is not able to walk with heel to toe action in a straight line. Broad based gait is normal up to the age of 2 years. It is also seen in cerebellar diseases.
- *Toe walking:* The child walks on toes. It is seen in children with spastic cerebral palsy and Duchenne muscular dystrophy.

Autonomic Nervous System

- Autonomic nervous system comprises the sympathetic and parasympathetic system and enteric nervous system, acting as an efferent system affecting vital signs, pupillary reaction, lacrimation, salivation, gastrointestinal motility, bronchodilation, sweating, and sphincter functions.

- *Manifestation of autonomic nervous system involvement:*
  - Temperature differences
  - Postural hypotension
  - Tache cerebrale
  - Punctuate erythematous spots on palms
  - Variation in perspiration, salivation, and tears
  - Paroxysmal hypertension
  - Sudden gross changes in vitals
- Conditions affecting autonomic system
  - Guillain–Barré syndrome
  - Thyroid disorders
  - Pheochromocytoma
  - Neuroblastoma
  - Autonomic neuropathies
  - Prematurity
  - Mitochondrial disorders
  - Chromosomal disorders

Examination of Skull (Head)

- *Shape of head*: Observe the head and see whether the shape is normal or abnormal. Abnormal shapes of skull are shown in **Box 22**.
- *Fontanels:* Palpate the anterior fontanel. It measures 2.5 × 2.5 cm at birth in a term baby. It may be elevated (bulging) and full in a case of raised intracranial pressure like hydrocephalus and meningitis. It gets closed from 9 to 18 months. There may be delayed closure due to several conditions, most common are

---

Box 22: Abnormal shapes of the skull.

- *Scaphocephaly (dolichocephaly):* Anteroposteriorly skull is elongated due to premature fusion of sagittal suture
- *Brachycephaly:* Anteroposterior flattened skull (square and short) due to premature closure of coronal suture
- *Plagiocephaly:* Skewing of skull due to premature unilateral fusion of coronal or lambdoid suture
- *Oxycephaly (towering of skull):* Elongation of skull like a tower due to premature closure of sagittal and coronal sutures
- *Trigonocephaly:* Pointed skull due to premature closure of metopic suture

hydrocephalus, rickets, Down syndrome, hypothyroidism, etc. It may be depressed due to dehydration.
- Posterior fontanels may be open in a preterm baby. It may remain open due to rickets, hypothyroidism, etc.
- Note any associated dysmorphism and anomalies.
- *Size of head*:
  - Measure the head circumference and compare with normal value expected for age of the child.
  - *Microcephaly:* It is defined as head circumference more than –3 SD below the median for age of child and gender. It may be primary or secondary. Secondary microcephaly (small head) is due to failure of brain to grow and it may be due to perinatal or postnatal brain insult. There may be sutural ridging and early closure of anterior fontanel.
  - *Macrocephaly:* Head circumference exceeds the median by more than 2 SD for the age of the child and gender. It may be due to hydrocephalus, megalencephaly, subdural effusion, etc. The megalencephaly occurs in Canavan disease, Alexander disease, etc.
- *Craniosynostosis:* It occurs because of premature closure of sutures and results in abnormal shape of head. There is early closure of sutures and brain is growing normally, there will be manifestations of raised intracranial pressure. It will result in different shapes of head. Various syndromes are known associated with craniosynostosis like Apert syndrome, Carpenter syndrome, Crouzon syndrome, etc.
- *Macewen sign (cracked pot sign):* In a child with closed fontanels and raised intracranial pressure, this sign is elicitable. Raise the head above the bed. Tap lightly on one side of the parietal eminence, and listen to the reverberating sound on the opposite parietal eminence by the stethoscope. A classical sound as if coming from a cracked pot indicates raised intracranial pressure.
- *Transillumination test:* Place a beam of bright torch light on the skull in a darkened room to look for halo around the light. If there is hydrocephalus, there will be generalized transillumination in the entire skull. It may also be positive in a case of subdural effusion.

Examination of Spine

Examination of spine is must in all cases of neurological diseases.
- Look for meningocele and meningomyelocele.
- A tuft of hair, dimple or pilonidal sinus may indicate an underlying neural tube defect.
- Check for any swelling or localized vertebral tenderness.
- Look for any spinal deformity like kyphosis, lordosis, scoliosis, etc. Scoliosis may be associated with cerebral palsy, Friedreich ataxia, Duchenne muscular dystrophy, etc.

Localization of Neurological Lesion

Detailed history, thorough clinical examination and analysis of positive findings will help to decide the area in the nervous system involved. Knowledge of neuroanatomy and clinical manifestations of each component following involvement in the disease process is the crux of an art of localization of neurological lesion. The following methodological approach is most practical.

Is it UMN or LMN lesion?

It can be decided as shown in **Table 10**.

Table 10: Upper motor neuron and lower motor neuron disease.

Lesion	Upper motor neuron	Lower motor neuron
Weakness	Present	Present
Paralysis causes	Affects movements rather than muscle: • Hemiplegia • Paraplegia • Diplegia • Quadriplegia	Single muscle or group of muscles affected
Muscle tone	Hypertonia (Spastic paralysis)	Hypotonia (Flaccid paralysis)
Deep tendon reflex	Exaggerated	Diminished or absent
Superficial reflexes	Absent	Absent
Plantar reflex	Extensor	Flexor
Muscle wasting	Absent	Present
Fasciculations	Absent	May be present
Peripheral sensations	Normal	May be affected

Localizing UMN

In a child presenting with features of UMN lesion (spasticity, hyperreflexia, plantar extensor), the next point is to decide whether the lesion is in the spinal cord or above it.

A common neurological deficit in UMN involvement is hemiparesis. If other associated features are involvement of higher functions, cranial nerves, seizures or loss of consciousness, it indicates lesion is above the spinal cord.

If the lesion is in the brain, is it in the cortex, corona radiata, cerebellum, thalamus, basal ganglia, internal capsule, mid brain, pons or medulla?

Cortex:
- Contralateral hemiparesis with contralateral facial weakness
- Impairment of consciousness
- Seizures
- Aphasia (with involvement of dominant hemisphere)
- Visual impairment

Basal ganglia:
- Involuntary movements like choreoathetosis
- Dystonia
- Hemiballismus

Corona radiata: In hemiparesis, due to corona radiata involvement, the clinical findings are same as cortical lesions except seizures and impairment of consciousness.

Internal capsule:
- Contralateral hemiparesis with contralateral facial weakness
- Hemiplegia is dense, arms and legs are affected equally
- No aphasia
- Impaired consciousness and seizures are uncommon.

Brain stem (mid brain, pons, and medulla):
- Contralateral hemiparesis along with ipsilateral cranial nerve involvement
- Involvement of 3rd and 4th cranial nerves suggests involvement of mid brain.
- Involvement of 6th and 7th cranial nerves indicates lesion in the pons.
- Involvement of 9th to 12th cranial nerves is the characteristic of involvement of medulla.

Table 11: Localization of lower motor neuron lesions.

Site	Signs
Anterior horn cells	• Loss of power • Flaccidity • Fasciculation • Atrophy • Loss of reflexes • No sensory loss
Nerve roots	• Pain and paresthesia in dermatomal distribution • Motor affection as per myotome
Peripheral nerves	• Mononeuropathy or polyneuropathy • *Pattern of motor sensory loss:* Numbness, paresthesia (gloves and stocking), loss of vibratory, and position sense • May be patchy, asymmetric, loss of power, flaccidity, loss of reflexes
Neuromuscular junction	• Weakness increasing with exercise • Fatigability (fluctuating) • Diplopia • Ptosis • Dysarthria
Muscles	• Proximal muscle involvement is more than distal • Deep tendon reflexes are well preserved • No sensory loss

Features of spinal shock: Acute paralysis as a result of spinal cord disease is accompanied by flaccidity and loss of DTR and superficial reflexes, caused by sudden withdrawal of activity descending to anterior horn cells from the cerebral cortex and brainstem. This stage of hypotonia and areflexia is known as spinal shock. Over several days to weeks, muscle tone and reflexes return. Later muscle become hypertonic and DTR gets exaggerated.

In a more slowly progressive weakness of spinal origin, there is no stage of spinal shock and child develops gradually progressively spasticity without intervening phase of hypotonia and hyporeflexia.

Localizing LMN Lesion

Involvement of anterior horn cells, root diseases, peripheral neuropathy, neuromuscular junction disorders, and muscle diseases have characteristic features as shown in **Table 11** which helps to decide the localization of LMN lesion.

CHAPTER 11

Examination of the Newborn

Rhishikesh Thakre

INTRODUCTION

The infant in the first 28 days of life is called a neonate. A neonate is vulnerable due to the structural and functional immaturity of various organs and systems and is therefore at increased risk of morbidity and mortality. Approach to a newborn is a unique challenge as to obtain proper history is difficult, symptoms and signs are nonspecific and examination also poses a great challenge. It is essential for us to know important definitions for neonates as given in **Box 1**.

NORMAL NEWBORN

It is defined as one who fulfills following criteria:
- Birth weight more than 2.5 kg and gestation of 37 weeks or more.
- Birth weight between 10th and 90th percentiles for the corresponding gestation age, as per intrauterine growth charts.
- Absence of maternal illness or intrapartum event that may put a newborn at risk of illness such as gestational diabetes and antepartum hemorrhage.
- Normal Apgar scores and no need of resuscitation at birth.
- No postnatal illness like sepsis, respiratory distress, hypoglycemia, polycythemia or dyselectrolytemia.

HISTORY TAKING IN NEWBORN

Maternal health and illness during the antenatal period, intrapartum events and immediate care at birth have significant effects on the health and wellbeing of the baby. The maternal history includes the following points:
- The basic information regarding the baby including age in hours/days after birth, gestational age, sex, birth weight, any perinatal insult, etc. should be noted.

Examination of the Newborn

> **Box 1:** Definitions in neonatology.
> - *Low birth weight (LBW):* A neonate weighing less than 2500 g at birth is termed LBW
> - *Very low birth weight (VLBW):* A neonate weighing less than 1500 g at birth is termed VLBW
> - *Extremely low birth weight (ELBW):* A baby weighing less than 1000 g at birth is termed ELBW
> - *Adequate for gestational age (AGA):* If the birth weight of a baby is between 10th and 90th percentiles for that gestational age, it is termed as AGA
> - *Small for gestational age (SGA):* If the birth weight of a baby is below 10th percentile for that gestational age, it is termed as SGA
> - *Large for gestational age (LGA):* If the birth weight of a baby is above the 90th percentile for its gestational age, it is termed as LGA
> - *Perinatal mortality rate:* It refers to number of deaths of babies after 28 weeks of gestation (or weight >1000 g at birth) and up to 7th day of life per 1000 live births (late fetal deaths + early neonatal deaths)
> - *Prematurity:* A baby born before completion of 37 weeks, is termed as preterm
> - *Postmaturity:* A baby born after 42 weeks of gestation is termed postmature (post-term)
> - *Birth asphyxia:* Gasping or ineffective breathing or lack of breathing at 1 minute of life
> - *Neonatal death:* It refers to death occurring in first 28 days of life
> - *Early neonatal death:* It refers to death occurring in first 7 days of life
> - *Late neonatal death:* It refers to death occurring after 7th day and in the first 28 days of life
> - *Perinatal period:* It extends from 28 weeks of gestation to 7th day of life

- The details of parents including their education, occupation, economic and social status should be collected and recorded. Mothers belonging to lower socioeconomical class are likely to give birth to small for date and preterm babies due to their poor nutritional status and iron deficiency anemia.
- It is important to note maternal age, as advanced maternal age (>35 years) is associated with increased risk of chromosomal anomalies especially Trisomy 21 (Down syndrome) and young mothers (<18 years) are likely to give birth to low birth weight and preterm babies.

Past Obstetric History

- Gravidity, parity, abortions, stillbirths and neonatal deaths, if any, should be recorded. Gravidity is defined as the number of all conceptions including abortions and stillbirths,

while parity means total number of pregnancies reaching to viable gestational age (live births and stillbirths).
- The interval between successive pregnancies and their outcome should be enquired.
- History of recurrent abortions and stillbirth is suggestive of incompetent cervical os, diabetes mellitus, syphilis, Rh isoimmunization, etc.
- Gestational maturity, birth weight, congenital malformations and mode of delivery of previous babies should be noted.
- The neonatal course, unusual manifestations and outcome of previous babies should be ascertained.

Prepregnancy Health Status

- Maternal nutrition before pregnancy should be known as malnutrition is one of the important causes of intrauterine growth retardation (IUGR). Criteria for maternal malnutrition are height less than 145 cm, weight less than 40 kg and mid arm circumference less than 20.9 cm.
- Chronic systemic illness in mother like anemia, heart diseases, chronic renal failure, urinary tract infections are associated with IUGR.
- History of maternal endocrine disorders such as diabetes mellitus, hypothyroidism, hyperthyroidism should be asked. Systemic lupus erythematosus may be associated with congenital complete heart block in the baby.
- Blood group of mother should be confirmed to predict status of Rh and ABO incompatibility between mother and baby.
- Tetanus—toxoid vaccination status of the mother should be assessed.

Antenatal History

Enquire about details of antenatal care for community purpose, 'minimum antenatal care' is defined as atleast four antenatal visits and two doses of injection tetanus toxoid received during pregnancy.
- First trimester of pregnancy is the time of embryogenesis and therefore diseases and drugs taken during this phase of

pregnancy are potentially teratogenic. History of fever with rash during this phase should be asked in detail as its presence may be suggestive of TORCH infection. Detailed history of medications during pregnancy is important. Inadvertently exposure of the fetus to the drugs may cause malformations or abnormal clinical manifestations **(Table 1)**.

- The diagnostic and therapeutic procedures performed during pregnancy should be noted.
- Blood group of the mother should be known as Rh and ABO incompatibility may lead to neonatal jaundice.
- Dietary intake especially during second half of pregnancy is very crucial to ensure optimal growth of the fetus. During an uncomplicated pregnancy, most Indian mothers gain the weight between 6 and 11 kg. Less weight gain may be

Table 1: Common neonatal disorders due to maternal medications during pregnancy.

Neonatal disorder	Drugs
Vitamin K-dependent bleeding manifestations	Phenobarbitone, phenytoin, salicylates, INH, rifampicin, etc.
Thrombocytopenia	Quinine, salicylates
Seizures	Narcotic withdrawal syndrome, accidental injection of local anesthetic agent into fetal scalp, propranolol
Jaundice	Vitamin K, nitrofurantoin, primaquine, oxytocin
Deafness	Quinine, chloroquine, aminoglycosides like streptomycin
Cerebral depression and hypotonia	Pethidine, morphine, diazepam, magnesium sulfate, phenobarbitone, etc.
Drug withdrawal syndrome	Alcohol, morphine, addictive drugs, etc.
Intrauterine growth retardation	Smoking, alcohol, addictive drugs, etc.
Cretinism	Antithyroid drugs
Congenital malformations	Thalidomide, haloperidol, hormonal therapy, clomiphene, valproic acid, streptomycin, corticosteroids, etc.

due to undernutrition and weight gain in excess may suggest some complication like edema due to pregnancy-induced hypertension, hypothyroidism, etc.
- Undernutrition, anemia and pregnancy-induced hypertension may be associated with placental dysfunction, IUGR, perinatal hypoxia and birth asphyxia.
- History of bleeding per vaginum during pregnancy may be due to abruptio placentae or placenta previa.
- The quantity of amniotic fluid assessment by ultrasound study during pregnancy is important. Oligohydramnios (amniotic fluid <500 mL) is associated with placental dysfunction, postmaturity, renal agenesis, obstructive uropathy, etc. Polyhydramnios (amniotic fluid >2 L) is associated with open neural tube defects, esophageal atresia, duodenal atresia, twins, hydrops fetalis, maternal diabetes mellitus, etc.
- Meconium-stained liquor amnii in a vertex presentation is indicative of fetal distress or listeriosis.
- History of maternal immunization especially inj. tetanus toxoid, number of doses and at what interval should be noted.

Natal History

Evaluate for any risk factor for potential perinatal insult and sepsis.
- History of amnionitis (Fever and abdominal tenderness), prolonged rupture of membrane (>24 hours) and frequent vaginal examinations are considered as markers of sepsis.
- Prolonged labor (>18 hours for first stage and >6 hours for second stage) and difficult delivery are considered as risk factors for birth asphyxia and birth trauma.
- Ascertain whether the baby was delivered by vaginal route following spontaneous labor or after induction or augmentation with oxytocin. Enquire for history of instrumentation or operative delivery, elective or emergency cesarean section.
- Check for any evidence of fetal distress during labor, cephalopelvic disproportion, cord around the neck, cord prolapse, etc.
- Analgesics and anesthetic agents used during labor can adversely affect the baby.

Postnatal History

- Enquire whether baby cried immediately after birth or required neonatal resuscitation. Check the Apgar score.
- Ask whether the baby was kept with the mother or required neonatal intensive care unit (NICU) admission.
- Details of feeding and activity should be confirmed.
- Ascertain the passage of first urine (upper limit 48 hours) and stool (upper limit 24 hours) after birth. History of delayed passage of meconium may be associated with cystic fibrosis or Hirschsprung's disease.
- An occasional vomiting on first day of life is common and may not be of any significance. But bilious vomiting should not be missed as it may be due to some surgical condition or intestinal obstruction.
- History of neonatal jaundice, seizures and feeding problems during neonatal period should be checked.
- Confirm whether baby was given inj. vitamin K or not and if not given, inj. vitamin K should be given. Check whether baby received BCG, OPV and hepatitis B vaccines.

History of Present Illness

- Listen to mother or caretaker attentively for any complaint, contributory information, observation or concerns regarding illness of the baby. Their complaint or observation should never be overlooked.
- If the baby is referred by the obstetrician or pediatrician who attended labor call, one should go through the referral notes and if requires talk to the medical person.
- The illness of the neonatal should be correlated with gestational age, birth weight, perinatal insult, prolonged rupture of membrane, etc.
- Most of neonatal illnesses present with few common symptoms (**Box 2**) which are nonspecific.
- Early identification of a sick neonate is the key to successful management and good outcome. Very often it is difficult for the clinician to decide whether it is normal or sick baby. If you are in dilemma, best way is to observe the baby for sometime.

> **Box 2:** Common symptoms of sick neonates.
> - Refusal of feeds
> - Vomiting
> - Lethargy
> - Excessive crying
> - Convulsions (abnormal movements)
> - Remains cold
> - Fast breathing
> - Chest indrawing
> - Jaundice
> - Bleeding from any site
> - Blue lips and nails
> - Weight loss or not gaining weight

- The common neonatal problems are birth asphyxia, respiratory distress syndrome, jaundice, septicemia, bleeding manifestations, convulsions, congenital malformations, etc.
- Preterm babies are vulnerable to develop hyaline membrane disease, hypothermia, septicemia, necrotizing enterocolitis, intraventricular hemorrhage, patent ductus arteriosus, retinopathy of prematurity, etc.
- Neonates are known to manifest a large number of minor developmental peculiarities, physiological problems and minor illnesses which need to be identified and managed properly along with reassurance to mother.

Family History

Ask for family history of developmental and metabolic disorders. History of bleeding disorders and neonatal deaths in family should be asked. History of similar disorder in a previous sibling should be enquired.

Immunization History

Maternal status of tetanus toxoid vaccination should be enquired. Her status for hepatitis B, tuberculosis and other infections should be confirmed. Check whether BCG, OPV and hepatitis B vaccines are given to the baby.

NEWBORN EXAMINATION

The purpose of newborn examination is to identify normal from abnormal. It is a vital diagnostic tool and therefore the examination must be systematic, objective, and thorough. It needs to be flexible taking into account the newborn status and response. A well-baby evaluation usually takes 5–10 minutes with practice. The purpose of examination differs based on timing and place of examination **(Table 2)**. Common errors in diagnosis are more frequent due to lack of proper diagnostic process, i.e., history and/or clinical examination. The art and science of newborn examination involves inspection (look), palpation (feel), auscultation (listen), and percussion (tap, if necessary). By far, majority of information is derived by good observations.

Essential tools for examination:
- Stethoscope
- Measuring tape
- Infantometer
- Digital scale

Table 2: Purpose of newborn examination.

Age	Place	Purpose
Birth	Delivery room	• Identify need for resuscitation • Identify major congenital anomalies • Identify high risk newborn • Support physiologic transition
24–48 hours	Hospital discharge	• Identify high risk newborn • Assess gestation/growth • Identify major-minor-occult congenital anomalies • Respond to parental concerns
Day 3–7	OPD clinic	• Identify high risk newborn • Assess gestation/growth pattern • Identify physiologic variations • Perform clinical and metabolic screening • To assess growth, health, and behavior
Any	Emergency room	• Identify life-threatening event • Identify sick newborn • Identify physiologic derangements • Identify severity of illness

- Spatula
- Ophthalmoscope
- Appropriate growth charts.

Getting ready for examination:
- Wash and warm hands
- Draft free area with adequate light
- Neutral thermal environment
- Gather equipment
- Introduce and greet the parents/caretaker
- Ask the baby's name and confirm gender
- Ask about any concerns
- Inform the purpose of examination.

SEQUENCE OF EXAMINATION

Clinical evaluations that cause the least disturbance should be done first. The examiner may then proceed to the more disturbing maneuvers that are not so dependent on a quiet state for accurate interpretation.

The sequence of examination is not important but it should cover general assessment of wellbeing and body measurements, vital parameters, gestational assessment and growth status, moving from top to bottom examining the head, face, mouth, palate, nose, ear, eyes, chest, abdomen, arms, hands, legs and feet, and the skin. It is vital not to miss the genitals, anus, and spine.

PHYSICAL EXAMINATION

The examiner's hands should be warm and cleaned before examination.

Apgar Scoring System

Despite its limitations, Apgar scoring system is used to assess the condition of the baby at birth **(Table 3)**. Time taken by the baby to produce first cry after birth should be noted.

Anthropometry

The weight taken in first 24 hours is considered as birth weight and it is 2.5–3 kg. Average birth weight of an Indian baby is reported

Table 3: Apgar scoring system.

Criteria	Score		
	0	1	2
Breathing	Nil	Slow, gasping	Crying
Heart rate/min	Nil	Up to 100	>100
Muscle tone	Flaccid	In between	Flexed
Reflex response	Nil	Grimace	Cry
Color	Pale or blue	Peripheral cyanosis	Pink

to be 2.9 kg. Occipitofrontal head circumference, chest circumference at nipples and crown—heel length on an infantometer are recorded. The head circumference should be preferably measured after 24 hours of birth when caput succedaneum and over riding of sutures would have been disappeared. In a term baby, head circumference is around 34–35 cm with length of 48–50 cm.

Temperature

The normal body temperature of newborn is 36.5–37.5°C. Hypothermia is a more common response rather than fever in sick neonates. The low reading thermometer (30–40°C) is used to measure rectal temperature in neonates.

Heart Rate and Pulsations

In newborns, the normal heart rate is 120–160/min. One must look for femoral pulsations. Diminished or absent femoral pulsations suggest the possibility of coarctation of aorta.

Respiration

The normal respiratory rate of the neonatal is 40–60/min. Tachypnea in a newborn is defined as respiratory rate >60/min. Respiration should be assessed in a quiet baby and 30 minutes after the feed. Periodic breathing should not be mistaken for irregular respiration. Signs of increased work of breathing like tachypnea, chest retractions and abnormal sounds should be checked.

Blood Pressure

Normal blood pressure of a neonate is 60/40 mm Hg. Noninvasive methods for measuring blood pressure in neonates should be adapted.

GENERAL PHYSICAL EXAMINATION

Head

- Look for head size, shape of skull and symmetry.
- Check for any evidence of molding, caput succedaneum or cephalohematoma. Examine for sutural separation, sutural ridging or forceps marks.
- Caput succedaneum is fluid collection in subcutaneous plane over scalp. It is soft, boggy swelling on presenting part of the head. It is not restricted by sutural lines. It is present at birth and usually disappears within 24 hours.
- Cephalohematoma is collection of blood under periosteum and is soft, cystic on palpation. It does not cross the sutural lines. It appears 24–48 hours after birth and may persist for 4–6 weeks. From soft swelling, it becomes firm and hard in consistency. It may take few months to disappear. It should not be aspirated. It may be responsible for exaggeration of physiological jaundice.
- Sutural over-riding in first 2–3 days may be normal.
- Examine anterior fontanelle, which is 2.5 × 2.5 cm in size. It is diamond shaped. Bulging anterior fontanelle is seen in conditions with raised intracranial pressure like acute bacterial meningitis, hydrocephalus, intracranial hemorrhage, etc. Depressed fontanelle is seen with dehydration.
- Posterior fontanelle is small in size between sagittal suture and lambdoid sutures. It is closed usually in full term babies. It may be open in preterm babies physiologically. Persistent open posterior fontanelle may be due to hypothyroidism, vitamin D deficiency or raised intracranial pressure.
- Look for dysmorphic facial features.
- Check for bruising or forceps marks. Facial asymmetry, more obvious on crying, suggests facial nerve palsy.
- Patency of nostrils should be checked to exclude choanal atresia.

- Look for cleft lip, cleft palate, micrognathia, retrognathia, etc.
- Look for shape of ears, low set ears, preauricular skin tags, slanting of eyes, hypertelorism (increased distance between two eyes), lips, philtrum and chin. Hairy pinna is characteristic of an infant of diabetic mother.
- Examination of eyes in neonates requires patience as they keep the eyes closed due to physiological photophobia and trial to open the eyes forcibly fails. The baby can be rocked gently in the mother's lap or head is propped up on the mother's shoulder to make him eyes open spontaneously. Look for coloboma, subconjunctival hemorrhage, cataract and corneal haziness. Blue sclera may be normal in preterm babies. Check for conjunctivitis which is very common in neonates.
- Milia (yellow white papules on the nose due to retention of sebum) is very common in newborns and disappear spontaneously.
- Salmon patches and capillary hemangioma may be present over face.
- Sternomastoid tumor is a hard swelling over the middle of anterior border of sternocleidomastoid muscle due to calcified hematoma which may cause torticollis. It requires physiotherapy for correction.

Skin

- Look for jaundice, pallor, cyanosis, petechiae, birth marks, hemangioma, skin rashes, etc.
- Postmature neonates often have wrinkled and desquamating skin especially over the creases of hands and soles.
- Toxic erythema or urticaria neonatorum is common in term babies during first week of life. Erythematous skin rash with central pallor appears on face on second or third day of life and spreads to the trunk and extremities. It disappears spontaneously after 2–3 days without any treatment. The rash should be differentiated from pyoderma, transient pustular melanosis and congenital syphilis. Look for congenital ichthyosis.

- Pallor is seen with anemia, hypoxia and decreased perfusion, while newborns with polycythemia appear plethoric. Polycythemia may be associated with small for gestational age (SGA) and infants of diabetic mothers.
- Acrocyanosis (cyanosis of hands and feet) is common in newborns and may be normal, associated with environmental cold. Central cyanosis indicates some serious systemic disorders like cyanotic heart disease.
- Icterus is visible on the skin. There is cephalocaudal progression of yellow discoloration as the serum bilirubin level increases. The yellow staining of trunk indicates serum bilirubin 10–15 mg/dL and yellow soles and palms 15–20 mg/dL.
- Capillary refill time (CRT) indicates the status of perfusion. To assess CRT, press over forehead or sternum for 5 seconds and note the time by which blanched area becomes normal. Normal CRT is <3 seconds, indicates baby is well perfused. If CRT is >3 seconds, it suggests poor perfusion, may be shock.
- Umbilical stump and nails should be examined for meconium staining. If it is present, it indicates intrauterine hypoxemia.

Genitalia

- Look for genitals, inguinal hernia and hydrocele.
- If the genitalia are ambiguous, it is essential that the assignment of the gender should be deferred till genetic, endocrinal and genitourinary investigations have been performed. It should be considered as social emergency.
- In a male child, look for urethral opening to exclude hypospadias or epispadias. Prepuce in newborn is normally nonretractile, one should not attempt to retract the foreskin. It is called as physiological phimosis. It becomes retractile in due course of time by its own. Micropenis (stretched penile length <2.5 cm) is seen hypopituitarism.

Usually, both the testes are located in scrotum in term male babies at birth. In preterm babies, there may be undescended testis at birth, but it comes down by its own and may not require any treatment. If they are not palpable or abnormally located, it requires proper workup. In term female newborns, the labia majora should completely cover the labia minora. A mucous or bloody vaginal discharge is normal in first few days following withdrawal of maternal hormones.

Normal Variations in Newborn

- *Erythema toxicum:* It is a benign condition found in term newborns, less common in preterm babies. It is characterized by the appearance of small, papular lesions with surrounding intense erythema, appearing first on face on first or second day of life. Gradually, the lesions are found on trunk and extremities sparing palms and soles. Its etiology is not known, but scrapping of the skin lesions show eosinophils. The condition is self-limiting and does not require any treatment, lesions disappear in a week time.
- *Milia:* They are yellowish white spots found over nose, forehead, chin and cheeks, found in almost all newborns and disappear spontaneously. They are epidermal inclusion cysts of about 1-2 mm in diameter.
- *Mongolian spots:* They are commonly found in lumbosacral area and buttocks but also can be found on thighs and arms. They are bluish or slate gray macular lesions of variable size. They are considered due to accumulation of melanocytes within dermis. These lesions are benign and disappear gradually.
- *Epstein pearls:* They are epithelial inclusion cysts found on either side of medium raphe of hard palate and are of no significance.

Identify Pathologic Signs

Presence of any of the following is pathological and demands evaluation for its cause—pallor, plethora, cyanosis, jaundice up to soles, edema, asymmetry of movements, and abnormal posture or movements.

Identify Danger Signs (Box 3)

At any time, if you notice any of the danger signs, one skips the assessment and moves for urgent stabilization.

> **Box 3:** Danger signs.
> - Hypothermia
> - Hyperthermia
> - Cyanosis
> - Chest indrawing
> - Grunt
> - Seizures
> - Decreased feeding
> - Decreased activity

If the mother happens to breastfeed during examination, note the position and attachment of the baby.

FOCUSED SYSTEMIC EXAMINATION

Cardiovascular System

- *Inspection:*
    - Look for growth pattern, dusky hue or cyanosis, and work of breathing
    - Note the precordial bulge, precordial pulsations, symmetry of chest, and apical impulse.
- *Palpation:* Note the heart rate, pulse volume, femoral pulses, rhythm, and symmetry of pulses.
- *Auscultation:* Note the first and second heart sound (split), abnormal heart sounds, and murmur.
- Assess for signs of cardiac failure (tachypnea, tachycardia, gallop rhythm, hepatomegaly).
- Ask for pulse oximetry check.

Respiratory System

- *Inspection:*
    - Note the chest symmetry, movement, rate, depth, and work of breathing.
    - Note the color, cry, and activity pattern.
    - Note audible sounds if any—grunt, stridor, etc.
- *Auscultation:*
    - Listen to the air entry and note the quality of breath sounds
    - Note if any abnormal sounds, crackles, grunt, etc.

Abdomen

- *Inspection:*
    - Observe for shape of abdomen, visible loop, and lump or peristalsis.
    - Note the position of umbilicus. Look for any discharge or periumbilical redness.
    - Evaluate the hernial orifices.
- *Palpation:*
    - Palpate gently across the abdomen; feel for any lump.
    - Note the consistency, size, and extent of swelling.
- *Auscultation:* Note the quality of bowel sounds.

Neurologic System

- *Inspection:*
    - Assess alertness, interaction with mother, and behavior
    - Note the posture—extended, flexed, scissoring or frog legged
    - Note the quality of cry
    - Note the symmetry and spontaneous movements of all limbs
    - Note if there are any abnormal movements of limbs, body or eyes
    - Look for symmetry of face on crying
    - Note the position of thumb in response to hands, i.e., cortical thumb.
- *Tone:*
    - Assess tone by posture.
    - Note the resistance to passive movement in both the upper and lower limb.
    - Hold the newborn by placing the hands in both the axilla and allow to suspend (Axillary suspension) **(Fig. 1A)**. Note the tone and slipping out through the examiner's hands.
    - Bring the newborn from supine position to sitting position holding both the elbows (Traction response) **(Fig. 1B)**. Note the curvature of spine and position of head.
    - Hold the newborn by supporting the abdomen and allowing the body to be in horizontal position (Ventral suspension) **(Fig. 1C)**. Note the position of head, limbs, and trunk.
    - Place the newborn on the tummy. Note the position of head, trunk, and limbs.

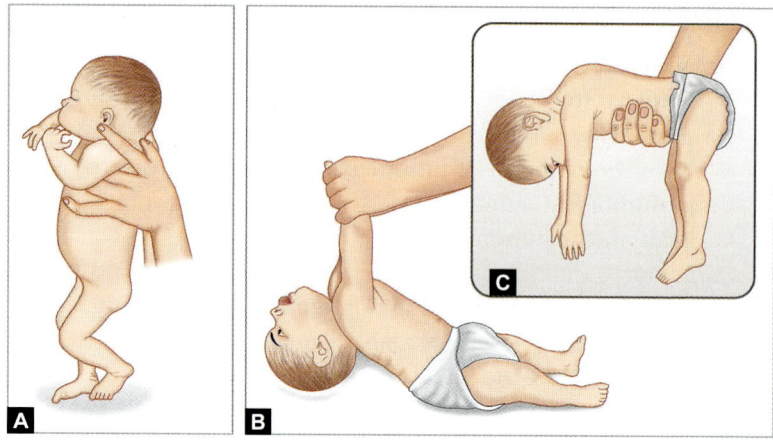

Figs. 1A to C: Assessment of hypotonia. (A) Axillary suspension; (B) Traction response; and (C) Ventral suspension.

- *Power:* Note the movement against gravity.
- *Neonatal reflexes (**Table 4**):* There are several primitive reflexes (>73) in neonates. It is practically difficult and not necessary to elicit all these reflexes. The following reflexes are important and useful for clinical purposes and one should know how to elicit them and their clinical applications.
  - *Moro reflex:* Moro reflex or startle response is the most important reflex in newborn examination. The baby should be held supine over the right hand and arm. The head is flexed to 30° and allowed to drop suddenly. The normal response consists of rapid abduction and extension of upper limbs along with opening of hands followed by slower adduction and flexion or embrace equivalent **(Fig. 2A)**. The infant may cry. It can also be elicited by pulling a supine infant by both hands. When angulation occurs between the head and trunk, the hands are sharply released to cause sudden extension of neck.

    The response may be depressed or absent in babies with cerebral depression. It is exaggerated in babies with cerebral irritability.
    - *Incomplete Moro reflex:* The Moro reflex is incomplete in preterm babies, where the arms tend to fall backwards

Table 4: Neonatal reflexes.

	Technique	Assess	Disappearance
Palmar/ plantar grasp	Place your finger on the infant's palm/soles and stroke	Infant's fingers/toes close and grasp the finger	3 months
Rooting reflex	Stroke the cheek or corner of the mouth by your finger	Infant's head turns toward the side of stroking and opens the mouth	4 months
Sucking reflex	Touch the roof of the mouth with your finger	Infant starts sucking on the finger	
Moro reflex	Drop the infant from semisitting posture with the head supported and catch midway before touching the ground with hands supporting the back and head	The legs and head extend while the arms jerk up with the fingers extended followed by adduction of both the upper limbs, clenching of fist and cry	6 months
Stepping reflex	Touch the shin across the edge of the table	The infant raises the opposite foot as if trying to walk	2 months
Tonic neck reflex	Turn the head to one side	There is extension of the hand in the direction of face with flexion of the opposite extremity	

(flexion component is absent) on to the table during adduction phase because the antigravity muscles are weaker than in the full term infants.

- *Asymmetric Moro reflex:* Asymmetric response suggests brachial plexus palsy, fracture of clavicle or humerus.
- *Reverse or exaggerated Moro reflex:* In babies with kernicterus, the Moro response is often characteristic. The sudden extension of arm is not followed by flexion component but often accompanied with downward rolling of eyeballs, lid lag and a peculiar grin. Reverse Moro reflex is also seen in basal ganglia damage due to kernicterus and other reasons. In this condition, there is no response in the first 5 days and then child responds by extending and externally rotating the arms and then fixing the rigidity in same position.

Moro reflex appears at 28 weeks of gestation, completes at 32 weeks of gestation and disappears at 3 months of age. Persistent Moro reflex beyond 3 months of age may be due to cerebral palsy.
- *Rooting and sucking reflexes:* Stimulation of angle of mouth or lips by nipple of mother's breast or a finger of the examiner would initiate rooting and sucking **(Fig. 2B)**. The mother's report regarding feeding behavior of the baby is more informative.
- *Glabellar tap:* Tapping the nasion is followed by closure of eyes.
- *Palmar and plantar grasp:* The finger is placed on the palmar surface of fingers or plantar surface of toes **(Fig. 2C)** of the baby to elicit grasp or flexion of digits.
- *Asymmetrical tonic neck reflex* **(Fig. 2D)**: Passive rotation of head in supine position leads to extension of limbs on same side and flexion of contralateral side. It appears at birth and disappears by 3 months of age. Its persistence beyond 3 months of age suggests cerebral palsy. It prevents baby from rolling, therefore it must disappear when the baby learns to turn prone voluntarily.
- *Symmetrical tonic neck reflex:* Passive extension of head in prone position leads to extension of both upper limbs and flexion of both lower limbs. It appears at 3 months of age and disappeared by 6 months of age. Its persistence is seen in cerebral palsy. When the baby learns to turn to prone position, choking over bed may asphyxiate him. So if the baby lifts the chin by extension of neck, automatically both upper limbs are extended and choking is avoided. However, this reflex must disappear if the baby has to crawl as that will require voluntary flexion and extension of upper and lower limbs. Therefore, it must disappear by 6 months of age.
- *Placing and stepping reflex:* When the dorsum of foot of the baby is stimulated at the undersurface of the table, he lifts the stimulated foot and places it on the surface (placing reaction).

Examination of the Newborn

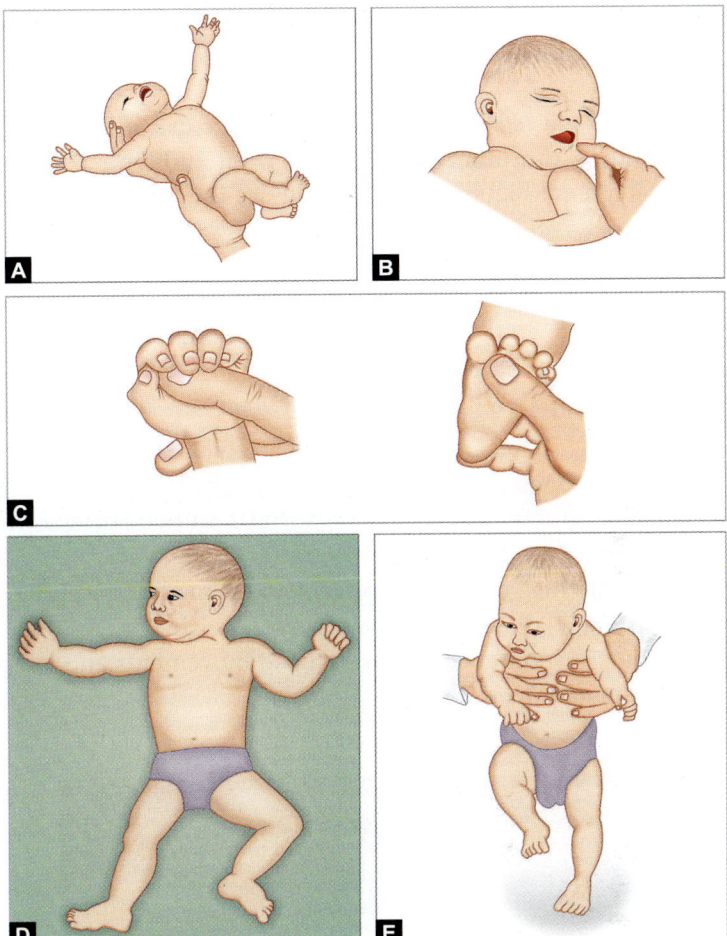

Figs. 2A to E: Neonatal reflexes. (A) Moro's reflex; (B) Suck reflex; (C) Palmar/plantar grasp; (D) Tonic neck reflex; and (E) Stepping reflex.

When the examiner allows the plantar surface of the other foot to a table top, the infant makes crude sequential walking movements (stepping reflex) **(Fig. 2E)**.

- *Landau reflex (position reflex):* Passive extension of neck in ventral suspension leads to extension of spine, lower and upper limbs. Passive flexion of neck leads to flexion of

spine, lower and upper limbs. It appears at 6 months of age and disappears at 9 months of age. It is absent in cerebral palsy.
- *Parachute reflex:* The parachute reflex can be evoked by holding the infant's trunk and then suddenly lowering the infant as if he or she were falling. The arms will spontaneously extend to break the infant's fall. This reflex is a prerequisite to walking. It appears at age of 9 months and persists for lifetime.

Musculoskeletal System

- *Arms and legs:*
  - Note the shape, posture, and symmetry of extremities. Look for asymmetry of knees (Galeazzi's sign) **(Fig. 3)**. With the infant supine, place the sole surface on bed surface with hip and knee flexed at 90°. Normally, both knees should be at same height. If one hip has developmental dysplasia of hip (DDH) that knee will be at shorter height.
  - Note for spontaneous and induced movements and if any, limitations of movements

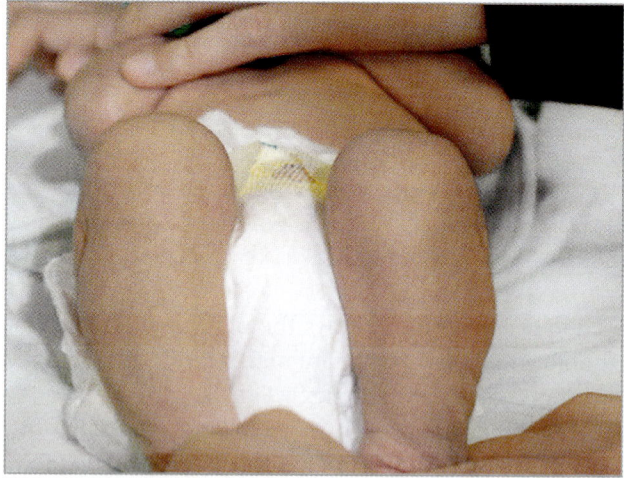

Fig. 3: Asymmetry of knees (Galeazzi's sign).

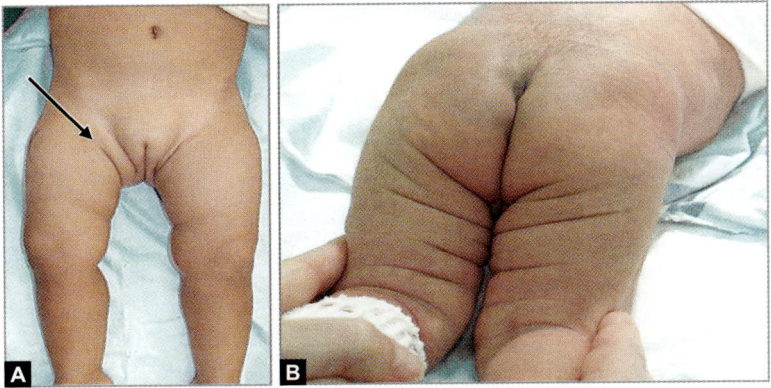

Figs. 4A and B: Examination of hip and asymmetry of thigh creases.

- Count the digits of hands and feet
- Note if there is any foot deformity.
- *Hips:*
  - Note the proportions and symmetry of the lower limbs and skinfolds before testing hip stability **(Figs. 4A and B)**.
  - Following gentle abduction, the hips are tested using both the Barlow and Ortolani's tests to ensure they are neither dislocated nor dislocatable **(Fig. 5)**.
- *Spine:*
  - Note the spine curvature. Look for integrity of spine.
  - Note if there is any cleft, dimple, sinus, tuft of hair, or meningomyelocele **(Fig. 6)**.
- *Clavicle:* Run hands over the clavicle and note for any break or swelling.

  Throughout the examination, the baby's behavior and posture can be noted to complete the assessment of the central nervous system.

Examination of Eye

With one hand holding a flashlight, gently rock the newborn which causes the newborn to open the eyes. If required, the eyelids are gently separated with the examiner's index finger and thumb.

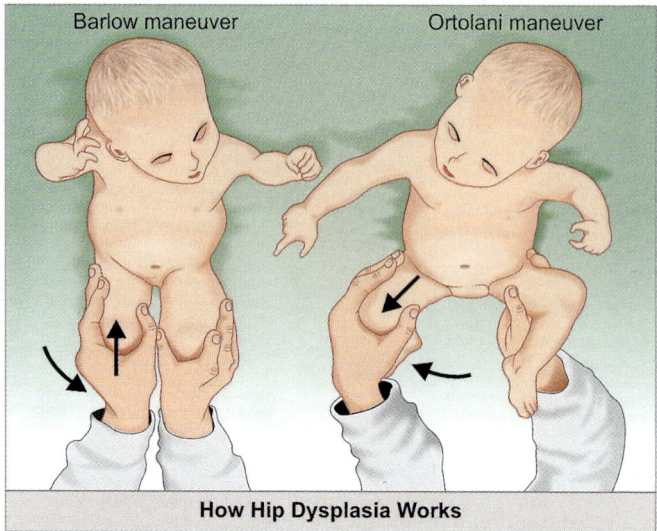

Fig. 5: Clinical tests for congenital dislocation of hips.

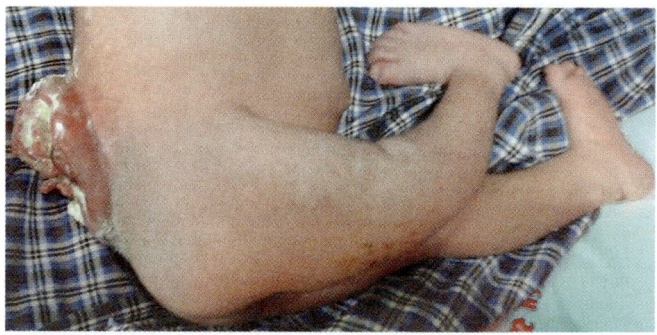

Fig. 6: Lumbosacral meningomyelocele.

Light is shined tangentially into the eyes to rule out corneal lesions and visible cataracts, and the examiner should ensure that a red reflex is seen bilaterally **(Table 5 and Figs. 7A to C)**.

COMMUNICATION AND DOCUMENTATION
- Listen to the mother. Do not interrupt or ignore her concerns.
- Use simple words while providing information and counseling.

Examination of the Newborn

Table 5: Red reflex test.

Use an ophthalmoscope, with the lens power set at 0. Project light on eyes simultaneously with 15–20 cm away from the patient. The test is done in OPD during routine visit and needs no eye drops. Ensure that the eyes are open.

Note	Interpret
Symmetric red reflex	Normal
Normal red reflex in one eye but diminished in another eye	Refractory error, retinoblastoma
Normal red reflex in one eye but absent in another eye	Cataract

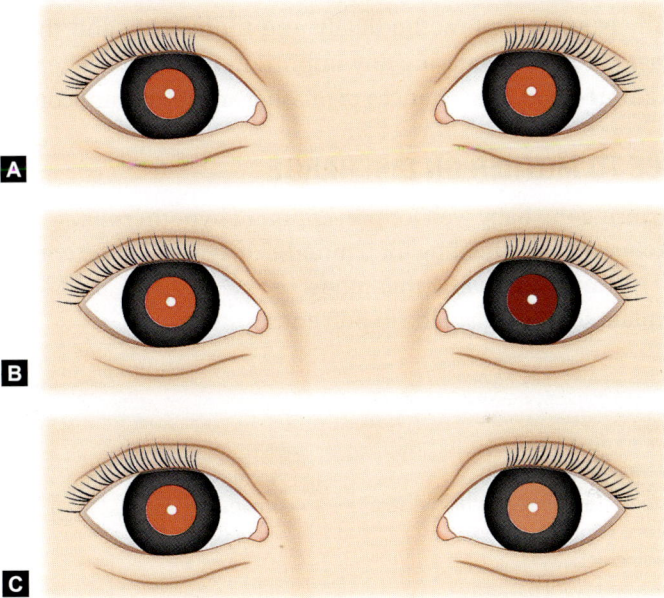

Figs. 7A to C: Red reflex and asymmetry of color.

- Use of nonverbal means of communication (gestures, facial expressions, tone, and body language).
- Discuss the findings with the parents and answer any queries.
- Ensure that the findings of the examination are appropriately and accurately recorded.

LIMITATIONS OF PHYSICAL EXAMINATION

- Metabolic disorders, hearing deficits are missed as there is a window period when the newborn is likely to be asymptomatic. Hence, screening for congenital hypothyroidism, phenylketonuria, cystic fibrosis, etc., and the hearing screening, is offered in the neonatal period.
- One-time assessment may not be enough. A trend is far more informative.
- Newborn evaluation in a nutshell can be described as shown in **Table 6**.
- Checklist for newborn examination **(Table 7)**. It should be routine to follow this checklist for newborn examination so that baby is examined methodically and thoroughly and there are least chances of missing any important condition. The baby is examined and least chances of missing any important condition.

ADVICE TO MOTHER ON DISCHARGE

- Covering the baby well for prevention of hypothermia.
- Exclusive breastfeeding for 6 months of age and to be continued till 2 years of age with other foods.
- Explain for good hygiene to prevent sepsis.

Table 6: Newborn evaluation in a nutshell.

Ask	Look
• Parental concerns • Maternal, antenatal, perinatal, family history • Feeding activity • Urine and stool pattern • Vaccination	• Appearance (posture, activity) • Breathing • Color (Cry)
Examine	Document
• Vitals • Head-to-toe: Normal variations, physiologic variants, pathologic signs, anomalies, spine, genitals • Gestational age • Anthropometry • Neonatal reflexes • Systemic examination	• Age in hours (For first week) • Risk factors • Anthropometry on growth chart • Abnormal findings • Specific instructions/tests

Table 7: Checklist for newborn examination.

No.	Assessment	Tick here
1.	Washes hands	
2.	Ensures room is well lit, draft free and temp of 36°C	
3.	Gathers all instruments	
4.	Introduces, informs, and greets parents	
5.	Takes brief history of pregnancy, birth, newborn	
6.	Observes the newborn, dressed/undressed	
7.	Notes vital parameters	
8.	Assesses gestation	
9.	Inspects head for size, shape, and swelling	
10.	Opens mouth and checks patency of palate	
11.	Notes the eyes, face, and ears for symmetry, position, and anomaly	
12.	Inspects eyes for opacity, red reflex	
13.	Palpates femoral pulse	
14.	Inspects spine and looks for tags, pits, dimple or sinus	
15.	Inspects the genitals, confirms testis in scrotum	
16.	Identifies physiologic variations	
17.	Assesses key primitive reflexes	
18.	Inspects and palpates abdomen, hernia orifice	
19.	Inspects chest and checks for air entry, breath sounds	
20.	Notes precordium, apical impulse, and heart sounds, murmur	
21.	Demonstrates maneuvers for hip stability	
22.	Demonstrates pulled to sit, ventral suspension, prone placement, and axillary suspension	
23.	Measures and interprets weight, length, and head circumference	
24.	Clothes the baby and hands over to mother	
25.	Thanks the parents	
26.	Washes hands	

- Nothing should be applied over umbilical cord, eyes, ears or at BCG site.
- Regular follow-up for growth, development and immunization.
- To report immediately if child develops any of danger signs like refusal of feed, inactivity, fast breathing, convulsions or yellow palms and soles.

CHAPTER 12

The Musculoskeletal System

Chandrika S Bhat, Anand Rao

INTRODUCTION

The musculoskeletal system (MSK) is a dynamic organ system that provides mechanical support and allows movement of the body. The major components of this complex system are muscles, bones, cartilage, ligaments, and tendons. In children, a large number of conditions can present with MSK symptoms. Recognition of such disorders with the help of a thorough clinical history and systematic examination would reduce the need for unnecessary investigations.

The history plays an important role in the children with disorders of the musculoskeletal system. Joint swelling and pain are one of the important symptoms, which bring the child to the attention of a pediatrician. It is important to inquire about the duration, progression, and presence of other associated symptoms, which might give a clue to the diagnosis. The pattern of arthritis also might help to reach the diagnosis. Additive arthritis in which arthritis involves new joints with persistent arthritis in the already existing joints is commonly seen in subtypes of juvenile idiopathic arthritis (JIA). Migratory arthritis is classically seen in acute rheumatic fever where previously affected joints settle down when new joints become involved.

Acute arthritis with duration in hours or days is commonly seen in viral arthritis, septic arthritis, acute rheumatic arthritis, arthritis associated with vasculitis, autoinflammatory disorders, and reactive arthritis. Chronic arthritis where duration of illness is more than 6 weeks is typically seen in JIA, juvenile spondyloarthropathy, tuberculous arthritis, and arthritis associated with connective tissue disorders [e.g., systemic lupus erythematosus].

It is important to differentiate articular from extra-articular disease on the basis of history. Articular diseases tend to have symptoms localized to the joint alone. While this is an easily discernible fact for older children and adolescents, it proves to be a challenge in an infant or a toddler. Inflammatory articular diseases are usually associated with swelling, tenderness, and reduced range of motion. Articular diseases, which are inflammatory in nature, typically tend to be associated with early morning stiffness and gelling. Early morning stiffness is the stiffness felt in the joints in a child when he or she wakes up from bed and tries to ambulate. This is thought to be due to accumulation of proinflammatory cytokines in the joint during the period of inactivity. It can last from a few minutes to a few hours. It tends to mirror the overall disease activity. Gelling is the nomenclature used for the stiffness after shorter periods of inactivity. Inflammatory back pain refers to stiffness in latter half of night or early morning in the back, which tends to get better with activity and worsens with rest.

Musculoskeletal system examination in children can be challenging as they may appear well even in the face of a serious or chronic illness and the history may not be localizing. Often, the diagnosis is made using a constellation of symptoms and signs that is referred to as "pattern recognition". Thus, examination in rheumatology involves a detailed general physical examination, screening, and focused MSK examination followed by examination of other systems.

HISTORY

- Presence of antecedent events such as sore throat (acute rheumatic fever) must be inquired.
- Certain conditions like sickle cell disease predispose the child to osteomyelitis due to vascular occlusion and infarcts of the long bones.
- Age and sex of the child can point certain conditions:
  - Acute rheumatic fever is common between the age of 5 and 15 years.

- Kawasaki disease is common in children less than 5 years of age.
- Scurvy is more common in infants and young children.
- Systemic onset juvenile idiopathic arthritis is more common at younger age.
- Hemophilic arthropathy is common in boys. Girls are more likely to have polyarticular JIA.
- A sick neonate with neonatal sepsis can develop osteomyelitis by hematogenous route.

- History of trauma is important as it can cause transient synovitis or post-traumatic effusion in the joint.
- Limping gait may be painful or painless, acute or chronic. The different mechanisms for limping are elaborated in **Table 1**.
- Limb pains occurring during night are bilateral, improving with massage and disappears in the morning, are frequent in child and are referred as growing pains.
- The child with musculoskeletal involvement may initially present with difficulty in walking or limp. The painful limp may be due to osteomyelitis, transient synovitis, trauma, acute leukemia, etc. and painless limp due to developmental dysplasia of hip, Duchenne muscular dystrophy, cerebral palsy, Perthes disease, etc.
- The mode of onset and progress helps in reaching the diagnosis. An acute and migratory onset of arthritis or arthralgia is the characteristic of acute rheumatic fever, while slow,

Table 1: Mechanisms of limping.

Pain	• Child takes minimum support on the painful joint and there is compensatory increase in weight bearing on the opposite limb • It can be due to trauma, infection, inflammation, neoplasm, etc.
Structural abnormality	Asymmetrical limb length, deformity and muscle contractures, may be congenital or acquired
Neuromuscular disease	May be due to muscle disease (dystrophy) or due to lesion in nervous system causing loss of proprioception or muscle control (cerebellar disease)

gradually progressive and persistent is suggestive of juvenile rheumatoid arthritis.
- Other conditions which can lead to acute onset of arthritis in children include septic arthritis, trauma, hemophilia, sickle cell disease, reactive arthritis, Kawasaki disease, inflammatory bowel disease, etc.
- Single joint involvement may be due to tuberculous arthritis, oligoarticular rheumatoid arthritis, septic arthritis, etc.
- Pain of rheumatoid arthritis improves with activity, while pain increases following trauma and hemarthrosis.
- History of remissions and relapses suggests immune disorders.
- Pain in the knee joint may be referred from the hip joint and pain to the hip from the lower back.
- Other important points include presence of rashes such as erythema marginatum in rheumatic fever, macular and malar rashes in systemic lupus erythematosus (SLE), nodular rash in erythema nodosum, in inflammatory bowel disease, etc. Renal manifestations like hematuria and hypertension may be due to Henoch-Schönlein purpura, etc. Hepatosplenomegaly and lymphadenopathy may suggest leukemia.

GENERAL EXAMINATION

It includes assessment of peripheral pulses (pulse volume, presence of all pulses, audible bruit); blood pressure (hypertension); skin including nails, hair and nail fold capillaries; eyes; cartilaginous structures (ears, nasal cartilage); mucous membrane; oral cavity (dentition, tonsils, tongue, and buccal mucosa); and lymph nodes. The symptoms and signs found during general examination in a case of arthritis provide important clues for diagnosis as shown in **Table 2**.

PHYSICAL EXAMINATION

- Sparing some time just to observe the child for its appearance, well looking or sick, posture and gait is quite rewarding. Always observe the active movements before any attempt to make a passive movement to avoid causing pain.

Table 2: Associated symptoms and signs with arthritis which can give a clue to the diagnosis of various forms of arthritis.

Condition presenting with joint pain	Associated symptoms and signs
Systemic onset JIA	Evanescent rash, generalized lymphadenopathy, hepatosplenomegaly, chest pain due to pleurisy or pericarditis
ANA positive oligoarticular JIA (ANA positive) which would include ANA + oligoarticular and polyarticular disease	Anterior uveitis in the form of inflammatory cells in the anterior chamber, irregular pupils, band-shaped keratopathy, cataract
Rheumatoid factor positive polyarticular JIA	Rheumatoid nodules
Enthesitis-related arthritis	Presence of entheseal tenderness, sacroiliac involvement, acute anterior uveitis
Reactive arthritis	Uveitis, urethritis
Systemic lupus erythematosus	Nonerosive polyarthritis (distal > proximal), malar rash, discoid rash, photosensitivity, mucosal ulcers, nonscarring alopecia, generalized lymphadenopathy, vasculitic rashes, serositis, hypertension, and pedal edema due to nephritis
Juvenile dermatomyositis	Proximal muscle weakness (Gower's sign), malar rash, heliotrope rash, Gottron papules, vasculitic ulcers, calcinosis cutis
Inflammatory bowel disease associated arthritis	Chronic diarrhea, dysentery, erythema nodosum
IgA vasculitis (Henoch–Schönlein purpura)	Palpable purpura predominantly over the lower limbs, abdominal pain, dorsal fullness of hands and feet
Kawasaki disease	Conjunctival congestion, strawberry tongue, limb edema, polymorphic generalized rash, periungual desquamation

(ANA: antinuclear antibody; JIA: juvenile idiopathic arthritis)

- The important points to be noted on general assessment of skeletal system on physical examination is shown in **Box 1**.

> **Box 1:** Important points on general assessment and examination of the skeletal system.
> - The sequence of examination should be look (inspection), feel (palpation), move (gait)
> - Look for any redness, swelling and subcutaneous nodules
> - Look for any deformity of joint like flexion deformity, spinal deformity, knock knees, muscle wasting, contractures, etc.
> - Check for shortness of a particular limb by measuring its length from any fixed anatomical land mark
> - Observe whether the child can get up from floor and stand up. If child requires support to do so or not able to get up, it indicates proximal muscle weakness
> - Check the joint for temperature, swelling and tenderness
> - Confirm for any restricted movement of joint
> - Check the spine for any deformity like scoliosis, kyphosis, lordosis, etc.

MUSCULOSKELETAL EXAMINATION

A thorough MSK examination can be time consuming and requires patience. To overcome this limitation in routine clinical assessment, pGALS (pediatric Gait, Arms, Legs, Spine) was designed. pGALS is a simple validated tool that is used for MSK screening in school-aged children and has been particularly designed for non-MSK specialists. It is an adaptation of adult GALS with a few additional maneuvers that help discern normal from abnormal in children. pGALS should be performed in any child with muscle, bone, joint pain or when a rheumatological illness is suspected based on the clinical history. As the name implies, pGALS consists of examination of the gait, arms, legs, and spine. The order of examination can be altered in a non-weightbearing child and prior to performing pGALS, the child should ideally be undressed. The components of pGALS are outlined in **Table 3**.

While performing pGALS, the pediatrician should carefully note the joint range of movement (decreased or increased); asymmetry of joint movement, muscle bulk, or joint swelling; muscle wasting (would indicate chronicity of illness); referred pain (e.g., pain in the hip can be referred to the knee); and nonverbal cues (e.g., wincing while moving a joint or refusal to being examined). It is also important to be aware of age appropriate milestones and normal

Table 3: The pGALS assessment.

Screening maneuver	What is being assessed?
Observe the child standing (from front, back, and sides)	• Posture and habitus • Skin rashes • Deformity*
Observe the child walking and make the child walk on their heel and tiptoes	• Ankles, subtalar, midtarsal, and small joints of feet and toes • Foot posture#
Ask the child to hold their hands straight out in front	• Forward flexion of shoulders • Elbow extension • Wrist extension • Extension of small joints of fingers
Ask the child to turn hands over and make a fist	• Wrist supination • Elbow supination • Flexion of small joints of fingers
Ask the child to pinch their index finger and thumb together	• Manual dexterity • Coordination of small joints of index finger and thumb and functional key grip
Ask the child to touch the tips of their fingers	• Manual dexterity • Coordination of small joints of fingers and thumbs
Squeeze the metacarpophalangeal joints for tenderness	Metacarpophalangeal joints
Ask the child to put their hands together palm to palm (Namaste or namaskar posture) followed by joining the back of the hands in the form of "inverted Namaste or namaskar posture"	• Extension of small joints of fingers • Wrist extension and flexion subsequently • Elbow flexion
Ask the child to reach up, touch the sky, and look at the ceiling	• Elbow extension • Wrist extension • Shoulder abduction • Neck extension
Ask the child to put their hands behind the neck	• Shoulder abduction • External rotation of shoulders • Elbow flexion
Ask the child to try and touch their shoulder with the ear	Cervical spine lateral flexion
Ask the child to open wide and put three (child's own) fingers in the mouth	Temporomandibular joints (and check for deviation of jaw movement)

Contd...

Contd...

Screening maneuver	What is being assessed?
Feel for effusion at the knee (patellar tap, or cross-fluctuation)	Knee effusion (small effusion may be missed by patella tap alone)
Active movement of knees (flexion and extension) and feel for crepitus	• Knee flexion • Knee extension
Passive movement of hip (knee flexed to 90° and internal rotation of hip)	Hip flexion and internal rotation
Ask the child to bend forward and touch their toes	Forward flexion of thoracolumbar spine (and check for scoliosis)

*e.g., varus or valgus deformity, scoliosis, alterations in limb alignment
#Flat feet—arch should be visible when a child is walking on tiptoes.
Source: Adapted from http://www.arthritisresearchuk.org.

variations in children. Normal variants in gait patterns and leg alignment include habitual toe walking up to 3 years of age, in-toeing between 3 and 8 years of age, bow legs up to 18 months, knock knees till 7 years, and flat feet up to 6 years of age. Persistent changes beyond the expected age should be investigated.

Abnormalities detected in pGALS should be followed up with a more detailed and targeted examination. pREMS (pediatric Regional Examination of the Musculoskeletal System) is also based on adult REMS principle of "look, feel, move, function". For instance, if hypermobility is detected while performing pGALS, this should be followed by targeted examination to determine generalized joint hypermobility using the Beighton scoring system. Further information is available on https://www.versusarthritis.org/.

WHEN TO SUSPECT RHEUMATOLOGIC DISORDER?

Try to derive the following information while taking history and physical examination which will provide an important clue to reach the diagnosis:
- Is it arthritis or arthralgia?
- Is any associated muscle involvement present?
- Is there any evidence of vascular involvement?
- Is it associated with organomegaly and/or lymphadenopathy?

- Is it primary disease or musculoskeletal manifestations following some secondary diseases like leukemia?
- Is it congenital or acquired?

Joint Examination

- Joint pain should be differentiated, is it due to arthritis or arthralgia?
  Arthritis is an inflammation of the joint and inflammation includes swelling, pain, redness and restricted joint movement. Arthralgia refers to joint pain without inflammation and therefore there is no swelling or redness.
- The following points are helpful for further analysis in a case of joint swelling:
  - Duration of joint swelling.
  - The number of affected joints during the first 6 weeks. JIA has to be more than 6 weeks old.
  - Presence of any extra-articular sign.
  - Onset before the age of 16 years.

Is it acute arthritis or chronic arthritis?
The defining criterion for chronic arthritis is persistence of symptoms in the joint should be for more than 6 weeks.

Is the involvement is articular or nonarticular?
Articular structures include synovium, synovial fluid, articular cartilage, intra-articular ligaments, joint capsules and juxta-articular bones. Nonarticular structures include supportive ligaments, tendons, bursa, muscles, fascia, bones, nerves and overlying skin.

Pain, restricted movement of joint and joint tenderness indicates articular disease. Associated swelling due to synovitis, joint effusion, bony enlargement, instability and locking of joint, crepitus and deformity suggest articular involvement. Hyperpigmentation indicates long standing deformity.

Nonarticular pain (periarticular pain) has point tenderness and pain on active movement rather than on passive movement. The range of movement is preserved. Associated joint instability, deformity and crepitus are absent.

Is it inflammatory or noninflammatory?
Inflammatory disorder may be due to infection, immune mediated or idiopathic. Noninflammatory conditions have usually mechanical causes. Inflammatory diseases have systemic manifestations with laboratory evidences of inflammation, while noninflammatory conditions have variable clinical findings usually no positive laboratory findings. Mechanical causes will lead to more pain after physical activity, worsening as the day progresses and improves with rest swelling, warmth and systemic manifestations are absent.

Again for deciding the cause, relevant information is important.

What is the onset?
Acute arthritis needs urgent treatment, likely septic arthritis. Hemarthrosis in a case of hemophilia may present as acute arthritis. Chronic arthritis is defined as arthritis of more than 6 weeks duration. JIA is the most common cause of chronic arthritis. Tuberculosis, brucellosis and other uncommon disorders should be excluded.

Is axial peripheral joint involvement present?
Axial joint involvement is rarely seen in SLE and vasculitis. It is one of the important manifestations of enthesitis-related arthritis.

Is it oligoarticular or polyarticular?
Oilgoarticular juvenile arthritis refers to arthritis with involvement of not more than four joints and polyarticular arthritis means arthritis with involvement of at least five joints. This refers to joint involvement in the first 6 months of disease onset.

Is the involved joint characteristic of some disease?
Site of involvement is characteristic of many diseases like distal interphalangeal in psoriatic arthritis, bilateral temporomandibular joint in RF negative polyarthritis, hip joint in reactive arthritis, etc.

Is the involvement additive, migratory or intermittent?
It is an important diagnostic clue. Additive involvement means already one joint is affected and now another joint is involved. This is the characteristic of reactive arthritis. In migratory or fleeting joint pain, from one joint, the inflammation spreads to another joint. In this type, the first joint may start to improve before the

other joints are involved. This is seen in rheumatic fever. In intermittent involvement, after an episode of arthritis, there is a phase of remission and after a few months, again relapse develops. It is the characteristic of rheumatologic disorders.

What is the distribution of joint involvement?
- *Symmetrical:* It includes systemic, polyarticular JIA, SLE, sarcoidosis, viral infections, etc.
- *Asymmetrical:* This includes oligoarticular idiopathic arthritis, septic arthritis, infective endocarditis, etc.

Is the arthritis deforming or nondeforming?
Deforming arthritis is seen in RF positive polyarticular JIA, oligoarticular JIA, etc. Nondeforming arthritis is seen in SLE, inflammatory bowel disease, etc.

Extra-articular Manifestations
Any systemic examination finding may be an important clue for the diagnosis. For example, uveitis is an important finding suggesting oligoarticular JIA, vasculitis, skin rash, arthritis and abdominal pain are characteristics of *Henoch-Schönlein* purpura. In a sick child presenting with hepatosplenomegaly and lymphadenopathy, leukemia should be excluded. Pain while walking, intermittent claudication, vascular rashes, gangrene changes, nonhealing ulcer are features of involvement of vascular system.

EXAMINATION OF OTHER SYSTEMS
- Cardiovascular system for the presence of pericardial friction rub or other murmurs.
- Respiratory system for crackles, wheeze, and reduced chest expansion.
- Central and peripheral nervous system for muscle weakness and neuropathy.

Examination of Skin and Its Appendages

CHAPTER 13

Vijay Bhaskar, R Madhu

INTRODUCTION

The skin is the largest organ of the human body with many vital functions. It has been observed that about 30–40% of children seen in pediatric office practice, present with dermatological problems. Many a times, skin condition offers a visual clue to the underlying systemic disorders. It is essential to look at the patient as a whole and not restrict to only dermatological examination. Detailed history and thorough clinical examination are mandatory to arrive at a correct diagnosis. Skin over the entire body has to be examined including palms, soles and mucosa. It is important to examine the hair and nails. The age, morphology and distribution of skin lesions always give a clue to the diagnosis of dermatological conditions.

HISTORY ELICITATION

A good history and astute clinical examination will help in accurate diagnosis. One has to find out whether the disease is of acute or chronic in nature. Any constitutional and prodromal symptoms have to be elucidated. Various questions that have to be asked include onset of disease, site of onset, evolution and associated symptoms such as itching, burning sensation or pain. If the symptoms are recurrent, then the number of episodes, frequency, duration of each episode and triggering factors such as food, heat, cold, sunlight, exercise, drug, physical activities, contact with animals and seasonal variation have to be noted. History of any allergies in the form of drug, atopy, allergic rhinitis and asthma will give clue to allergic disorders. Past history of similar illness, previous hospitalization and surgeries have to be inquired. Elicitation of proper family history is very important in children with genodermatoses and allergic disorders. History of sexual contact and intravenous drug abuse has to be elicited as per the clinical scenario.

EXAMINATION

Dermatological examination has to be always done in a well-illuminated room. Magnifying hand lens and torch light are simple, but very important tools which aid in the diagnosis. Examining pediatrician should observe the type, morphology, arrangement and distribution of the skin lesion.

A few terminologies have to be understood for examination of skin in children.

A lesion is any area of altered skin which may be single or multiple. Skin lesions can be primary, secondary or special which will give a clue to the diagnosis.

Primary Lesions

Primary lesions are the most characteristic lesion for a particular or a group of diseases and need not appear in the early part of the disease. It is a basic reaction pattern of skin with definite morphology. Similar primary lesion may occur in different diseases. Examples include macule, patch, papule, nodule, vesicle, blister, etc.

- *Macule (Latin: macular means spot):* It is a circumscribed area of change in skin color which is flat, measuring less than 0.5 cm. It appears white in vitiligo and brown in café au lait macules **(Fig. 1)**.
- *Patch:* It is similar to macule which is more than 0.5 cm. Sometimes multiple macules may coalesce to form patch **(Fig. 2)**.
- *Papule (Latin: papula means pimple):* It is an elevated solid lesion less than 0.5 cm **(Fig. 3)**.
- *Nodule (Latin: nodulus which means small knot):* It is an elevated solid lesion more than 0.5 cm **(Fig. 4)**.
- *Plaque:* It is a well-demarcated area of abnormal skin which is either raised above or sunken below the skin surface **(Fig. 5)**.
- *Vesicle (Latin: vesicular which means a little bladder):* It is a circumscribed elevated cavity filled with fluid and measuring less than 0.5 cm **(Fig. 6)**.

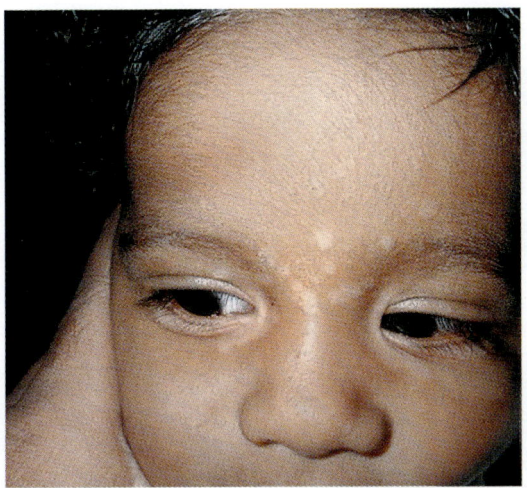

Fig. 1: Macule over the face in pityriasis versicolor.

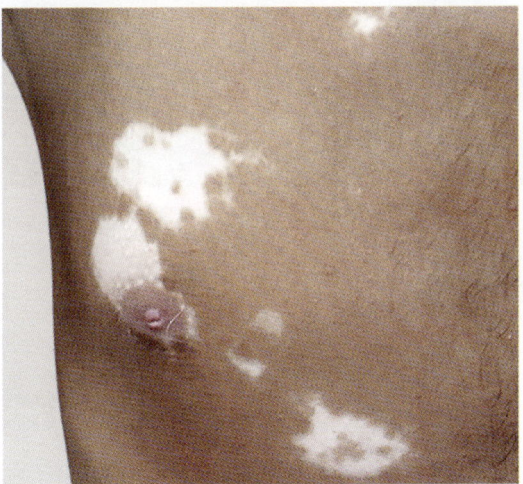

Fig. 2: Patch over the trunk in vitiligo.

- *Bulla (Latin: bulla which means bubble):* It is similar to vesicle but measures more than 0.5 cm **(Fig. 7)**.
- *Pustule (Latin: pustula which means inflamed sore, blister):* It is a vesicle which contains pus.

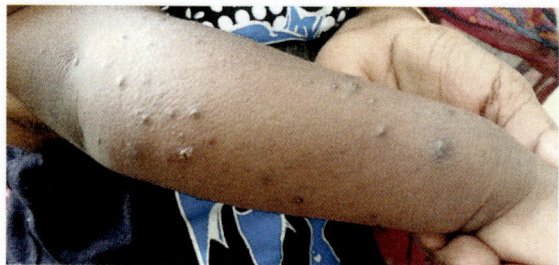

Fig. 3: Papules over the forearm in miliaria rubra.

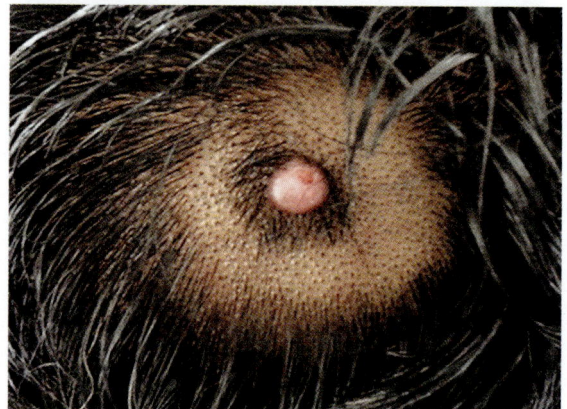

Fig. 4: Nodule over the scalp.

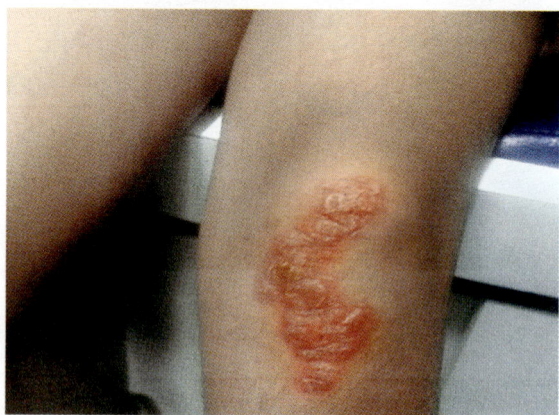

Fig. 5: Plaque in psoriasis vulgaris.

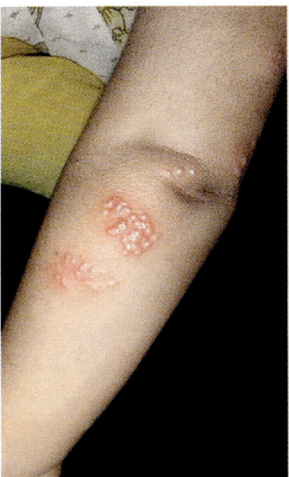

Fig. 6: Vesicle in herpes zoster.

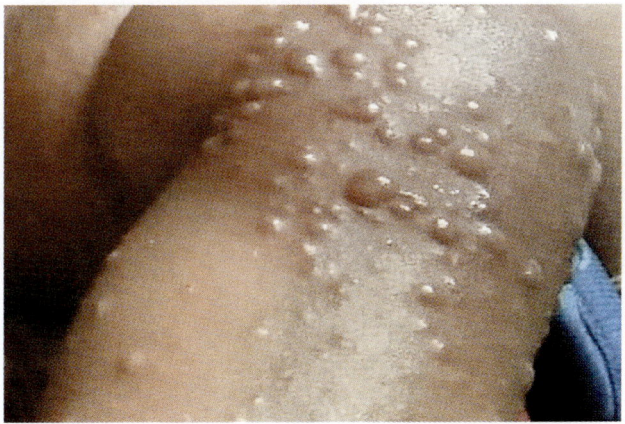

Fig. 7: Bulla—hand-foot-and-mouth disease.

- *Wheal:* It is an area of dermal or hypodermal edema, erythema and pallor which is evanescent. Urticaria is the classical example **(Fig. 8)**.
- *Cyst:* It is a closed cavity or sac with an epithelial, endothelial or membranous lining containing fluid or semisolid material. Examples include epidermal cyst, etc.

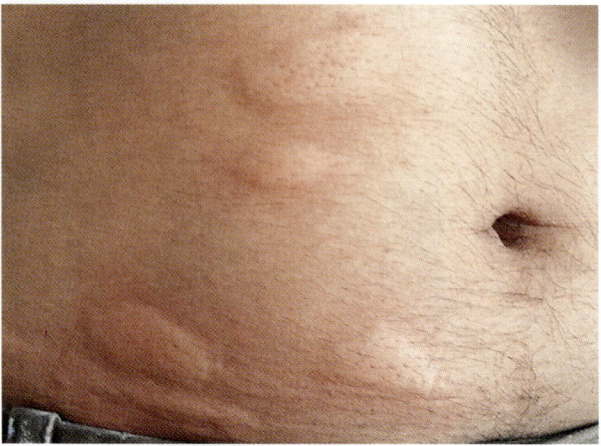

Fig. 8: Wheal in urticaria.

Secondary Lesions

Secondary lesions are lesions that develop during the evolution of skin disease or that may result due to scratching or secondary infection. Following are the examples of secondary lesions:
- *Scale:* It is visible exfoliation of stratum corneum in the form of flat plate or flake. The various types are furfuraceous in pityriasis versicolor, lamellar in ichthyosis, silvery scales in psoriasis and collarette in pityriasis rosea **(Fig. 9)**.
- *Crust:* It consists of dried serum and exudates commonly seen in impetigo **(Fig. 10)**.
- *Excoriation:* It is loss of skin surface produced by scratching which may be linear or circumscribed.
- *Erosion:* It is due to loss of whole or part of epidermis which heals without scarring. Commonly follows a blister and is typically seen in impetigo.
- *Ulcer:* It is due to loss of epidermis and part of dermis and may involve the underlying tissues. Commonly seen in trauma and stasis ulcer.
- *Scar:* It is defined as replacement of tissue that has been destroyed by injury or disease by fibrous tissue. These can be atrophic, hypertrophic, cribriform, varioliform and pitted.
- *Lichenification:* It is thickening of epidermis and to some extent of the dermis, pigmentation and accentuation of skin markings

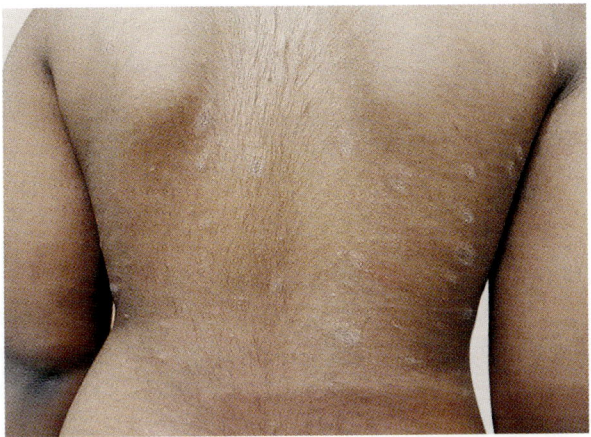

Fig. 9: Scales in pityriasis rosea.

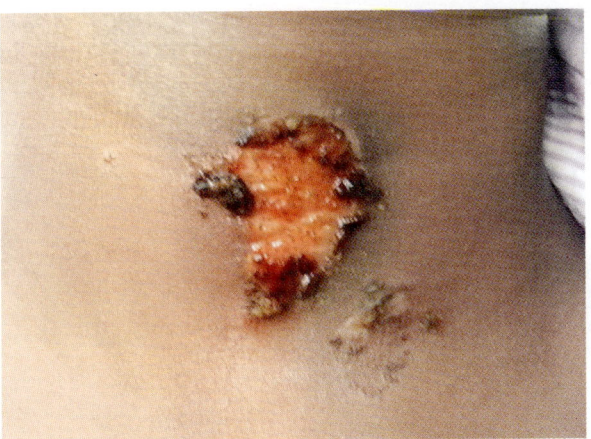

Fig. 10: Crust in impetigo.

in response to prolonged rubbing. Example is lichen simplex chronicus.
- *Induration:* It is thick skin due to dermal involvement.
- *Sclerosis:* It is a diffuse or circumscribed induration of the subcutaneous tissues and may involve the dermis. Sclerosis is better felt than seen as in scleroderma.
- *Atrophy:* It is loss of tissue characterized by loss of normal skin markings.

Special Lesions

Special lesions are specific for certain diseases.
- *Burrow:* It is a tunnel in the skin which houses the parasite like itch mite in scabies.
- *Comedo:* It is a special lesion with a plug of keratin and sebum in a dilated pilosebaceous orifice as seen in acne **(Fig. 11)**.
- *Telangiectasia:* It is a visible and permanent dilatation of capillaries.
- *Target lesions:* It has three zones, a central zone of dusky erythema or purpura, middle pallor zone of edema and an outer ring of erythema with a well-defined edge which is commonly seen in erythema multiforme.

Distribution and Morphological Patterns

- Dermatological diagnosis can be made depending on the distribution of the skin lesion and the morphology. The distribution and the disease associated are given in **Table 1**.
- Some dermatological conditions have predilection for certain sites of body **(Table 2)**.

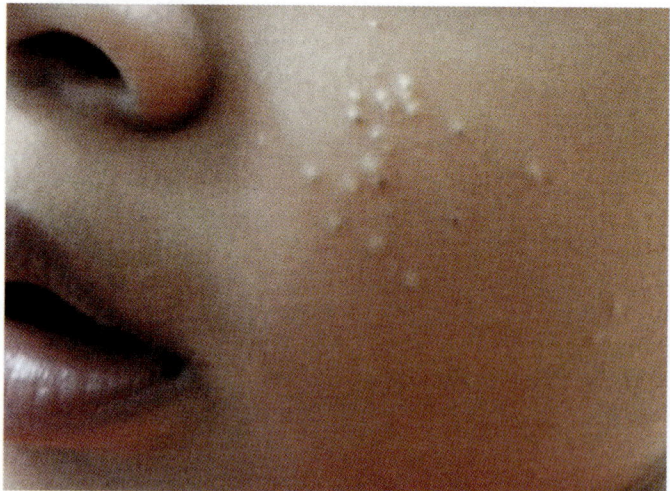

Fig. 11: Comedone in acne.

Table 1: Dermatological condition versus characteristic pattern of distribution.

Distribution	Dermatological condition
Segmental	Vitiligo **(Fig. 12)**
Dermatomal	Herpes zoster **(Fig. 13)**
Seborrheic	Acne, seborrheic dermatitis
Christmas tree pattern	Pityriasis rosea
Follicular	Keratosis pilaris, phrynoderma **(Fig. 14)**
Grouped	Herpes zoster
Photoexposed area	Polymorphous light eruption
Bizarre	Dermatitis artefacta

Table 2: Dermatological condition versus common site of occurrence.

Trunk
- Pityriasis versicolor
- Tinea corporis
- Pityriasis rosea
- Pityriasis rubra pilaris
- Vitiligo
- Leprosy
- Scabies
- Psoriasis vulgaris **(Fig. 15)**
- Lichen planus

Scalp
- Aplasia cutis congenital
- Nevus sebaceous **(Fig. 16)**
- Tinea capitis
- Alopecia areata
- Psoriasis

Groin/genitals
- Intertrigo
- Tinea cruris
- Acrodermatitis enteropathica

Nails
- Psoriasis
- Lichen planus
- Alopecia areata

Acral
- Erythema multiforme
- Pellagra

Extremities
- Scabies
- Psoriasis
- Lichen planus
- Granuloma annulare **(Fig. 17)**
- Gianotti-Crosti syndrome

Face
- Pityriasis alba **(Fig. 18)**
- Pityriasis versicolor
- Polymorphous light eruption
- Acne
- Milia
- Atopic dermatitis
- Contact dermatitis
- Perioral dermatitis
- Hansen's disease

Flexors
- Intertrigo
- Atopic dermatitis **(Fig. 19)**
- Seborrheic dermatitis

Oral mucosa
- Lichen planus
- Stevens-Johnson syndrome
- Geographic tongue

Perioral
- Acrodermatitis enteropathica
- Staphylococcal scalded skin syndrome

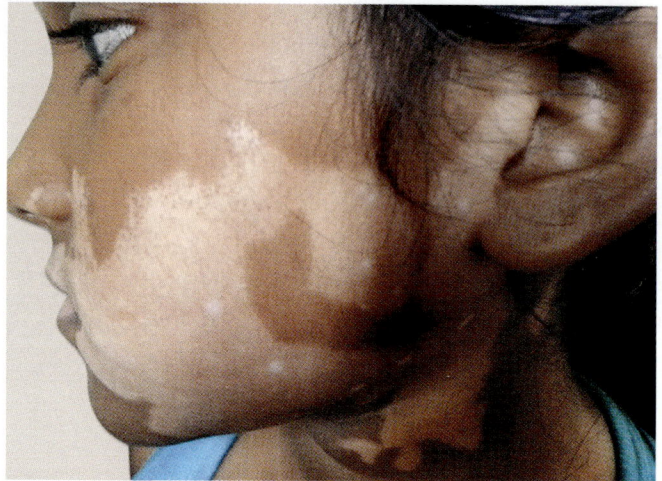

Fig. 12: Vitiligo in a segmental distribution.

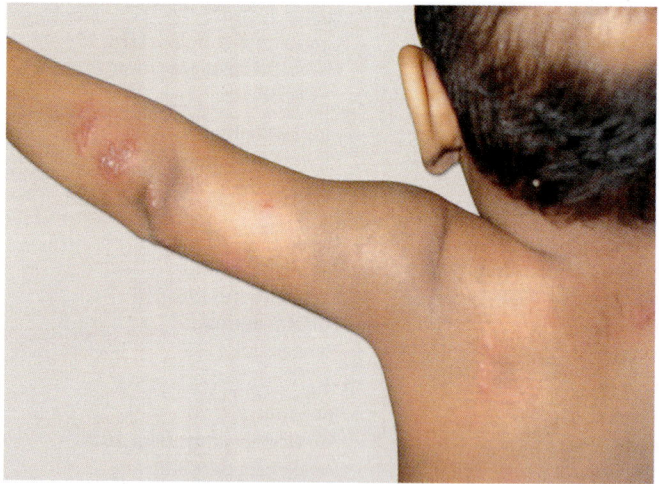

Fig. 13: Herpes zoster in a segmental pattern.

Changes in Skin Color

The color of the lesions also contributes to arrive at a diagnosis. Red lesions are vascular or inflammatory. Examples include

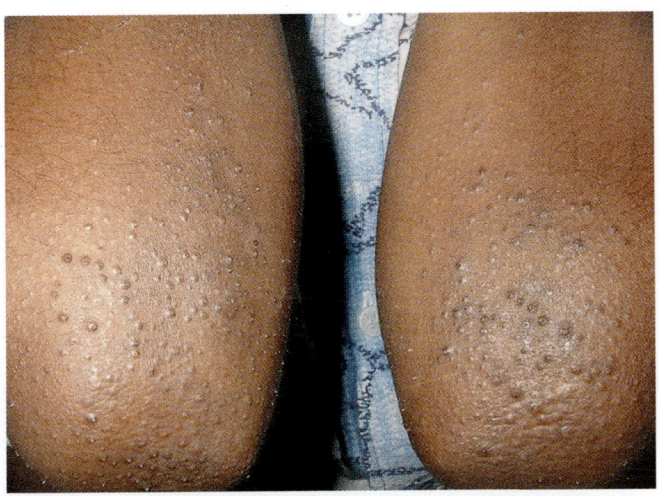

Fig. 14: Phrynoderma in follicular distribution.

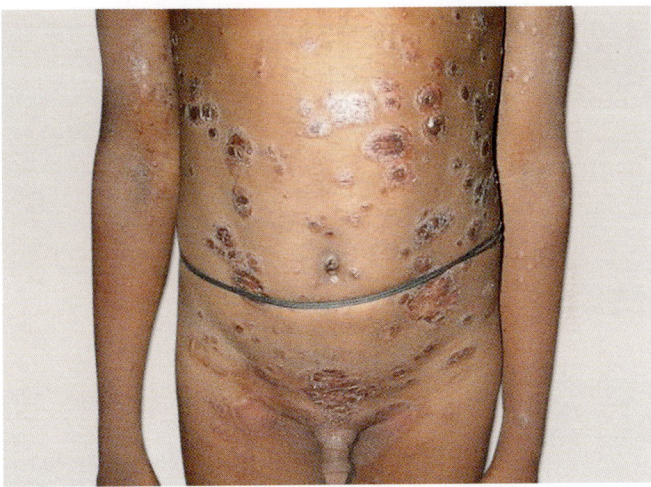

Fig. 15: Psoriasis vulgaris in truncal distribution.

hemangioma and psoriasis **(Fig. 20)**. Hypopigmented lesions are less pigmented as in pityriasis versicolor, pityriasis alba, Hansen's disease, nevus achromicus and postinflammatory hypopigmentation. Wood's lamp aids in the differentiation of nevus

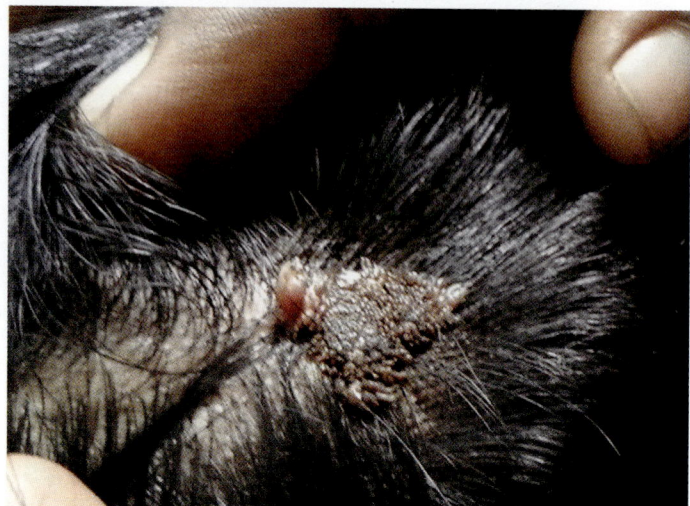

Fig. 16: Nevus sebaceous over the scalp.

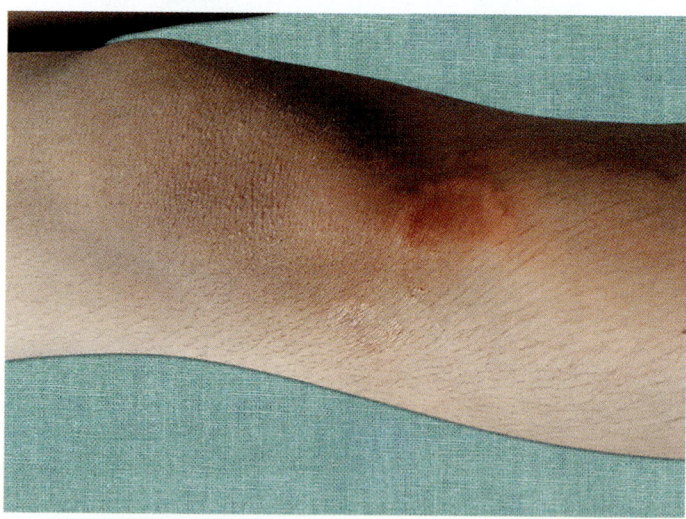

Fig. 17: Granuloma annulare over the extremities.

achromicus/anemicus and vitiligo. Erythrasma is diagnosed by the characteristic coral-red fluorescence, pityriasis versicolor by yellow orange fluorescence. Brilliant green fluorescence is seen in

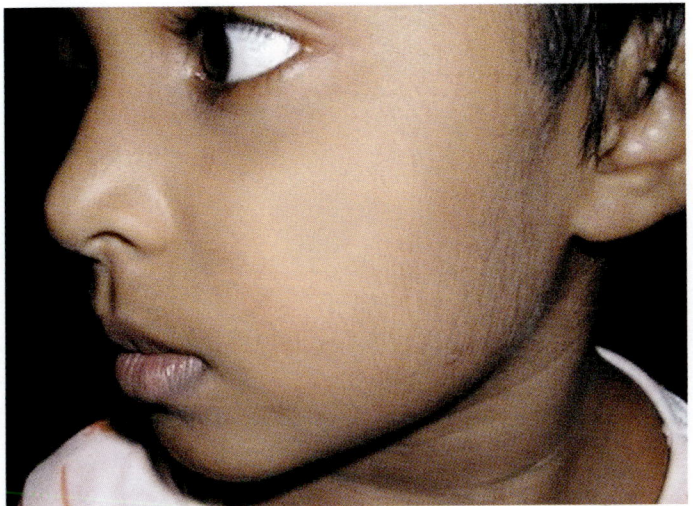

Fig. 18: Pityriasis alba over the face.

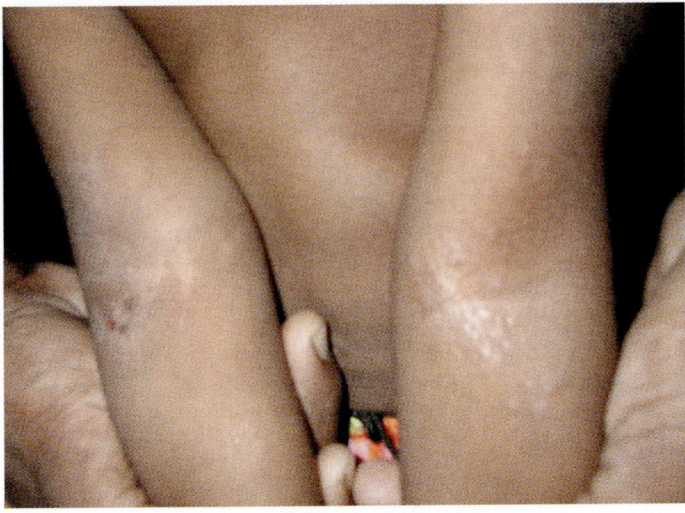

Fig. 19: Atopic dermatitis in flexors.

children caused by tinea capitis caused by *Microsporum* species. Nevi, fixed drug eruption, melasma and acanthosis nigricans present with hyperpigmentation.

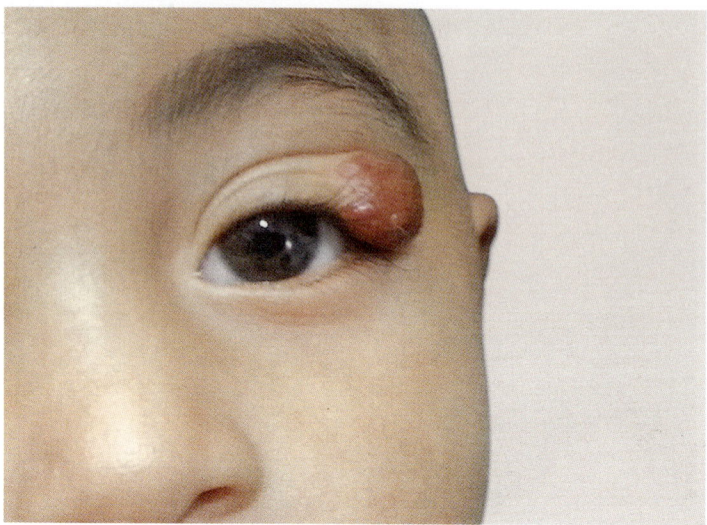

Fig. 20: Red vascular lesion in hemangioma.

EXAMINATION OF SKIN AND ITS APPENDAGES
Appendages of Skin

Hair and nails provide protection to the skin and have common embryologic origin, ectoderm. Many diseases of hair and nails may be associated with dermatologic and systemic disease. This emphasizes the importance of their thorough examination.

Hair

- *Hypertrichosis:* Growth of excessive hair which is coarser and more profuse than normal for age, sex and race of the individual is called as hypertrichosis. Hirsutism refers to growth of coarse terminal hair in the adult male sexual pattern in females. Systemic conditions associated with hypertrichosis are listed in **Box 1**.
- *Alopecia:* Alopecia refers to loss of hair, which can be localized or diffuse. Alopecia areata is a common, autoimmune disorder, characterized by round or oval patches circumscribed or diffuse hair loss. It is commonly-associated thyroid disorders, Down syndrome anhidrotic ectodermal dysplasia, etc.

> **Box 1:** Systemic conditions associated with hypertrichosis.
> - Familial or constitutional
> - Drugs like corticosteroids, phenytoin, etc.
> - Cushing's syndrome
> - Porphyria cutanea tarda
> - Coffin–Siris syndrome
> - Cornelia de Lange syndrome
> - Treacher–Collins syndrome (Hair on the side of face)

- *Trichotillomania:* It is seen in children above 5 years and most commonly involves the scalp and present as a compulsive pulling of hair resulting in irregular areas of partial hair loss.
- *Color of the hair:* Premature graying of hairs, especially of scalp hair, at an age earlier than physiologically accepted (20 years), is seen in vitiligo and alopecia areata. It is also described in pernicious anemia, hyperthyroidism, ataxia telangiectasia, tuberous sclerosis, progeria and drugs like chloroquine.

Nail

- Nail pitting is a common problem and present as small punctuate depressions. Large and irregular pits are characteristic of psoriasis. Regularly spaced, fine pits in rows are seen in alopecia areata.
- Beau's line is a transverse groove that develops as a reaction to stress and it temporarily interrupts nail growth. They may occur due to trauma, acrodermatitis enteropathica and chronic antibiotic usage. Recently, it has also been observed in Kawasaki disease.
- Koilonychias is a thin, depressed, concave nail. It is considered as pathognomonic sign of iron deficiency anemia. Platynychia may be an early stage of koilonychia.
- Paronychia is the inflammation of nail folds resulting from infection. It may be bacterial or fungal infection. History of thumb sucking or finger sucking is common with paronychia. Disruption of cuticle is seen in systemic lupus erythematosus (SLE) and dermatomyositis.
- Clubbing of nails is seen in variety of conditions and described in details in Chapter 3.

Some Common Skin Conditions

Impetigo

Impetigo is the most common skin infection in children. There are two classic forms of impetigo, bullous and nonbullous. Nonbullous impetigo is most commonly due to Group A β-hemolytic streptococci, but *Staphylococcus aureus* can also cause it. Bullous impetigo is always caused by *Staphylococcus aureus* that produce exfoliative toxins.

Nonbullous impetigo accounts for more than 70% of cases. Lesions are typically begin on the skin of face or on extremities have been traumatized. The most common lesions that precede nonbullous impetigo are insect bites, abrasions, lacerations, chickenpox or scabies. A tiny vesicle or pustule forms initially and rapidly develop into honey-colored crusted plaque that is generally <2 cm in diameter. The infection may be spread to other parts of the body by the fingers and clothing. Lesions are associated with no pain and constitutional symptoms. Pruritus may occur occasionally. Regional lymphadenopathy is found in 90% cases.

Bullous impetigo is mainly an infection of infants and young children. Flaccid, transparent bullae develop most commonly on the skin of face, buttocks, trunk, perineum and extremities. Rupture of bulla occurs easily, leaving a narrow rim of scale at the edge of shallow, moist erosion. Unlike nonbullous impetigo, lesions of bullous impetigo are a manifestation of localized staphylococcal scalded skin syndrome and develop on intact skin.

Scabies

The characteristic lesions are linear burrows seen over axillae, flexor surface of extremities, wrists, interdigital areas of palms and soles and genital areas. Usually, the face is spared. There is intense and intractable itching especially during night. There is secondary excoriations, eczematous areas, pustules and crusting due to itching, rubbing and secondary bacterial infection. Scabies is highly contagious and several family members are affected simultaneously.

Seborrheic Dermatitis

Seborrheic dermatitis is usually associated with dandruff and has predilection for infants and adolescents. It starts from scalp with greasy-yellowish scales and extend down the forehead to involve the eyebrows, nose and ears. Loss of scalp hairs and depigmented skin lesions are seen during the course of disease. It should be differentiated from atopic dermatitis and histiocytosis.

Papular Urticaria

It is a common, intensely pruritic condition caused by an allergic response to insect bites, most common due to mosquito and flea bites. It may be manifestation of scabies in infants.

Atopic Dermatitis

The distribution of skin rash in atopic dermatitis varies depending upon the age. In infancy cheeks, extensor surfaces of the arms and legs typically develop papulovesicular, often weeping or wet lesions which may develop fine scabs or lichenification. The scalp and postauricular areas are often affected while diaper area is usually spared. Secondary infection and traumatic lesions may develop due to scratching and rubbing. In older children, dry maculopapular lesions are commonly distributed over the flexor aspects of extremities. Raised serum IgE and eosinophilia support the diagnosis.

Zinc Deficiency

Skin manifestations due to zinc deficiency are commonly seen over perioral, periorabital and perinasal areas. Involvement of hands and feet is also common. The vesiculobullous skin lesions become dry, scaly and crusted with sharply demarcated borders. The vesicles rupture, revealing a moist, red base and then dry. Diarrhea failure to thrive and alopecia are common other features of zinc deficiency.

Pityriasis Alba

It is a common, asymptomatic skin condition of unknown etiology in infants and children. The skin lesions are well demarcated, hypopigmented, round or oval patches with minimal fine scales. The lesions are commonly seen over face, but may be present on the neck and upper trunk.

Tinea Versicolor

It is characterized by appearance of asymptomatic ovoid or coin-shaped brown colored or whitish macules over the neck, chest and back. The lesions have fine adherent scales. Pruritis is minimal or absent. It is more common after puberty through young children.

Tinea Capitis

It often presents as a kerion with an inflammatory, boggy, pustular patch with localized alopecia of scalp. The typical scaly circular lesion with raised edges and central clearing that is seen in tinea corporis is uncommon in tinea capitis. There is eczematization, scab formation and formation of scales. It should be differentiated from seborrheic dermatitis.

Tinea Corporis

It is characterized by annular erythematous ring lesions with active elevated margins and central clearing. The border is scaly, slightly elevated and often studded with microvesicles and tiny pustules.

Candida Infection

Candida infection of skin has special predilection for moist areas like diaper area, neck, axillae groin, perioral and perianal regions. It produces confluent erythema with maceration and fissuring. There are vesiculopustular lesions over an erythematous base. Oral thrush and paronychial candidal infection may coexist. Beyond neonatal period, development of recurrent candidiasis should alert the pediatrician to look for an underlying condition like HIV, diabetes mellitus, DiGeorge syndrome, etc.

Erythema Multiforme

It is characterized by erythematous lesions of pleomorphic morphology. The lesions begin as erythematosus macules and evolve into papules, vesicles, bullae, urticarial plaques or patches of confluent erythema. The symmetric crops of skin lesions usually occur on extensor surfaces of arms and legs often involving palms and soles. The skin lesions may heal over 4–6 weeks with hypopigmentation, without any scarring. When skin lesions are associated with involvement of two mucous membranes, the condition is called as Stevens–Johnson syndrome.

Toxic Epidermal Necrolysis

Toxic epidermal necrolysis (TEN) is characterized by loosening of large sheets of epidermis with formation of flaccid bullae. The bullae rupture leading to exposure of intensely pink, underlying epidermis or dermis which gives an appearance scalded skin. Nikolsky sign is positive, epidermis can be readily peeled by rubbing the skin at normal sites. It may occur due to certain drugs or bacterial infections.

TORCH Infections

Intrauterine infections may manifest as petechiae and ecchymoses over trunk and extremities due to thrombocytopenia. 'Blueberry muffin' spots are characteristic skin lesions of congenital cytomegalovirus (CMV) infection. Congenital syphilis is characterized by maculopapular rash initially pink and subsequently turning to coppery brown with desquamation especially over palms and soles.

INVESTIGATIONS

Scraping of skin lesion in the characteristic sites could be done to visualize the mites in children with scabies **(Figs. 21 and 22)**. Diagnosis of dermatophytosis and pityriasis versicolor is usually clinical. But, when in doubt, superficial fungal infections can be diagnosed by microscopic examination of the scrapings of the lesion in 10% potassium hydroxide **(Fig. 23)**. In children with tinea capitis, 40% potassium hydroxide is used for hair root examination **(Fig. 24)**.

Tzanck smear is a bedside investigatory tool to diagnose viral infection or bullous disorders. Vesicle or bulla is to be opened

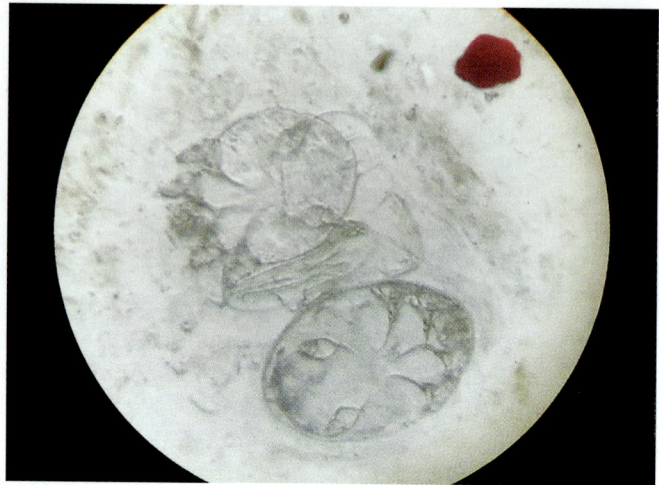

Fig. 21: Low power view of *Acarus* mite.

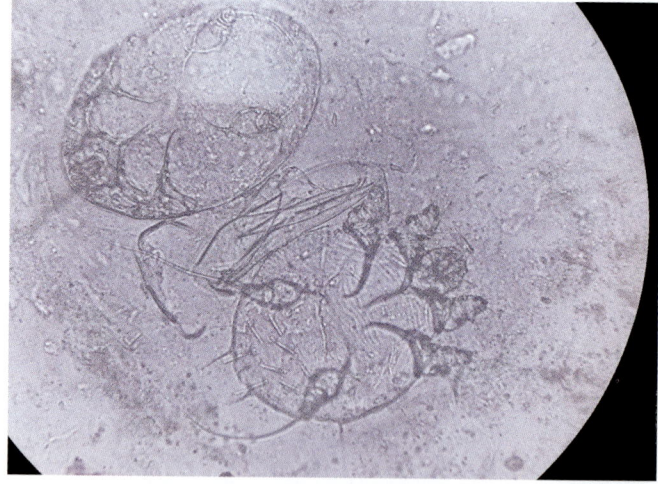

Fig. 22: High power view of *Acarus* mite.

with a scalpel and the fluid is let out. The floor of the lesion is scraped with the blunt end of the scalpel and smear is made on the glass slide and Leishman's staining is done and viewed under the microscope. Multinucleate giant cells are seen in viral

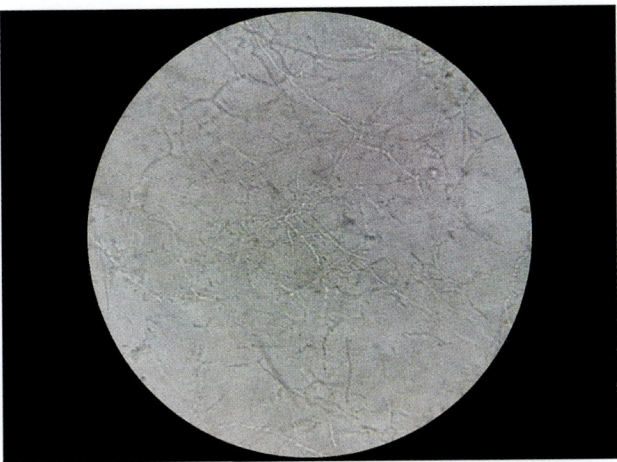

Fig. 23: 10% potassium hydroxide (KOH) wet mount showing dermatophytes with long branching septate hyphae.

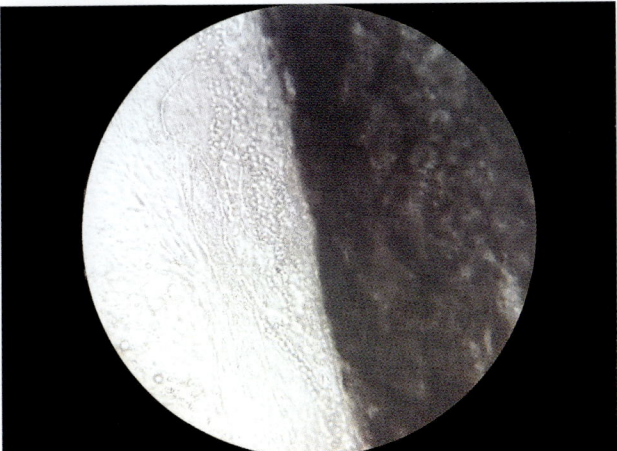

Fig. 24: 40% potassium hydroxide (KOH) wet mount of hair root showing endothrix invasion.

infections, while Tzanck cells are seen in bullous disorders. Tzanck cells are large keratinocytes with hypertrophic nucleus and hazy or absent nucleoli with abundant basophilic cytoplasm with a perinuclear halo.

CONCLUSION

Skin being a visual specialty, the examining physician should have an eye for details. Head to foot examination in a well-illuminated room and use of magnifying lens are mandatory. Systematic observation of the type, morphology, color, distribution and site of involvement will throw light on diagnosis. It is a known fact that skin lesions, many a times, give a clue to the underlying systemic disorders and this only goes to further stress the significance of astute dermatological examination.

Examination of Eye

CHAPTER 14

Aloka Santosh Hedau

INTRODUCTION

The human eye is a precise system, which comprises components that must be optimally maintained so that a clear image is seen. Eye undergoes a lot of dynamic changes in its anatomy and functionality in the first few years of the child's life.

They are born farsighted and slowly the vision gets adjusted. Depth perception, focus, tracking, color vision, and other aspects of vision continue to develop throughout the childhood. Between the ages 1 and 3, coordination between hands, eyes, and body allows children to pick up objects, walk or run, and throw and catch a ball. Overall cognitive development and physical development are largely dependent on vision. It is for this reason that eye examination is of utmost importance for any baby.

The World Health Organization (WHO) reports that there are approximately 19 million visually impaired children in the world, and 1.4 million are blind. In India, by the 2017 published study, 0.8 per 1,000 children are estimated to be blind. About half of the causes of blindness and visual impairment are potentially preventable or treatable.

Timely and periodic screening is critical for the detection of visual impairment and its etiology and to plan early intervention. Protocols vary from country to country. A Joint Policy Statement by the American Academy of Pediatrics, American Academy of Ophthalmology, American Association for Pediatric Ophthalmology and Strabismus, and American Association of Certified Orthoptists emphasizes that vision assessments and screening eye examinations are critical for the detection of conditions that result in visual impairment, lead to problems with school performance, harbinger serious systemic disease, and, in some cases, threaten the child's life. There are no formal Indian national guidelines for vision and eye screening in children.

ANATOMY OF THE EYES

The human eye is divided into adnexa, which includes the orbital area, lid and lacrimal system, anterior segment comprising the cornea, conjunctiva, iris, lens and aqueous humor, and posterior segment comprising the vitreous humor, choroid, retina, and uvea **(Fig. 1)**. Optic nerve and optic pathway form the neurological part of the eye.

Common Symptoms Related to the Eye

- *Eye discharge:* Any discharge from the eyes of a child requires due attention. In newborn, it may be due to conjunctivitis or congenital dacryocystitis. In older children, it may be

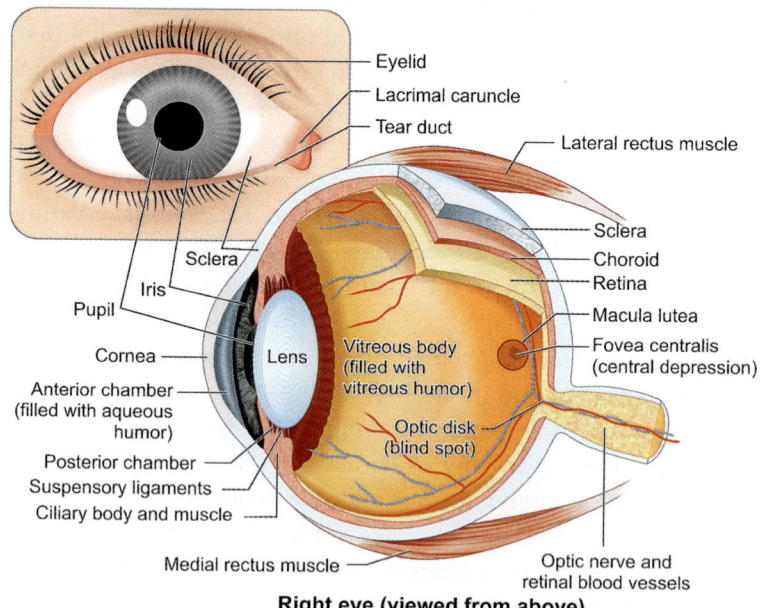

Fig. 1: Anatomy of the eye.

due to allergic or infective conjunctivitis, trauma or chronic dacryocystitis.
- *Red eye:* Congestion in the eye is always pathological. The reason may be trivial as rubbing due to itching but may be due to some serious condition which requires prompt attention. It may be due to conjunctivitis, conjunctival injury or foreign body. It may be due to viral infection like measles and Epstein-Barr virus (EBV) or systemic disorders such as systemic lupus erythematosus (SLE), Kawasaki disease, etc.
- *Itching of eye:* Itching of the eye is the hallmark of allergic conjunctivitis, but may be due to blepharitis.

Mass Lesions in the Vicinity of the Eyelid

The common mass lesions of their differentiating features are described in **Table 1**.

White Reflex in Pupil

This is also known as amaurotic cat's eye reflex or leucocoria and has ominous implications. In neonates, it may be due to congenital cataracts, retinoblastoma, endophthalmitis, etc. In older children, it may be due to congenital or traumatic cataract, retinal detachment, endophthalmitis, etc.

METHODS OF EYE SCREENING

It is essential to do eye screening at birth and again during infancy, preschool, and school years. An overview of the same is available in **Table 2**.

Screening of Child's Eyes

- *External examination:* Examine with torchlight and look for ptosis, corneal clarity, pupillary abnormality, lens clarity, iris abnormalities, and conjunctival evaluation **(Fig. 2)**.
- *Corneal light reflex test:* In a corneal light reflex test, the child's attention is attracted to a target (a light or a brightly colored object), while a light in front of the child is directed at the child's eyes. The light's reflection will be symmetric in each pupil by 4-6 months of age in patients with normally aligned eyes.

Table 1: Common mass lesions around the eyelids.

Lesion	Cause	Clinical features	Important clues
Chalazion	Blockage of meibomian gland opening with a granulomatous reaction to the lipid content in the gland	Firm, painless, slowly growing swelling in tarso-conjunctiva, free from overlying skin	Bluish or yellowish discoloration on the conjunctival side of lesion
Stye	Blockage of the duct of glands of Moll or Zeis with bacterial superinfection, commonly staphylococcal	Acutely inflamed, tender swelling of one of the glands associated with eyelashes	A pus point at the root of the lash
Distention of lacrimal sac	Obstructed nasolacrimal duct due to incomplete canalization	Soft swelling in the medial canthal region	Pressure over the swelling causes discharge of contents muco-purulent
Dermoid	Common in children, congenital, arising from ectoderm, can be pinched off	Soft cystic mass	Subcutaneous, overlying skin normal, fixed to periosteum
Hemangioma	Proliferation of vascular endothelial cells	Soft, red mass, grows rapidly, involutes later on	Blanches with pressure

A wide nasal bridge or epicanthal folds may give the appearance of eye deviation; however, on closer examination, the light reflection will be found to be symmetric. This is pseudostrabismus, a normal variant **(Figs. 3A to C)**.

- *The red reflex test or Bruckner's test:* The red reflex test is properly performed by holding a direct ophthalmoscope close to the eye with the ophthalmoscope lens power set at "0". In a darkened room, the ophthalmoscope light should then be projected onto both eyes of the child simultaneously from approximately 18 inches away **(Fig. 4)**.

Table 2: Age appropriate methods of eye screening.

Method	Indications for referral	Recommended age					
		Newborn to 6 months	6 months and until the child is able to cooperate for subjective visual acuity measurement	3–4 years	4–5 years	Every 1–2 years after 5 years of age
Red reflex examination	Absent, white, dull, opacified, or asymmetric	X	X	X	X	X
External inspection	Structural abnormality (e.g., ptosis)	X	X	X	X	X
Pupillary examination	Irregular shape, unequal size, poor or unequal reaction to light	X	X	X	X	X
Fix and follow test	Failure to fix and follow	Cooperative infant older than 3 months	X			
Corneal light reflex text	Asymmetric or displaced		X	X	X	X
Instrument-based screening*	Failure to meet screening criteria			X	X	X
Cover test	Refixation movement			X	X	X

Contd...

Contd...

Method	Indications for referral	Recommended age				
		Newborn to 6 months	6 months and until the child is able to cooperate for subjective visual acuity measurement	3–4 years	4–5 years	Every 1–2 years after 5 years of age
Distance visual acuity[†] (monocular)	20/50 or worse in either eye 20/40 or worse in either eye Worse than three of five optotypes on 20/30 line, or two lines of difference between the eyes			X	X X	X X X

Note: These recommendations are based on panel consensus. If screening is inconclusive or unsatisfactory, the child should be retested within 6 months; if results are inconclusive on retesting or if retesting cannot be performed, referral for a comprehensive eye evaluation is indicated.

*Subjective visual acuity measurement is preferred to instrument-based screening in children who are able to participate reliably. Instrument-based screening is useful for young children and those with developmental delays.

[†]Lea symbols, HOTV, and Sloan letter are preferred optotypes.

Source: Adapted with permission from American Academy of Ophthalmology Pediatric Ophthalmology/Strabismus Panel. Preferred practice pattern guidelines. Pediatric eye evaluations. San Francisco, Calif: American Academy of Ophthalmology; 2012:10.

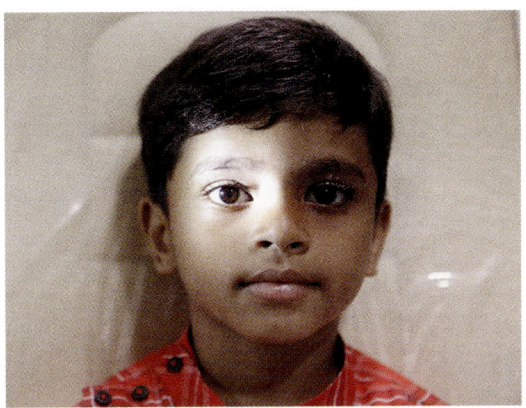

Fig. 2: External evaluation of the eye.

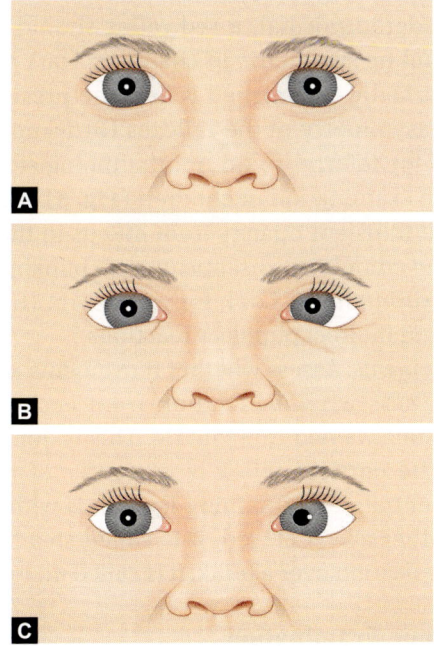

Figs. 3A to C: Corneal light reflex test. (A) Normal corneal light reflex in normally aligned eyes; (B) Pseudostrabismus. The child appears to be converging his left eye toward his nose because of the enlarged epicanthal folds; however, note that the light reflex is symmetric in each eye; (C) True strabismus. Note the light reflex is central in the fixating (the child's right) eye, but is displaced in the nonfixating (the child's left) eye.

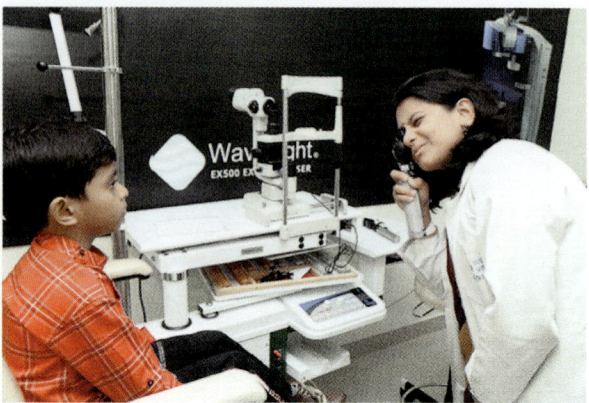

Fig. 4: Bruckner's test.

To be considered normal, a red reflex should emanate from both eyes and be symmetric in character. Dark spots in the red reflex, a markedly diminished reflex, the presence of a white reflex, and asymmetry of the reflexes (Bruckner reflex) are all indications for referral to an ophthalmologist who is experienced in the examination of children **(Fig. 5)**. The exception to this rule is a transient opacity from mucus in the tear film that is mobile and completely disappears with blinking.

- *Pupillary examination:* Look for anisocoria (unequal pupils) and direct and indirect pupillary reactions.
- *Ocular movements:* Assess whether movements are full and free.
- *Fixation:* Assess whether fixation from each eye is central, steady, and maintained uniocularly. This is done with penlight source. If the corneal reflex is in center of the pupil then fixation is central; if maintaining fixation is without wandering when the other eye is closed, it is called steady; and if eye is maintaining fixation over a blink, it is called maintained fixation.

Ophthalmoscopic Examination

Retina is the only structure in the body where one can directly see blood vessels and optic nerve. The examination of retina can detect several systemic diseases affecting central nervous system (CNS), cardiovascular system and hematological disorders. The etiology may be infective, vascular, nutritional or metabolic.

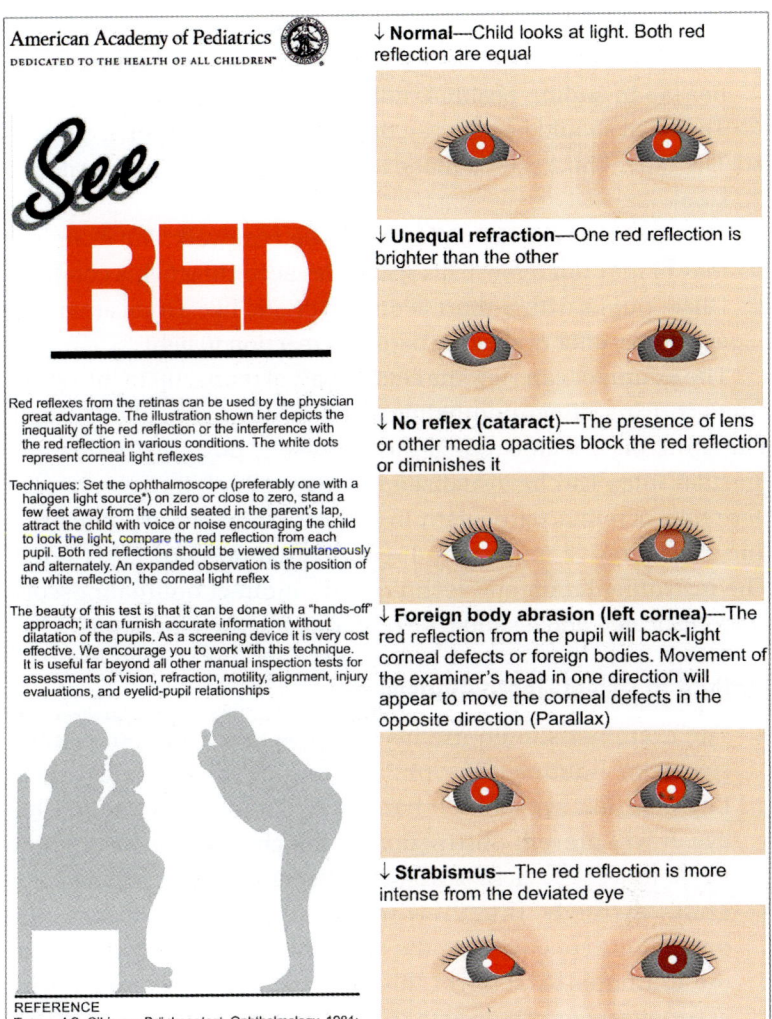

Fig. 5: Red reflex examination.
Source: Used with permission of Alfred G. Smith, MD, ©1991.

Direct Ophthalmoscopy

Prerequisites

- The room light should be dimmed.
- The examiner and patient should be comfortable.

- The examiner should wear a mask.
- The infant should not be hungry. The mother holds the child in her lap in supine position, holding the arms against the body. The head should be between the knees of the examiner.
- The older child can be made to lie down supine or can sit on a stool.
- The spectacles of the child should be removed. The examiner may or may not remove his spectacles according to his comfort.
- Dilate pupils with a short acting mydriatic like Tropicamide 1% eye drops, after evaluating papillary reaction to light.

The examiner can view the central part of retina, up to the retinal equator using direct ophthalmoscopy through the dilated pupil. The optic disc, major retinal blood vessels, posterior retina and macular lutea can be visualized by this method. But, to examine periphery of retina, particularly in case of retinopathy of prematurity and degenerative myopia, indirect ophthalmoscopy is required. The instrumentation and technique for indirect ophthalmoscopy is sophisticated and it should be performed by an ophthalmologist.

Method of Direct Ophthalmoscopy

- The examiner should use his right eye to examine the child's right eye holding the ophthalmoscope in his right hand. Likewise, left eye and left hand for examination of child's left eye. It will prevent obstruction by the child's nose as examine has to move very close to examine the fundus in more details.
- Look through the viewing aperture and center the ophthalmoscope light on the eye to be examined. It is easy for the examiner to perform this with his both eyes open. With experience, one can do with other eye closed.
- The first step is to perform a distant direct ophthalmoscopy which will give an idea of the transparency of the ocular media. The focusing lenses should be rotated first one way then the other till the pupil is in focus. At this point, the examiner can see a reddish-orange glow in the pupil. The glow is a reflection of the ophthalmoscope light from the vascular choroidal layer of the eye. It is absent or dull in conditions like cataract, vitreous hemorrhage and endophthalmitis. If there is any doubt,

it can be compared with another eye. The absent red glow is an indication for reference to an ophthalmologist.
- Keeping the light focused on the pupil, the examiner should go as close to the child as possible. Eventually, the middle finger of the hand holding the ophthalmoscope will be close to or resting on child's cheek. The fingers of examiner's other hand should rest on the forehead of the child and the thumb used to gently pull up the upper eyelid. The examiner should be angled slightly temporal of center while the child looks straight ahead. By this way, the examiner can avoid throwing light on the macula and dazzling the child. Rotate the focusing lenses with your index finger, clockwise and then counter clockwise, till retinal structure is seen. The appropriate lens is usually found by trial and error and will vary from patient to patient. It depends upon the refractive error of the examiner's and patient's eyes.
- The retina has a refractile, orange-red appearance, one can see only a small segment of the retina at any time. Usually, vessels are seen and one should trace then till he comes to optic disk.
- To view different areas, you will have to keep changing the angle of view by small degree at a time, in a systematic manner, up, down, left and right. Child should be reminded to look straight ahead, otherwise it will be impossible for the examiner to focus on anything long enough to make a judgment.
- *Optic nerve head:*
  - It should be examined for size, shape, color and margins. It is a vertically oval to round disk, pink in color with a pale center (optic cup) from which emerge of the central retinal artery and vein. It has distinct margins **(Fig. 6).**
  - In papilledema, the optic nerve head is hyperemic, the cup is full, margins blurred with peripapillary retinal edema and hemorrhages, the retinal veins at the disk are tortuous and dilated **(Fig. 7)**.
- *Retinal vessels:*
  - The retinal vessels should be examined next for their caliber, tortuosity and any changes at the sites where arterioles and venules cross each other. Arterioles are bright, pinkish-red,

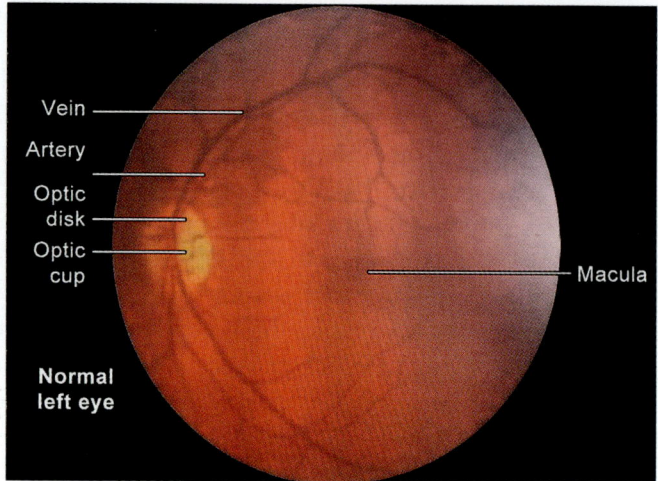

Fig. 6: Normal fundus examination.

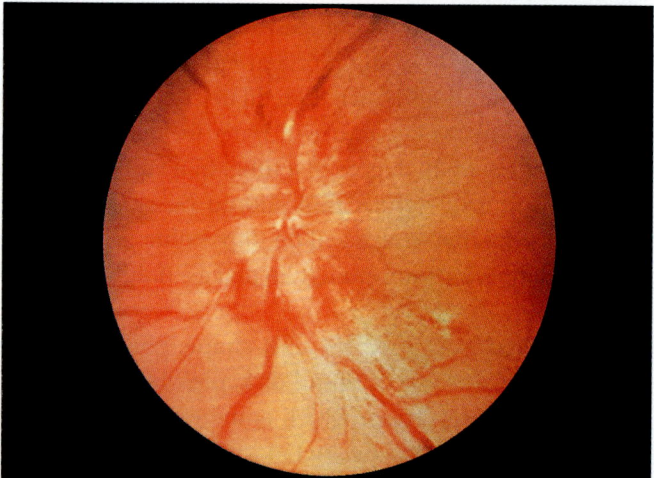

Fig. 7: Papilledema. Refer the text for details.

with a shiny reflex running down their center. They are thinner, being approximately two-thirds of the thickness of the venules. The latter are dark red vessels.
- In patients with hypertension and diabetes mellitus, the caliber of the vessels may change, there may be hemorrhages and exudation from leaky vessels. In malignant hypertension, there may be disk edema. The disk edema is

also seen in optic neuritis when the involvement is mainly of the optic nerve head (papillitis). In retrobulbar neuritis, on the other hand, the disk will not be edematous, but may show pallor on the temporal side in later stages.
- *Background of the retina:* It should be orange-reddish in color, the color depending on the degree of pigmentation in the choroid and retina. It is pale in anemia and with retinal edema. Superficial retinal hemorrhages and Roth's spots are seen in patients with severe anemia. Roth's spots are also seen in subacute bacterial endocarditis. They are small superficial hemorrhages with pale centers.
- *Macula lutea:* Ask the patient to look directly into the light of ophthalmoscope and you will see the macula lutea, the central retina which is darker in color due to luteal pigment. In its center, there is a small depression called the foveola. The light reflects off the walls of the foveola to produce a bright light reflex that helps in identifying this area. Absence of the foveolar reflex suggests a macular lesion. Subhyaloid hemorrhage is a characteristic boat-shaped hemorrhage in the macular area. It is seen in severe anemia. These hemorrhages immediately reduce visual acuity and take a longer time to resolve since the macula is relatively avascular.
- *Fundus evaluation:* It can be done by direct ophthalmoscope or indirect ophthalmoscope **(Figs. 8 and 9)**. Look for the posterior pole comprising of optic disk, macula, and central vessels. Optic disc color, shape, contour, cup, neuroretinal rim, and cup:disc ratio should be noted. To enhance visualization, dilation of the pupils may be done by tropicamide (0.8%) eye drops.
- *Vision screening:* Age appropriate vision screening methodologies should be applied where needed **(Table 3)**. Even if only torchlight is available, try to check the fixation pattern in each child possible. Also always check each eye vision individually, to screen for amblyopia **(Fig. 10)**.

Visual milestone according to the age of the child are shown in **Table 4**.
- Look for cataracts **(Fig. 17)** and accommodative esotropia which can be corrected by appropriate glasses **(Figs. 18 and 19)**.

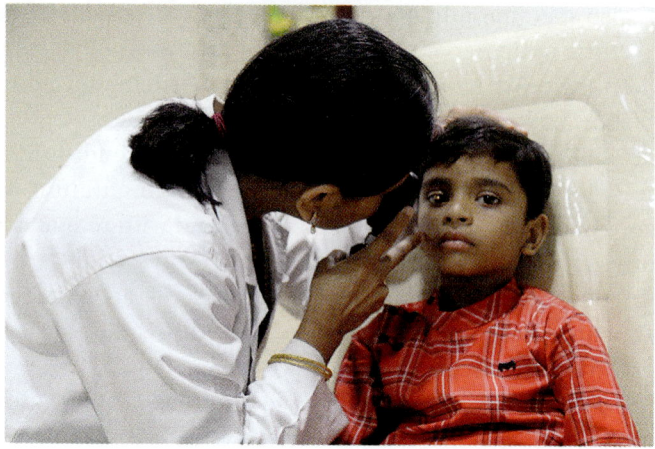

Fig. 8: Fundus evaluation with direct ophthalmoscope.

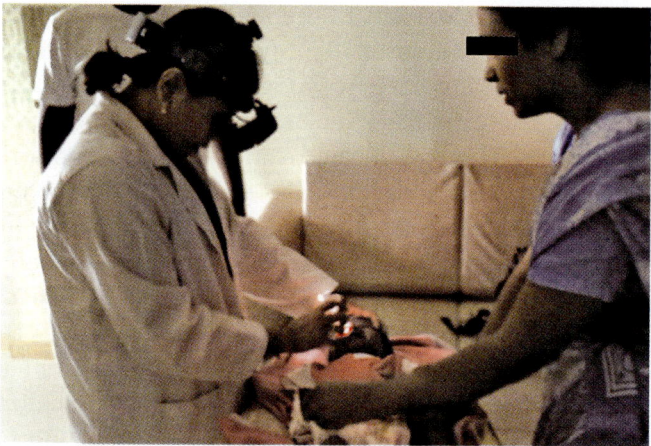

Fig. 9: Fundus evaluation with indirect ophthalmoscope.

Table 3: Age appropriate vision screening charts (Figs. 11 to 16).

Age	Vision screening method
Infancy	*Grating acuity:* Teller acuity, catford drum
Toddlers	*Preferential looking test:* Cardiff cards, allen cards
Preschool	*Recognition acuity:* HOTV matching cards, tumbling E chart
Schoolage group	Snellen chart, LogMAR chart

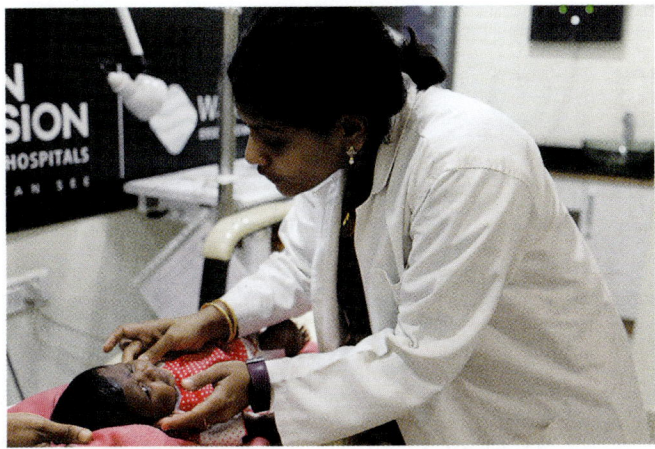

Fig. 10: Vision assessment in a newborn.

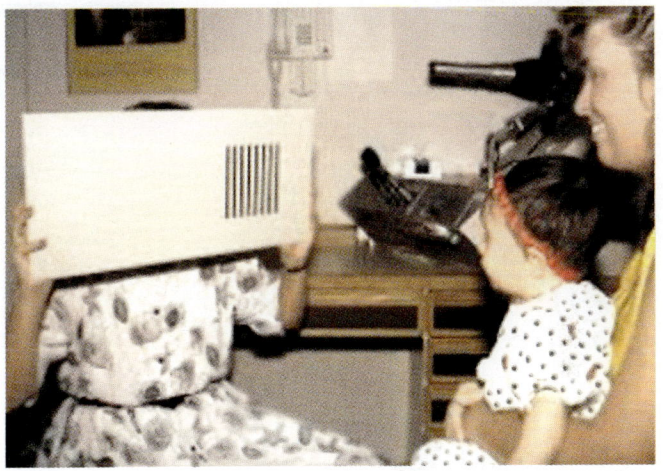

Fig. 11: Teller acuity chart.

REFERRAL TO PEDIATRIC OPHTHALMOLOGIST

Pediatric ophthalmologist and adult squint specialist is an ophthalmologist who had done 18-month fellowship in the field of pediatric ophthalmology and strabismus. Timely referral for care can go a long way in establishing a complete care for your patients **(Table 5)**.

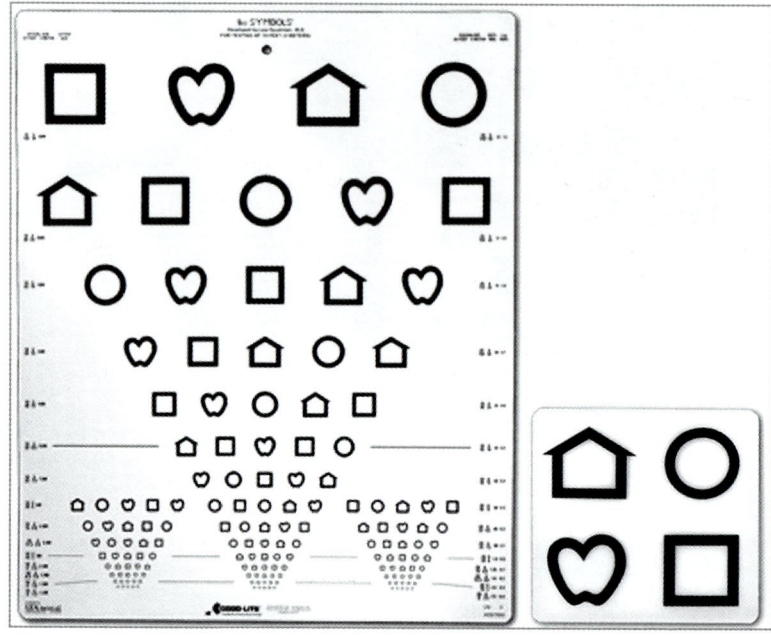

Fig. 12: Lea symbols.

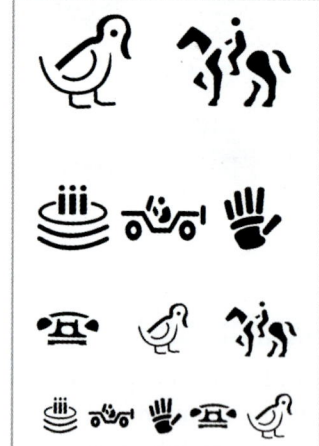 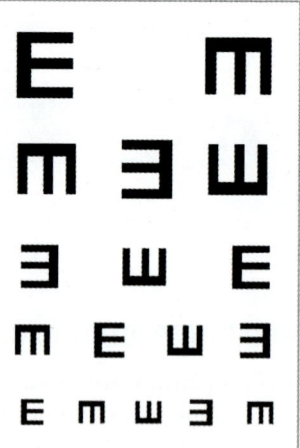

Fig. 13: Allen and tumbling E chart.

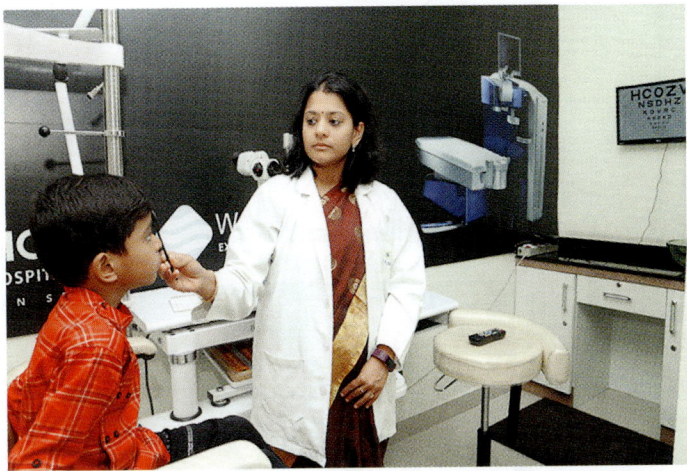

Fig. 14: Monocular vision assessment.

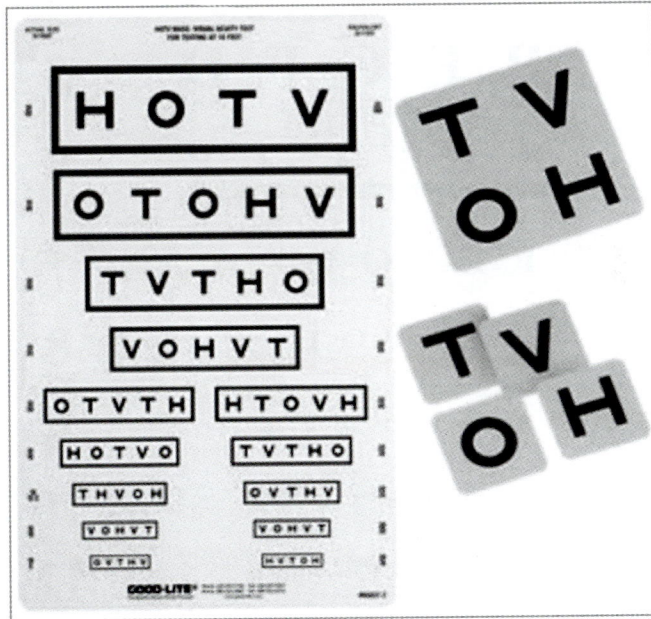

Fig. 15: HOTV matching cards.

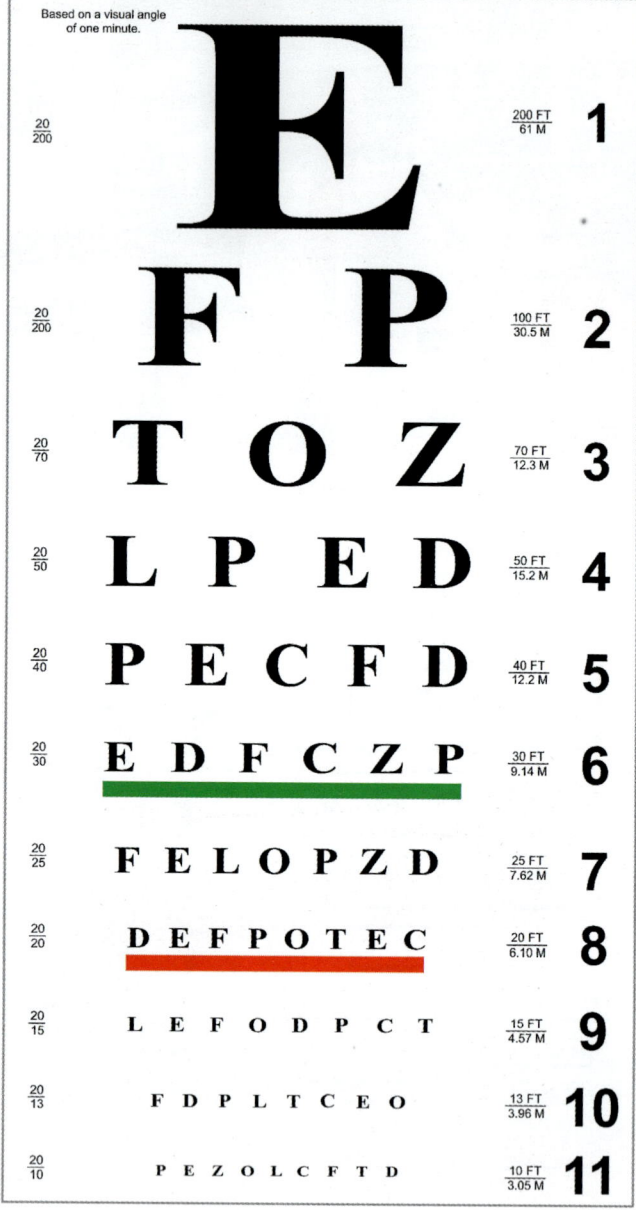

Fig. 16: Snellen's visual acuity chart.

Table 4: Visual milestones according to age of the child.

Age	Visual milestones
Birth to 1 month	Baby should fixate at bright light or faces. Black and white patterns more stimulating
1–3 months	Begins to watch parent's faces. Follow objects horizontally. Primary colors and lights most stimulating
3–5 months	Focusing, convergence, depth perception, and color vision develops. Reaches for nearby objects and looks at objects in hand
5–7 months	Eye hand coordination develops. Eyes should be straight and well aligned most of the time by this age
7–12 months	Imitation of social gestures like smiling and waving. Crawls or moves towards object of interest
12–18 months	More visually guided behavior. Hide-and-seek, Peek-a-Boo favorite visual games. Points at pictures in books
18–24 months	Can draw vertical and horizontal strokes
2–3 years	Imitate play. Copy a circle
4–5 years	Draw simple form, color within lines, describe visual experiences with people or places

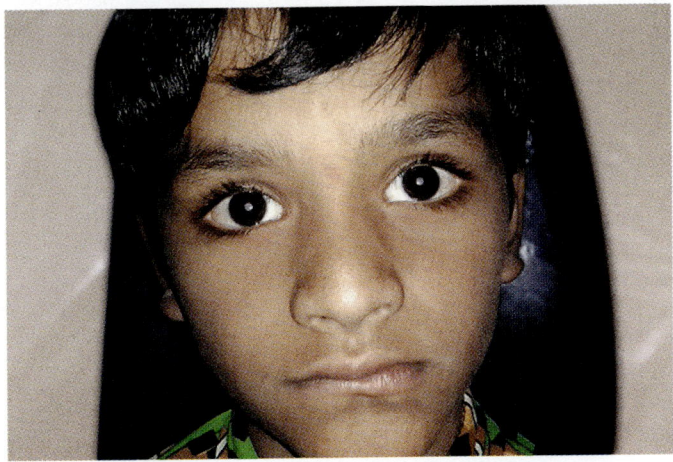

Fig. 17: A 6-year-old with bilateral cataracts.

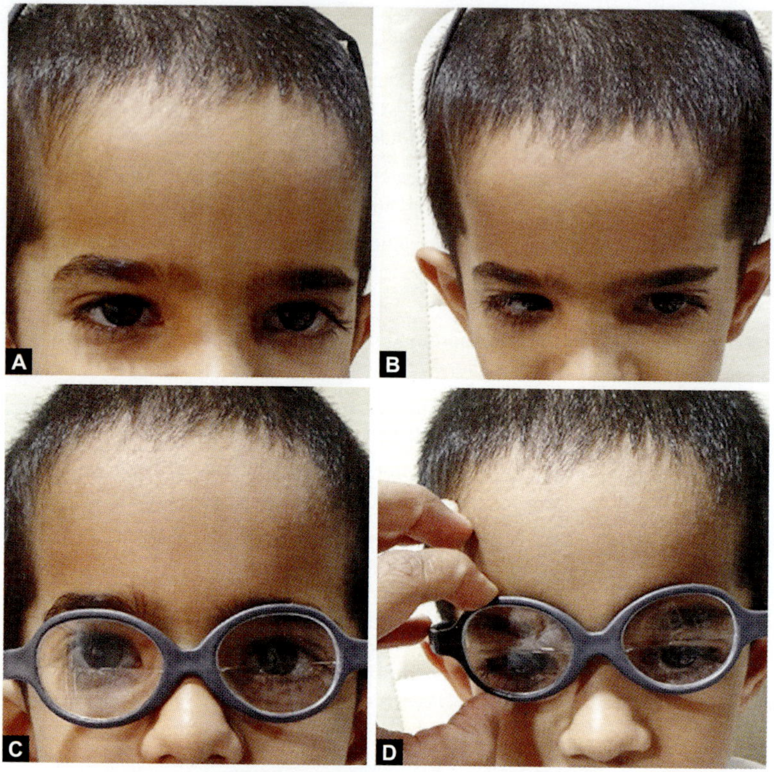

Figs. 18A to D: Child with accommodative esotropia corrected with glasses. (A and B) Squint for near; (C and D) Bifocal glasses with no squinting for near.

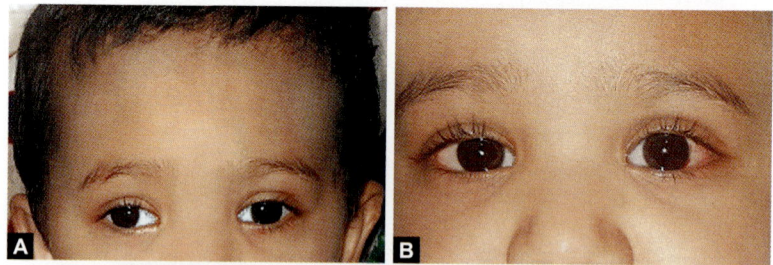

Figs. 19A and B: A 2-year-old child with intermittent exotropia corrected with bilateral surgical correction of squint.

Table 5: Need for referral to pediatric ophthalmologist.

Finding on screening	Need for referral
Visual behavior/acuity	Absence of social smile or eye contact by 3 months. Visual acuity <20/50 or difference of two lines or greater between two eyes. Intermittent or constant misalignment of eyes beyond 4 months
Eyelids	Any child with ptosis or eyelid mass lesion
Nasolacrimal system	Urgent referral in case of dacryocele or mucocele. Any persistent tearing beyond 10 months
Anterior segment	Congenital glaucoma—urgent referral. Chronic conjunctivitis—referral to rule out viral etiology causing corneal scarring
Ocular media opacities	Any white reflex, dull reflex, or asymmetric reflex needs urgent referral
Sensorimotor system (pupillary and ocular movements)	Dilated pupil to rule out 3rd nerve palsy. Constricted pupil to rule of Horner's syndrome, rarely associated with neuroblastoma any child with nystagmus any child with misalignment beyond 4 months of age
Prematurity	Preterm neonates who are born <34 weeks' gestation and/or <1,750 g birth weight; as well as in babies 34–36 weeks' gestation or 1,750–2,000 g birth weight, if they have risk factors for ROP. The first retinal examination should be performed not later than 4 weeks of age or 30 days of life in infants born ≥28 weeks' of gestational age. Infants born <28 weeks or <1,200 g birth weight should be screened early, by 2–3 weeks of age, to enable early identification of AP-ROP **(Flowchart 1)**
Systemic disorders	• *Aid to diagnosis:* Wilson's disease (Kayser–Fleischer ring), gangliosidosis (cherry red spot), mucopolysaccharidosis (corneal clouding) • Baseline evaluation needed in diabetes • Screening in juvenile rheumatoid arthritis and lupus • Sickle cell disease, albinism, Sturge–Weber disease, thyroid disorders • *Drug-related side effects:* Steroids in nephrotic syndrome, HCQ in rheumatoid arthritis
Congenital conditions	• Craniosynostosis, coloboma, any congenital anomaly affecting the optic nerve or ocular pathway • *Aid in diagnosis:* Lisch nodules in NF1, lens subluxation in Marfan syndrome

Contd...

Contd...

Finding on screening	Need for referral
Nonaccidental injuries	Any child with nonaccidental injury should have ocular evaluation to rule out "Shaken Baby syndrome"
Headaches	Chronic headaches, headache with projectile vomiting, headaches after prolonged reading

(HCQ: hydroxychloroquine; ROP: retinopathy of prematurity)

Flowchart 1: Scheme for following a child for retinopathy of prematurity (ROP).

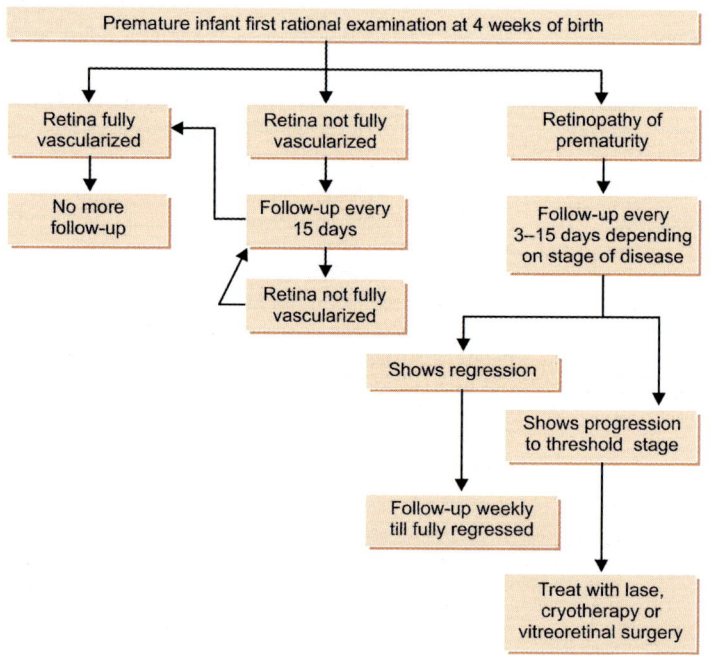

Examination of Ear, Nose, and Throat

CHAPTER 15

Suktara Sharma, Mukund Vaghela

INTRODUCTION
A wide range of ear, nose, and throat disorders affect children contributing to a fairly large number of patients seen in the pediatric outpatient department (OPD). Hence, broad-based knowledge of diagnosis and management of common disorders affecting ear, nose, and throat is essential. The history in very young patients is often provided by anxious parents. Establishing a rapport with the parents and the child is foremost for a good history and clinical examination thereafter.

SYMPTOMS RELATED TO THE EAR
- *Pain in the ear:* It is a common symptom for visit to a pediatrician. While older children may provide a clear history, very young children may present with just excessive crying or pulling of the ears. History of fever, upper respiratory tract infection (URTI), and refusing to feed may be present in cases of acute suppurative otitis media (ASOM). Associated hearing loss may be present in acute otitis media, serous otitis media, or impacted wax. Pain due to fungal infection (otomycosis) is common in the rainy season or in children with history of frequent swimming. Secondary cause of earache also known as referred otalgia may be due to pain originating from the teeth, pharynx, or the cervical spine. Common causes of pain in the ear are listed in **Box 1**.
- *Discharge from the ear:* Chronic suppurative otitis media (CSOM) is one of the most common chronic childhood infections worldwide and presents as chronic intermittent mucopurulent discharge from the ear. Preceding URI and earache may indicate ASOM. Amount, color, consistency, and odor of the discharge

> **Box 1:** Common causes of ear pain in children.
> - Acute otitis media
> - Otitis media with effusion
> - Otitis externa
> - Eustachian tube dysfunction
> - Cerumen or wax in the ear
> - Trauma to the ear
> - Foreign bodies of the ear
> - Referred ear pain can be from teeth, tongue, tonsil, and throat

must be noted. Profuse mucopurulent and nonfoul-smelling discharge is seen in the mucosal or safe type of CSOM. Scanty, purulent, and foul-smelling discharge is seen in squamous or unsafe variety of CSOM. Associated headache, vomiting, fever, and neck pain should be evaluated for intracranial complications of otitis media. Blood-stained discharge may be present in trauma, granulations, or foreign body in the ear.

- *Itching in the ears:* Itching in the ears is commonly due to otomycosis, otitis externa, dermatitis, or CSOM. It might be the only symptom of foreign body in the ear. Itching may be associated with pain and discharge from the ear. Itching with discharge may lead to excoriation of skin around the pinna and the external auditory canal.
- *Hearing loss:* Hearing loss may be congenital or acquired after birth and may range from mild to profound. Acquired hearing loss may be prelingual (happens before speech development) or postlingual (happens after speech development). In very young children, absence of startle response to loud sounds observed by parents might be the first sign of hearing impairment. Moving the eye in the direction of sound and responding to toys that make sound is seen in infants with normal hearing. In toddlers, delayed speech or reduced vocabulary for the age of the child must be investigated. Sudden hearing loss may follow viral infections or meningitis. CSOM and secretory otitis media are also associated with hearing loss. Early detection and intervention is critical for speech as well as social and cognitive development of children. The various causes of hearing loss are listed in **Table 1**.

- *Swelling in and around the pinna:* Mastoid abscess **(Fig. 1)**, hematoma of the auricle **(Fig. 2)**, infected preauricular sinus, and accessory auricular tags are some of the causes of swelling around the pinna.

Table 1: Causes of hearing loss in children.	
Conductive hearing loss	Sensorineural hearing loss
Congenital: • Anotia/microtia/atresia of external auditory canal • Ossicular malformations • Tympanic membrane malformations	Congenital: • Genetic factors (syndromic, connexin26, and mitochondrial) • *In utero infections:* CMV, rubella, and measles • Maternal rubella • Premature birth • Exposure to ototoxic drugs during pregnancy
Acquired infections: • Otitis media/otitis media with effusion • Foreign body including cerumen • Cholesteatoma • Trauma (ossicular disruption, tympanic membrane perforation	Acquired infections: Bacterial meningitis, measles, mumps, and Lyme disease Trauma: Physical or acoustic Neurodegenerative or demyelinating disorders (Alport syndrome, Usher syndrome, and Pendred syndrome
(CMV: cytomegalovirus)	

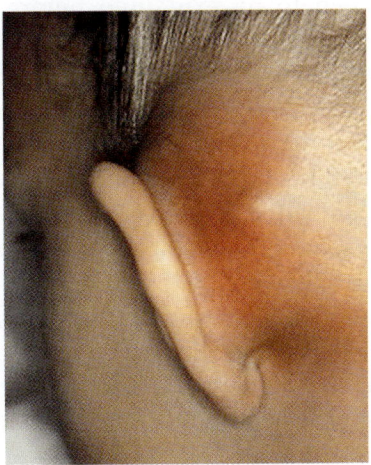

Fig. 1: Mastoid abscess.

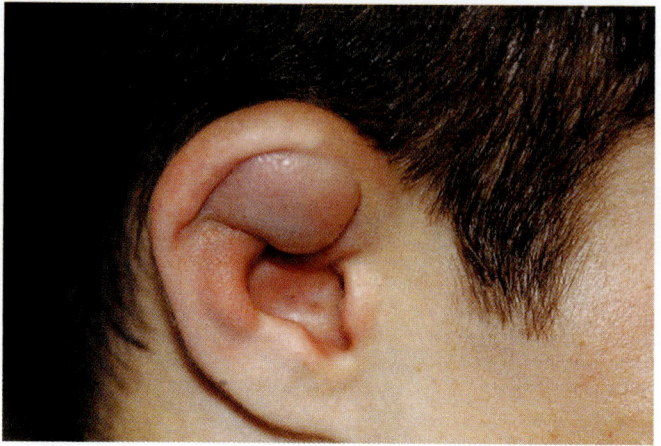

Fig. 2: Hematoma of the auricle.

- *Giddiness and tinnitus:* They are both rare in children. In the absence of other systemic disorders such as anemia, cardiac anomalies, hypothyroidism and central cause, child should be evaluated for CSOM, migraine, and benign paroxysmal positional vertigo (BPPV).

Examination of the Ear

Most children need to be explained before attempting any examination about the process unless the child is very young. Toddlers are best examined while sitting on the mother's lap with the child's head resting securely on the mother's chest **(Fig. 3)**. Place the child's legs between the parent's legs. While one arm is placed around the child's body, the other is used to hold the child's head firmly. If examination is done in the lying down position in very young children, have the parent hold the arms either extended or close to the sides to limit motion.

Approach the examination in a systematic way, starting from the outer parts of the ear before moving to the inner parts of the ear.
- *Pinna:* Deformities of the pinna, such as low set ears, bat ear, microtia (underdeveloped pinna) **(Fig. 4)**, anotia (absent pinna), preauricular appendages, preauricular pits, or sinuses **(Fig. 5)**, should be looked for. All such patients should be evaluated for

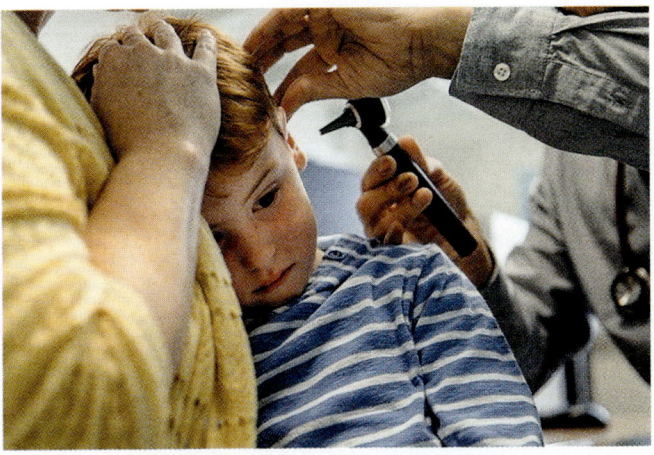

Fig. 3: Method of ear examination in a child.

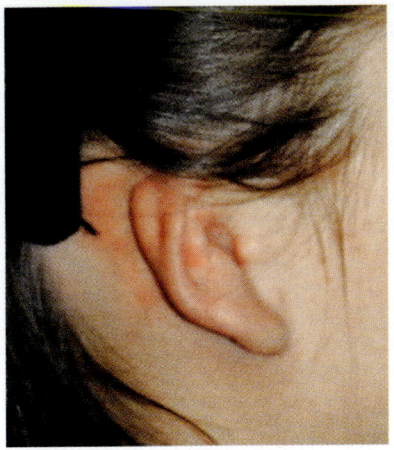

Fig. 4: Microtia or underdeveloped pinna.

other anomalies involving the middle ear and the inner ear as well as other genetic and developmental anomalies of the body. Pinna should also be examined for any scars, lacerations, hematoma, or keloids. Postauricular area should be palpated for any tenderness. An inflamed and tender mastoid with the pinna pushed forward indicates the possibility of mastoiditis. Postauricular area and the mastoid should be examined

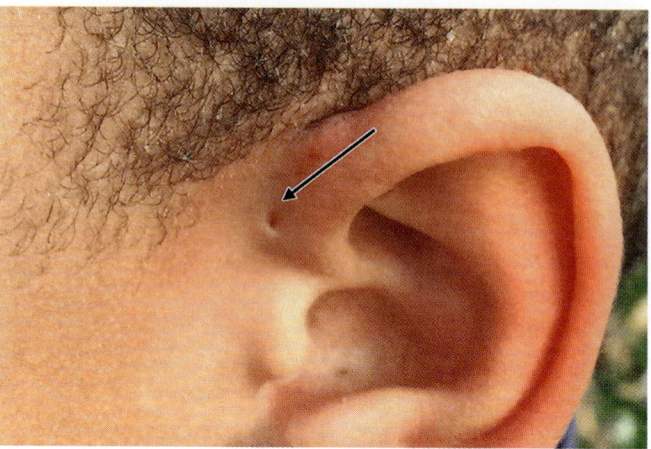

Fig. 5: Preauricular sinus.

> **Box 2:** Common congenital deformities of the pinna.
>
> - *Anotia:* Missing one or both ears
> - *Protruding ears:* More than 2 cm from the head
> - *Cryptotia:* Upper ear underneath the scalp skin
> - *Stahl's ear:* Pointed outer ear
> - *Ear tag (accessory tragus):* Cartilage bump in front of the ear
> - *Congenital earlobe deformities:* Duplicate earlobes or earlobes with clefts or skin tags
> - *Ear hemangiomas:* Small to large benign tumor

   for scars, swellings, abscess, and sinus. Tragal tenderness may be present in otitis externa. Common deformities of the pinna are listed in **Box 2**.
- *External auditory canal:* External auditory canal should be examined by pulling the pinna upward, backward, and laterally to bring the S-shaped external auditory canal in alignment. Most children allow a gentle otoscopic examination. The otoscope is held like a pen between thumb and index finger, left hand for left ear, and right hand for right ear. Speculum of appropriate size should be used to prevent pain and discomfort. External auditory canal should be examined for the following:
    - Stenosis or atresia of the meatus
    - Obstruction due to foreign body or wax that looks like brown or black debris and is a frequent cause of pain and deafness

- Pain, tenderness, swelling, redness, or furuncles
- Discharge mostly seen in cases of otitis media and sometimes in otitis externa. The amount, color, consistency, and odor of the discharge should be noted
- Otomycosis which appears like a wet piece of paper with black spores
- Polyps, granulations, and cholesteatoma flakes may be seen
- *Tympanic membrane:* Normal tympanic membrane is pearly white, translucent, and shiny. The tympanic membrane should be examined for color, presence of perforation, bulging, or retraction. A pneumatic otoscope helps in assessing the mobility of the tympanic membrane in Eustachian tube dysfunction. Appearance of the tympanic membrane in various ear disorders are listed in **Table 2 (Figs. 6 and 7)**.

Table 2: Appearance of the tympanic membrane in various ear disorders.

Red and congested	Acute otitis media
Bluish	Secretory otitis media and hemotympanum
Perforation	ASOM, CSOM, and traumatic
Retraction	CSOM and Eustachian tube dysfunction
(ASOM: acute suppurative otitis media; CSOM: chronic suppurative otitis media)	

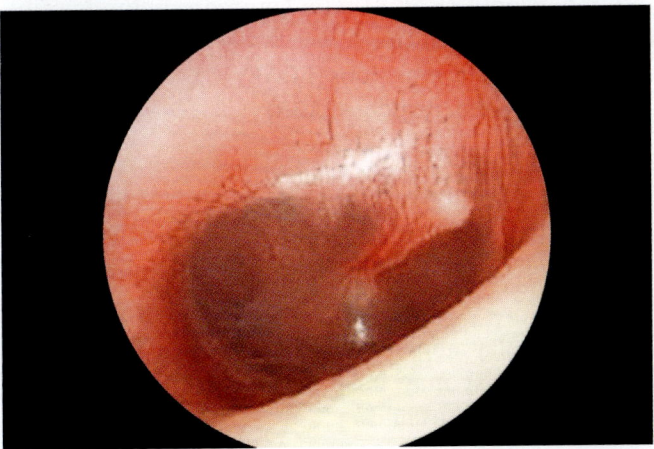

Fig. 6: Red and congested tympanic membrane in acute suppurative otitis media.

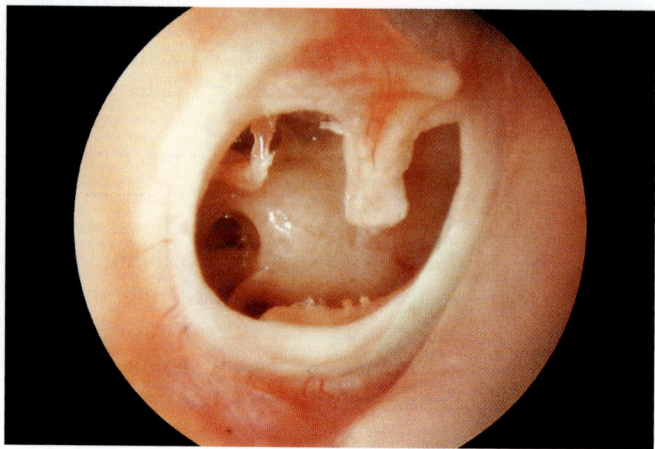

Fig. 7: Perforated tympanic membrane in chronic suppurative otitis media.

Hearing Assessment in Children

Several methods of assessment are available depending on the age and development of the child. Early detection and intervention is critical for speech as well as social and cognitive development of the child.

Newborn: It is recommended that all infants be screened for hearing loss prior to 1 month of age. High-risk neonates should compulsorily undergo targeted screening for early detection of hearing impairment **(Box 3)**. The common methods of hearing assessment in a newborn are:
- Evoked otoacoustic emissions (EOAE)
- Auditory brainstem response (ABR)

Infants:
- Behavioral audiometry
- Brainstem evoked response audiometry (BERA)
- Auditory steady state response (ASSR)

Toddlers:
- Conditioned play audiometry (CPA)
- Tuning fork test may be done according to the age and understanding of the child.

> **Box 3:** Conditions requiring screening and hearing assessment in children.
>
> - Birth weight <1,500 g
> - Consanguinity
> - Children in the neonatal intensive care unit (NICU)
> - Ototoxic drug
> - Sepsis
> - Mechanical ventilation ≥5 days
> - Low Apgar score <4 at 1 minute and <6 at 5 minutes
> - Hyperbilirubinemia
> - Stigmata with risk of deafness
> - Family history of hearing loss
> - Craniofacial abnormality
> - In utero infection (TORCH)

Older children:
- Pure tone audiogram (PTA)
- Tympanometry can be done in suspected cases of serous otitis media.

SYMPTOMS RELATED TO THE NOSE

Nasal obstruction: It may be unilateral or bilateral. While older children can express and describe their discomfort, for infant's family, provides the history of mouth breathing, disturbed sleep, and noisy breathing. Although not usually a severe condition, nasal obstruction may be life-threatening in neonates and infants. Family history of atopy is important in patients with history of asthma mucoid discharge and excessive sneezing. The common causes of nasal obstruction in children are as follows:
- *Adenoid hypertrophy:* Symptoms include nasal obstruction, sleep disturbances, and middle ear effusions with hearing loss. Size of the adenoid increases up to the age of 6 years, then slowly atrophies and completely disappears by the age of 16 years. Untreated adenoid hypertrophy may present with a characteristic facial appearance known as adenoid facies characterized a long face, open mouth, crowded teeth, high arched palate, and pinched nose **(Figs. 8 and 9)**.
- *Choanal atresia:* It can be one-sided (unilateral) or affect both sides (bilateral). Bilateral choanal atresia should be suspected

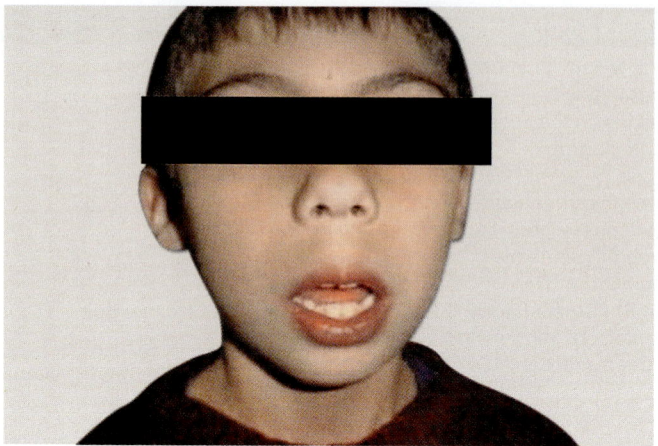

Fig. 8: Adenoid facies.

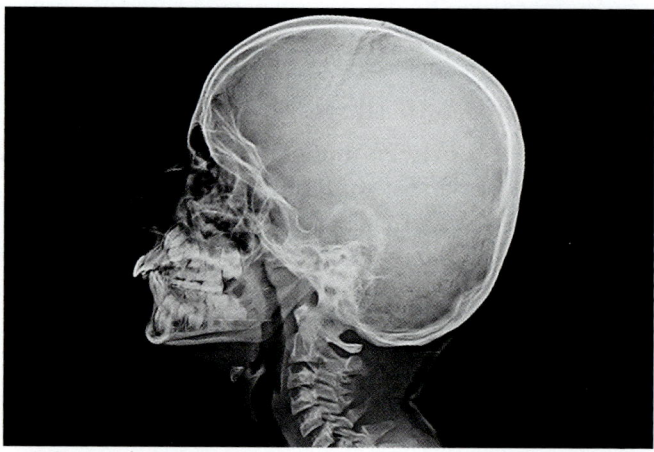

Fig. 9: X-ray showing enlarged adenoids in the nasopharynx.

in a neonate who turns cyanotic with feeding and improves with crying with the return of cyanosis with rest (paradoxical cyanosis). Unilateral choanal atresia commonly presents with purulent nasal discharge and obstruction on the affected side and may remain undetected for several years. Choanal atresia may be associated with various other anomalies; CHARGE syndrome is the most common of these and consists

of coloboma, heart disease, atresia choanae, growth and mental retardation, genital hypoplasia, and ear anomalies.
- *Deviated nasal septum:* Deviated nasal septum in children may be developmental or due to birth trauma during forceps delivery or caesarean section. They usually present as unilateral or bilateral nasal obstruction or epistaxis due to crusting.
- *Foreign bodies:* Children aged 2–5 years of age are most likely to insert objects into the nose. Nasal foreign bodies often present acutely but can be missed and remain for weeks, months, or even years after insertion. It is unusual to see nasal foreign bodies in children younger than 9 months as they are not capable of a pincer grasp. Longstanding foreign body produces local inflammation that can lead to pressure necrosis mucosal ulceration and epistaxis with history of offensive smell. Longstanding nasal foreign bodies can become calcified known as a rhinolith **(Fig. 10)**.
- *Hematoma:* Injury to the nose can also result in a hematoma that may obstruct the nasal passage. It must be treated immediately or may result in septal abscess and deformity.
- *Nasal polyps:* Nasal polyps in the pediatric population occur as inflammatory responses to bacterial infections and present as nasal obstruction. Most commonly unilateral antrochoanal

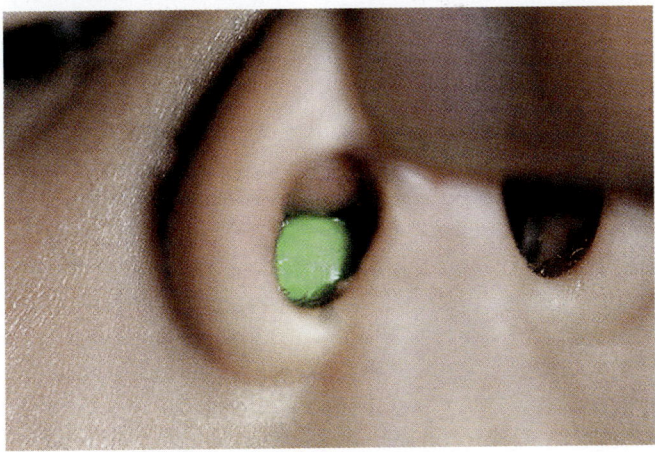

Fig. 10: Foreign body in the nose.

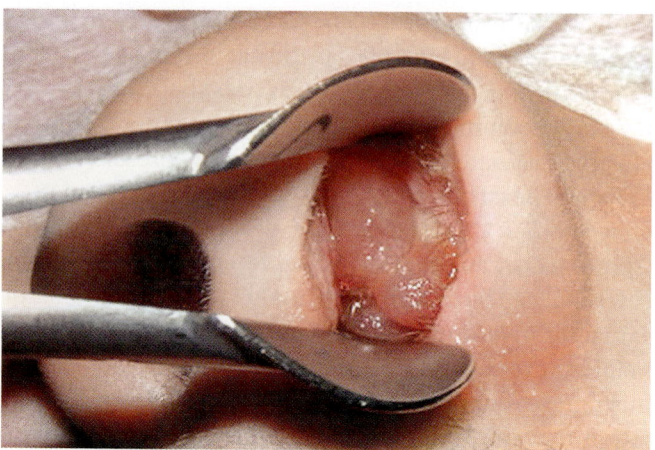

Fig. 11: Left-sided nasal polyp.

polyps are seen **(Fig. 11)**. Bilateral polyps are less common and often associated with cystic fibrosis. In very young children, meningocele and encephalocele must be differentiated from polyps.
- *Tumors:* Benign or malignant tumors are an uncommon cause of nasal obstruction in children. They are often noticed when one side of the nose is persistently stuffy, sometimes accompanied by bleeding, discharge, or swelling. Juvenile nasopharyngeal angiofibroma (JNA) is a specific type of benign tumor that is more common in prepubescent and adolescent males that can cause recurrent nose bleeding.
- *Epistaxis:* It is usually seen in 3–8 years of age. In children, epistaxis mostly occurs from the anterior part of the septum in the region of Little's area (Kiesselbach's plexus). Initiating factors include local inflammation, mucosal drying, and local trauma including nose picking. In recurrent epistaxis, systemic causes such as hepatic disorders, blood disorders, and coagulopathies such as immune thrombocytopenic purpura (ITP), thrombocytopenia, leukemia, and hemophilia should be ruled out. In pubertal males, torrential bleeding may be due to JNA. Common causes of epistaxis in children are listed in **Box 4**.

> **Box 4:** Common causes of epistaxis in children.
>
> *Traumatic:*
> - Digital trauma
> - Foreign bodies
> - Nasal fractures
>
> *Hematological:*
> - Thrombocytopenia
> - Hemophilia A and B
> - Von Willebrand disease
> - Liver failure
> - Leukemia
>
> *Inflammatory:*
> - Rhinitis
> - Acute infections and viral illness
>
> *Iatrogenic:*
> - Nasal intubation
> - Nasogastric tube
>
> *Neoplastic:* Juvenile nasopharyngeal angiofibroma

- *Rhinitis:* Acute rhinitis may be a symptom of common cold and is often associated with sore throat, fever, and cough. Rhinitis may also be caused by allergies and irritants. Allergic rhinitis is characterized by rhinorrhea, excessive sneezing, nasal obstruction, epiphora, and nasal itching. Rhinitis may be seasonal, pollen-induced hay fever, though numerous aeroallergens such as house dust mites may produce perennial symptoms, which can have an important impact on the child's quality of life. A purulent or mucopurulent discharge with fever, facial pain or swelling, and headache may be indicative of acute rhinosinusitis.

Examination of the Nose

Inspect the external nose, both anteriorly and laterally for the following:
- Size and shape
- *Obvious swellings or deformities:* Saddling or hump and dermoid cysts
- Scars, sinuses, or injuries

- *Redness or discharge:* Dermatitis/furunculosis
- *Crepitus and tenderness:* Nasal bone fractures

  The nasal cavity is examined using a headlight or a torchlight with the child in sitting position **(Fig. 12)**. The nose should be inspected from the front to examine the vestibule and anterior nares by lifting the tip of the nose up and looking inside without a speculum.

  The nasal cavity proper should be inspected gently by inserting a Thudichum speculum. The following structures are identified:

- *Nasal septum:* Check for perforation, septal deviation, hematoma, superficial vessels, or potential bleeding sites.
- *Turbinates:* Check the inferior turbinate for hypertrophy and middle turbinate is less commonly visible.
- *Entire nasal cavity:* Check for foreign bodies, discharge, and polyps.

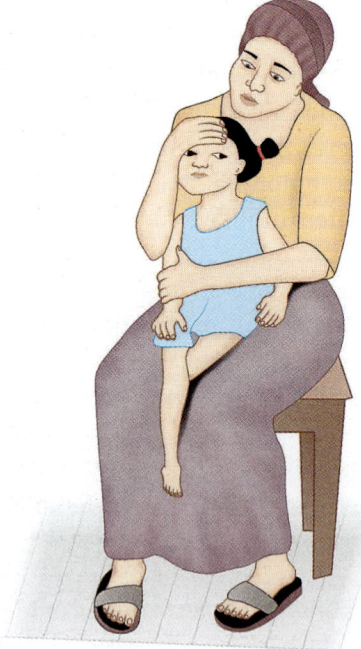

Fig. 12: Method of examination of nose in a child.

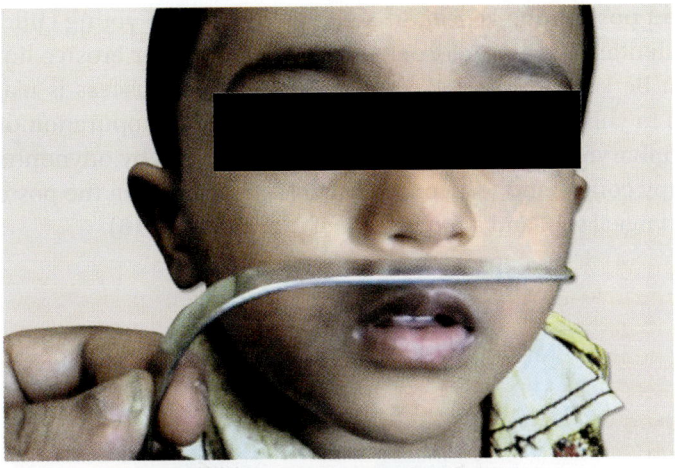

Fig. 13: Cold spatula test for nasal patency.

- *Mucosa:* Edematous and inflamed mucosa indicates an infective cause, while pale mucosa is seen in allergic rhinitis.
- *Cold spatula test for nasal patency:* Check patency of each side and ask the patient to sniff. To assess the nasal airway, hold a cold metal tongue depressor under the nose while the patient exhales and note the fogging over the tongue depressor under both nostrils, or occlude one nostril whilst the patient sniffs to give a reasonable idea of airway patency **(Fig. 13)**.

SYMPTOMS RELATED TO THE ORAL CAVITY, OROPHARYNX, AND LARYNX

Throat Pain

Pain in the throat is usually dull and aggravated on swallowing. Excessive crying and refusal to feed in a young child may be due to throat pain. Accompanying symptoms such as fever, vomiting, nasal blockage, or change in voice must be enquired into. Common causes include URI, pharyngitis, tonsillitis, and aphthous ulceration of the tongue or pharynx. Acute tonsillitis may have a recurrent history accompanied by high fever **(Fig. 14)**. Severe unilateral pain with a muffled voice may be seen in peritonsillar abscess. Acute dysphagia, drooling of saliva with inspiratory stridor, and a tripod positioning is seen in acute epiglottitis. In young children, accidental ingestion of foreign bodies **(Fig. 15)** or erosive liquids must be kept in mind. Acute retropharyngeal abscess is usually seen in children less than 3 years of age due to suppuration of the retropharyngeal lymph nodes and characterized by odynophagia, croupy cough, and torticollis. Diagnosis is by bulge in the posterior pharyngeal wall and a radiograph of the neck **(Fig. 16)**.

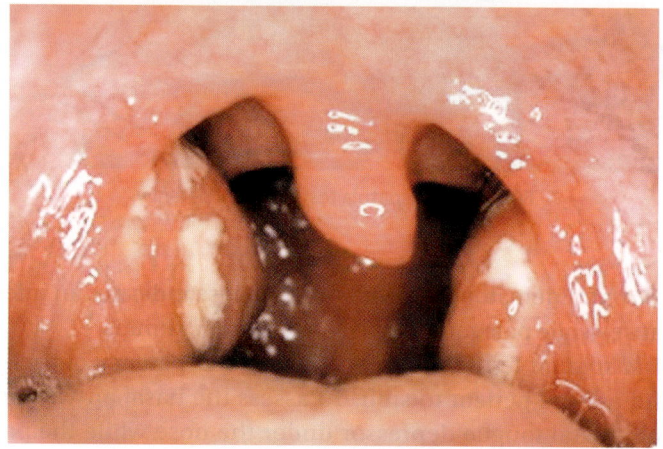

Fig. 14: Acute tonsillitis.

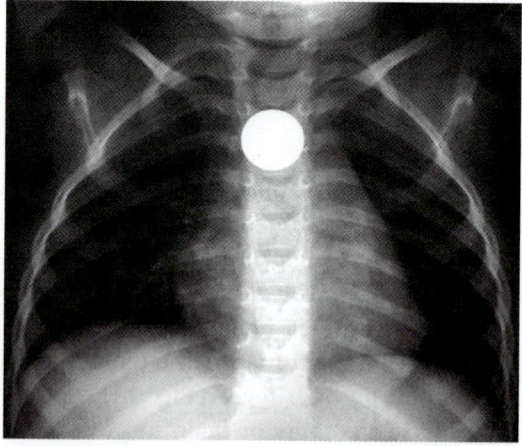

Fig. 15: Foreign body in the esophagus.

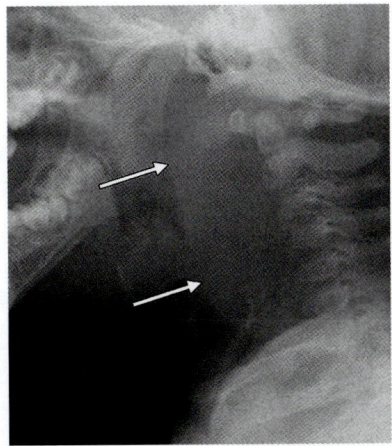

Fig. 16: X-ray showing retropharyngeal abscess.

Change in Voice

Hoarseness of voice or dysphonia in children may be due to a variety of causes which can be congenital, inflammatory, traumatic, neurological, and functional. Common causes of acute hoarseness include laryngitis or vocal abuse, while chronic and insidious causes include nodules, cysts, and papillomatosis. Laryngoscopy helps in correct diagnosis and treatment.

Noisy and Difficult Breathing

Enlarged adenoids and tonsils are associated with snoring and hyponasal speech. Enquiries about the child's voice or cry can provide valuable information about the airway. Hoarseness or diminished cry is a sign of laryngomalacia. Noisy breathing and stridor are high-pitched sound produced by turbulent airflow through a partially obstructed airway. Stridor may be inspiratory, expiratory, or biphasic depending on the site of obstruction **(Fig. 17)**.

Stridor

Stridor may also be acute or chronic. Acute stridor is most commonly infectious in origin. Croup or laryngotracheobronchitis is the

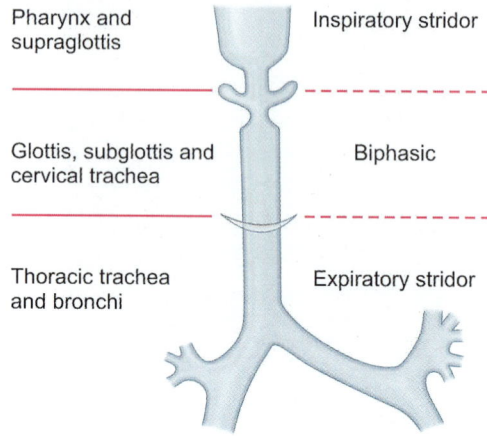

Fig. 17: Types of stridor and probable site of obstruction.

Table 3: Common causes of stridor in children.

	Acquired	
Congenital	Afebrile	Febrile
Laryngomalacia	Papillomatosis	Acute laryngitis
Laryngeal web	Injury	Epiglottitis
Subglottic stenosis	Foreign body	Laryngotracheal bronchitis
Hemangioma	Laryngeal edema	Diphtheria
Vocal cord paralysis	Vocal cord palsy	Retropharyngeal abscess
Tongue and jaw abnormalities		

number one cause of acute stridor in children followed by foreign body aspiration. Epiglottitis, though less frequently seen due to widespread vaccination with Hib vaccine, must be kept in mind in acute stridor.

Chronic stridor in infants is most often caused by anatomic defects such as laryngomalacia, subglottic stenosis, hemangiomas, laryngeal webs, and vocal cord paralysis. Stridor can be caused by rare anatomical malformations such as choanal atresia, lingual thyroid, thyroglossal duct cyst, macroglossia, micrognathia, and hypertrophic tonsil. Common causes of stridor are listed in **Table 3**.

Table 4: Causes of neck masses in children.

Inflammatory	Congenital
• Acute lymphadenitis: Bacterial/viral • Reactive lymphadenitis • Mycobacterial lymphadenitis • Abscess • Cat scratch disease • Salivary gland disorders	• Cystic hygroma • Dermoid cyst • Thyroglossal duct cyst • Branchial cleft cyst • Cystic hygroma • Teratoma
Benign tumors	Malignant tumors
• Lipomas • Sternomastoid tumor • Neurofibroma • Thyroid tumors vascular malformations	• Non-Hodgkins tumor • Hodgkins tumor • Metastasis (nasopharyngeal Ca) • Leukemias

Neck swellings: Neck swellings or masses in children can be developmental, inflammatory, reactive, or neoplastic. The most common neck swellings in children are enlarged neck nodes followed by congenital or developmental disorders. Fever, rapid enlargement, and pain usually indicate an inflammatory cause while fever, malaise, weight loss, and night sweats suggest a possible malignancy or tuberculosis. Midline neck masses are usually thyroglossal duct cyst, ranula, or dermoid cyst, while off midline lesions are more likely to be lymph nodes, branchial cleft cysts or lymphangiomas. Common causes of neck masses in children are listed in **Table 4**.

Examination of the Oral Cavity and Oropharynx

Oral cavity examination in a child is done in the sitting position either with a headlight or a torch. Often a tongue depressor is required to visualize the oropharynx. Oral cavity extends from the lips to the anterior tonsillar pillars. Structures included are lips, gingivae, teeth, hard palate, cheek mucosa, anterior two-thirds of tongue, and floor of the mouth. The palatine tonsils, soft palate, tongue base, and posterior pharyngeal walls are part of the oropharynx. Examination includes the following:
- *Lips:* Swelling, vesicles, ulcers, crusts, and clefts
- *Buccal mucosa, gums, and teeth:* Ulcerations, gingivitis, cysts, dental caries, crowded or maloccluded teeth, and growth
- *Palate:* Cleft palate and high arched palate oroantral fistula

- *Tongue:* It should be examined for size, large size seen in macroglossia, cretinism, lymphangioma, and edema. Bald tongue with irregular or complete absence of papillae seen in iron deficiency anemia or geographical tongue. Aphthous ulcers and traumatic bites must be looked for. Inability to protrude the tongue suggest ankyloglossia, while deviation suggest a XII cranial nerve palsy.
- *Tonsils and pillars:* The examiner should note the presence or absence of the palatine tonsils and their size. The tonsils have an irregular surface with deep crypts that are often filled with epithelial debris or food particles. In acute tonsillitis, they may appear enlarged inflamed with follicles or membrane over it. The examiner should also note the symmetry of the palato-tonsil area. Bulging of one side with contralateral shifting of the uvula may be indicative of a peritonsillar abscess or parapharyngeal tumor.
- *Soft palate and uvula:* Bulging may be seen in peritonsillar abscess. Uvula should be checked for symmetry and function. A bifid uvula may be seen with or without a cleft palate.

The posterior pharyngeal wall may show postnasal drip or a bulge in retropharyngeal abscess.

Laryngeal Examination

Examination of the child's larynx is mandatory in the management of pediatric airway problems. Laryngeal examination is usually done by otolaryngologist. In older children, an indirect laryngoscopy as done for adults can be done in the OPD. The techniques used to perform this examination have evolved over time and now present the airway specialist with choices that can be tailored to each specific situation. Traditionally, rigid direct laryngoscopy (RDL) has been used to evaluate the pediatric larynx. More recently, flexible fiber-optic laryngoscopy has been used to visualize the child's airway. Flexible fiber-optic laryngoscopy has become our technique of choice to evaluate the pediatric larynx, especially when airway dynamics are of concern. RDL remains the preferred technique when laryngeal/tracheal surgery is planned or establishment and protection of the airway with intubation or bronchoscopy is required.

Ethical and Legal Issues in Pediatric Practice

CHAPTER 16

Satish Tiwari

INTRODUCTION

The practice of medicine has evolved from arts to science and then to commerce. The commercialization and globalization of medical practice has resulted in newer and newer technologies, gadgets, medicines, instruments, etc. These advances have improved the healthcare, possibility of intact survival, quality of life, and overall outcome in the disease process. Paradoxically, these positive changes are also associated with deteriorating doctor–patient relationship, lack of ethical standards, commercialization, and corporate culture. The involvement of insurance companies, government schemes, and legal hurdles in practice added fuel to the fire. The overall situation is that the medical practice is at cross-roads where patients or relatives are bent upon settling the disputes with the hospitals/doctors by indulging in violence and the doctors or hospitals are shifting to defensive mode practice so as to remain free from the clutches of authorities or law-makers. The overall situation is appalling and there is need for major revamp and overhauling. There is need to create awareness about rights and duties of patients as well as medical practitioners. The advances in science and technology cannot be a substitute for good, evidence-based, academically sound clinical examination including the history taking.

HISTORY TAKING

A good history taking focused on the complaints of the patient still has potential to arrive at clinical diagnosis or differential diagnosis. A proper and detailed history from the informant (patient or relative) may be a cornerstone in the management

of the child. The following points in the history may be vital in specific situations:
- Keeping in mind the legal issues a history of drug allergy is very important so as to avoid litigations related to drug reactions or adverse effects.
- We are in the era of human rights including the rights of the fetus. History of LMP (last menstrual period) is important in cases of adolescent mothers, sexual abuse cases, or while dealing with the cases under The Protection of Children from Sexual Offences (POCSO) Act.
- Another important issue is to maintain the confidentiality. The information received during history and examination has to be kept confidential except in cases where it may be detrimental to other members of the society.
- Can we do the audiovisual recording of history, examination, or consent? Yes, in fact such recording should be promoted and encouraged, as it may help in the future. If we are recording some confidential or secret history or examining some internal or genital part, care should be taken that the same should not be misused in future by some miscreants.
- Many of our colleagues are saying that we should ask the history of relatives creating nuisance/violence or allegations by the relatives against the doctors/hospitals in the past. We feel that this is practically difficult. In the treatment history, we can ask history of receiving wrong treatment in past so that we can predict to some extent the behavior of the relatives in future.
- Follow principles of good communication skills during history taking and examinations.

The negative history is equally important in finalizing the clinical diagnosis. It is important to rule out many other differential diagnosis or associated diseases to prevent subsequent outcome in any patient. For any reason, if the patient is examined in hurry, ask him to come on next day. If the diagnosis is not confirmed, record other possibilities.

TELEPHONIC CONSULTATION

In the present era, many times the patient or relatives want to have suggestions telephonically. We should be very careful and preferably avoid telephonic consultations, as it is not possible to advise without examination of patient. If we want to give telephonic suggestions (in some extraordinary circumstances), please suggest the patient to consult nearby qualified doctor and then to go ahead with the treatment. We can also discuss the case with the available consultant on phone and then ask the patient to proceed with the treatment.

The Concept of Telemedicine

This mode of treatment is getting more and more acceptance in the present era, as a doctor based at remote center can communicate with a consultant at a developed center who can guide on computer or telephone. In this case, both the parties are officially involved in providing best possible care to the patient at a lesser equipped center. The legal liabilities of all concerned are also defined as per the law of the land.

EXAMINATION OF PATIENT

The examination of the patient shall be done with due care so as not to miss any obvious important clinical findings. Inadequate and improper examination may miss some of the findings, which may lead to improper diagnosis and ultimately improper treatment. Many times proper examination will rule out the differential diagnosis and will shorten the list of investigations, thus reducing the allegation of unnecessary investigations.

INFORMED CONSENT

A valid, proper, and informed consent is very vital aspect of medical treatment in present era. An informed consent means all information in comprehensible, nonmedical terms, and preferably in local language. The information should be about diagnosis, nature of treatment, risk involved, prospects of success, prognosis, if procedure not performed and alternative methods of treatment. Many case laws decided by Honorable Supreme Court, National Commission, and other authorities have upheld the importance of informed consent in deciding the medical negligence cases.

GUARDED PROGNOSIS

Medical science is not a perfect science. Some disease may be self-limiting while others may not respond even to best possible treatment. Unfortunate outcome can occur even in fully equipped healthcare setup with all latest gadgets/instruments and in best possible hands. Many of us have now started believing that life and death is in the hands of God. Hence, never guarantee for cure. Give guarded prognosis and guarantee for care.

THE CONCEPT OF DUTY

The duty of doctor toward patient starts once we accept the patient for treatment. If, for any reasons we have not accepted or started to treat the patient the duty does not start. Once we have started the treatment, it has to be as per the accepted norms, standards, and protocols followed by a group of consultants or experts with average skill, knowledge, and experience.

WHAT IS NEGLIGENCE?

Negligence is deficiency in duty (an Act of Commission or an Act of Omission), which directly results in damage to the patient or the relatives. The negligence is to be proved by the patients/relatives by submitting the expert evidence or references from another experts or standard textbooks or standard journals. In very obvious or visible case of negligence, there is no need for such evidence and principle of *"Res Ipsa Loquitur"* is applied. Most of the cases of medical negligence are decided under civil law and compensation is allowed. According to Honorable Supreme Court, the Criminal Liability should not be imposed on doctors routinely as no sensible professional will have "Mens Rea" (i.e., guilty mind or intension). The "4D" of negligence includes—(1) duty toward patient, (2) deficiency in that duty, (3) directly resulting in, and (4) damage to the patient or relatives. The cut throat competition in modern society has resulted in deterioration of moral and human values. Since the patient is paying money and going for "doctor shopping", his expectations are soaring and the end result is naturally frustration, if something unexpected happens. We have developed a scoring system to assess the risk of medicolegal cases in your day-to-day practice **(Table 1)**. The scoring

Table 1: Scoring system for risk of medicolegal or negligence case.

Criteria	Score				
	1	2	3	4	5
Access to medicolegal consultant (help and guidance)	All possible help	Written help/guidance discussed		No guidance	No help
Behavior (communication skills)	Communication with proper skills	Communication with relatives	Communication with "so-called social worker"	With patient but not with relatives	No communication
Consent	Informed	Written	Implied	Blanket	Not taken
Doctor–patient relationship	Excellent	Good	Average	Poor	Very poor
Expertise in the field	Proper qualification/experience	No experience	No qualification	Crosspathy	Quacks
Facts/documentation	Clear, correct comprehensive, and chronological	Record of other colleagues	Improper	Manipulated	Not available

Source: Medico-legal Issues in Pediatrics. Textbook on Medico-legal Issues related to Various Medical Specialties, 2nd edition. New Delhi: Jaypee Brothers Medical Publishers (P) Ltd.; 2019.

(Dr Tiwari's Score) or grading can be interpreted, analyzed, and calculated as follows:
- *High risk:* If the score is 25–30
- *Moderate risk:* If the score is 19–24
- *Average risk:* If the score is 13–18
- *Minimal risk:* If the score is 7–12
- *Negligible risk:* If the score is <7

DOCUMENTATION AND RECORD MAINTENANCE

A properly maintained record and well-preserved documents can prove to be friends in the hours of crisis. Proper record must be maintained for outdoor, indoor patients, intake-output charts, drugs prescribed or administered to the patient. The other record includes preanesthetic check-ups, details of surgical procedure (including the names of surgeons/anesthetists), postoperative care, etc. Discharge certificate should be patient friendly and not just mechanical.

ETHICAL ISSUES AND DILEMMAS

The ethical issues in practice of medicine have been discussed since ancient time. The Hippocratic Oath, which is almost 25 centuries old, recognizes the rights of patients and ethical principles in the treatment of patients. It was supposed to be service to humanity with nobility and dignity. The aim was "never do harm to anyone". The practice was highest standard of professional conduct without motive of profit. There are many ethical dilemmas for sincere and dedicated practitioners. The authorities and community have badly failed in protecting the ethical doctors.

A, B, C, D....... of medical practice:
- Attend the patient carefully and properly.
- Behavior (human vs. inhuman).
- Consent and communication.
- Documents shall be maintained as per the recommendations.
- Expertise and efficiency in management of patient.
- Finances, bills shall be explained properly to the concerned relatives.
- Guarded prognosis helps in cases of unexpected outcome.
- Hospital staff should behave properly with the patient/relatives.
- Insurance (individual/hospital) shall be helpful, if the compensation is awarded by court.
- Juniors and other staff shall be qualified whenever possible.
- Knowledge shall be updated regularly.
- Latest instruments shall be available as per the scope of practice.
- Medicolegal association must be joined, so that medicolegal consultation is available in hours of crisis.
- No manipulations should be done in records/documents.
- Opinion "second"—may be helpful and shall be taken especially in complicated cases.

The Diagnosis of Death

CHAPTER 17

Sudhir Mishra, Satish Tiwari

INTRODUCTION

Death is defined in dictionary as "A permanent cessation of all vital functions: The end of life" (Merriam Webster dictionary). Oxford dictionary defines death as "The end of life of a person or an organism, or permanent ending of vital processes in cell or tissues". In past, the diagnosis of death was usually made when respiration and heart beat were absent in an individual. It became more difficult with the availability of technology to support the respiration and consequent presence of circulation. This led to the advent of concept of "Brain Death"; this further gained ground with organ transplant coming in picture. Continued circulation supported by mechanical ventilation helps in preserving the cellular functions of organs thus making them suitable for transplantation. This also gives more time (hours or even days) compared to a state where cardiac and respiratory functions stop, for harvesting the organs after due consent from the next of kin for organ donation.

BRAIN DEATH

The World Health Organization, after discussions at an invitational forum, sponsored by Canadian Blood Services, held at Montreal Canada on 30th and 31st May 2012, defined brain death as "Diagnosis and confirmation of death based on the irreversible cessation of functioning of the entire brain, including the brainstem". They also defined brainstem death as "diagnosis and confirmation of death based on the irreversible cessation of functioning of the brainstem, predominantly but not exclusively secondary to a supratentorial brain injury (this forum supports the movement away from this traditional and imprecise terminology in favor of the cessation of neurological function)".

Another definition of brain death is "The irreversible loss of all functions of the brain, including the brainstem. The three essential findings in brain death are coma, absence of brainstem reflexes, and apnea".

The Diagnosis of Brain/Brainstem Death

These terms can be used interchangeably for the clinical purposes. The diagnosis of brain death is clinical as long as all the requirements are fulfilled. Investigations are not required. However, in the event of difficulties, investigations may be used to supplement clinical observations.

Importance of Diagnosis of Brain Death

The importance of diagnosis of death has two aspects. First and foremost is the knowledge that the result of organ transplant from brain dead patient while heart is still beating (better than the organs harvested from asystolic donors). Second is related to futility of care in situation of brain dead that prevents optimal utilization of resources, more so in resource-limited settings. Another related aspect is futile expenditure (more so when it comes out of family pocket) in a situation where outcome is known. Therefore, it is of utmost importance that a precise diagnosis of brain death is made and communicated to the next of kin.

Requirements for Diagnosis of Brain Death

It is a precondition that the patient should be deeply unconscious, apneic, and mechanically ventilated. There are four prerequisites to diagnosis of brain death that are enumerated in **Table 1**.

In Indian context, determination of cause of deep coma may remain clinical as extensive investigations for viral and metabolic etiology may not be possible or practical at most centers. Performance of complete neurological examination by a competent clinician however remains a minimum requirement. This should include detailed history and neurological examination to ascertain the cause. Description of detailed neurological examination is beyond the scope of this chapter.

The Diagnosis of Death

Table 1: Oculovestibular and oculocephalic response.

	Oculovestibular response	Oculocephalic response
Procedure	Patient is kept in semi-reclining position at 30°. It is important to ensure that tympanic membrane is intact and is unobstructed by presence of wax. About 50 mL iced water at about 50°C is poured slowly and external auditory canal is irrigated	Sudden and fast rotation of head by 90° to one side
Response	The eye will move to the opposite side	• Normally conjugate deviation of eyes to opposite side • Absent reflexes indicate brain stem lesion/function
Difficult if:		Inability to open eyes due to presence of ecchymosis or edema or injury to eye(s)
Contraindications if:		• Presence of cervical spine injury • Presence of severe hypertonia • Neck retraction

Potentially reversible causes for deep coma that need to be excluded are:
- Hypothermia.
- Use of therapeutic hypothermia prior to testing.
- Central nervous system (CNS) depressant drugs like narcotics, barbiturates, tranquillizers, and benzodiazepines. Especially in children, where they are commonly used as anticonvulsants or sedatives to synchronize ventilation, they may have markedly cumulative and persistent effect.
- High cervical spine injury (that may lead to apnea).
- Evidence of acquired neuromuscular paralysis like Guillain-Barré syndrome and residual neuromuscular blockade.

- Severe acid–base, electrolyte, and endocrine abnormalities that may contribute to presence of coma.
- Shock.

Clinical Methods for Assessment of Brain Death

Clinical examination is usually sufficient for the diagnosis of brain death. It should be performed by two clinicians; one of them should not be involved in day-to-day care of the patient. Apnea test should be performed at the end of second clinical examination. There are no definite guidelines on the time interval between two clinical examinations. We suggest that it should be at least 1 hour apart. Time of death is when apnea test is completed.

Cessation of brain function is assessed based on following:
- Coma (excluding spinal cord mediated reflex)
- *Brainstem reflexes:* Absence of following reflexes is considered definitive for diagnosis of brain death:
  - Mid dilated or fully dilated pupils, absent pupillary light reflex
  - Corneal reflex
  - Gag or pharyngeal reflex
  - Cough or tracheal reflex
  - Vestibulo-ocular reflex
  - Loss of capacity to breath.

Apnea test is done at the end of second clinical examination.

METHOD OF EXAMINATION
Examination of Pupil

In ideal situation, patient should be in a room where background light can be dimmed. However, in the current situation being discussed, it may be difficult to achieve. Dim the lights to the extent possible. Open the eyes; record the size of pupils; and bring a bright light either from below the nose or from the side. As the light intensity increases, constriction of pupil is observed. Constriction of pupil in the eye being illuminated is called direct response and in the eye not being illuminated, it is called consensual response. Record both.

Examination of Corneal Reflex

Take a wisp of cotton and twist it into a point. Then gently but firmly touch the cornea at its junction with the sclera. Sensitivity to pain increases medially from this point and decreases laterally. The junction of the cornea and sclera is a good compromise between causing pain to the patient and obtaining the reflex. There is a rapid blink of the eye being tested and a consensual blink of the other eye. If there is 7th nerve weakness on the side being tested, then observe the consensual reflex.

Gag or Pharyngeal Reflex

Pharyngeal reflex is tested by two methods. There is poor reproducibility of pharyngeal reflex in normal population. However, it is a definitive test with 100% specificity for the diagnosis of brain death as presence of pharyngeal reflex precludes diagnosis of brain death as it reflects presence of brainstem (medulla) activity. It can be tested by two methods:
1. First is by touching the posterior part of tongue on lateral side by a tongue spatula. This will lead to upward movement of uvula. This is called palatal reflex.
2. Second is by touching posterior pharyngeal wall with a spatula. This leads to retching and a sound in normal individuals.

While testing gag reflex for confirmation of brain death, it is important to ensure that the patient is not accidentally extubated. For this, one assistant should stabilize the head and another should stabilize the endotracheal tube manually. The procedure should be performed with utmost care and abandoned at the first sign of presence of gag or palatal movement or desaturation of patient.

Cough or Tracheal Reflex

In normal individuals, cough reflex is tested by nebulizing some irritant like tartaric acid. However, for the diagnosis of brain death, cough reflex is performed by passing a catheter through endotracheal tube (ET) up to carina, making sure that the catheter has gone beyond the length of the ET. This should elicit a cough in a live individual. Before proceeding to test the cough reflex, it is always good to ask the staff nurses who did suction last time about the presence of cough while suctioning, although while doing endotracheal suction, we are not supposed to go beyond the length of ET. If it is reported that patient had coughed during last suction, it should obviate the need for a formal test. Otherwise, the whole procedure should be performed as in ET suction. Patient should be preoxygenated with 100% oxygen. ET should be secured manually to avoid accidental displacement. If a side port for inline suction is available, suction tube can be passed through it without disconnecting ventilator, otherwise ventilator should be disconnected and a suction catheter be passed to elicit a cough response.

Oculovestibular and Oculocephalic Response

Oculovestibular response is preferred over oculocephalic response (**Box 1**). For oculovestibular reflex, it may be difficult to observe minimal eye movement. For this, some experts suggest making a pen mark at the level of pupil, which can be compared with deviated eye. The eye should be observed for at least 1 minute after finishing irrigation. An interval of 5 minutes is required before testing the other ear.

Apnea Test

This should be performed only once and after the second clinical examination and confirmation of absence of other signs of brainstem death. This test is performed by several methods. However, most commonly used method is "apneic oxygenation method". The other method is called "artificial CO_2 augmentation procedure".

In apneic oxygenation method, patient is disconnected from ventilator; a catheter is passed through ET and kept at the level of carina. 6 L/min oxygen is administered. Disconnection is maintained till $PaCO_2$ reaches a level of 60 mm Hg and patient does not

---

Box 1: Prerequisites for diagnosis of brain death.

- Determination of the cause of deep (apparently irreversible) coma
- Exclusion of potentially reversible cause (or confounding factors)
- Exclusion of potentially reversible causes of apnea
- Competence of persons performing the tests and competence of interpreting ancillary tests

have a spontaneous breath. The test is terminated if patient shows presence of spontaneous breath at any time during the procedure and patient is reconnected to ventilator.

For artificial CO_2 augmentation procedure, pure CO_2 is administered through inspiratory limb at the rate of 1 L/min without altering ventilator parameters (except oxygen) and patient is disconnected from ventilator for 1 minute. Arterial CO_2 level is expected to rise to 60–100 mm Hg. If the patient does have spontaneous breath during this 1 minute of disconnection, patient is considered brain dead. Availability of pure CO_2 is not a routine in Indian intensive care units (ICUs) and therefore, this test is more difficult to perform. It was noted in the study that complication rate was lower in artificial CO_2 augmentation method.

The death is declared at the time of completion of apnea test.

Ancillary Testing

Brain death is a clinical diagnosis and does not entail great difficulty in day-to-day practice except that sometimes parents may not be willing to accept it and desire a longer period of observation and repeat clinical examination. In some situations, where all tests required as part of clinical examination cannot be performed owing to injury, swelling or ecchymosis in local area, e.g., pupillary light reflex and corneal reflex cannot be performed due to inability to open eyes, these tests may be required.

There are two basic premises on which confirmatory tests are based. First is loss of cerebral blood flow and second is based on neuronal electrical activity. The tests that are most commonly used are transcranial Doppler (considered operator-dependent) and CT angiography. SPECT (single photon emission computed tomography), 1H-MRS (proton magnetic resonance spectroscopy), and positron emission tomography (PET) can also be used to demonstrate absence of metabolism. Tests for loss of neuronal activity include electroencephalogram (EEG) or evoked potentials and electroretinography. However, use and availability of these tests in Indian ICUs is extremely rare.

CHAPTER 18

Common Procedures in Pediatrics

Baldev Prajapati

INTRODUCTION

It is very essential for every medical student and practicing pediatrician to learn performing common pediatric procedures. The procedures are best learnt by observation, performing the procedure under supervision and repetitive performances. It should be practical, methodological, and safe for both patients as well as for the individual who perform the procedure.

GENERAL CONSIDERATIONS

Counseling

Explain the parents in detail regarding the procedure including its indications, technique of the procedure, possible complications, etc. If the child is older and able to understand, talk to him also, in simple language. By this, cooperation is available from parents as well as the child. It decreases the anxiety of all and the procedure can be performed smoothly.

An informed consent is must for all the procedures. In certain procedures like lumbar puncture, pleural and pericardial tapping, liver biopsy, renal biopsy, exchange transfusion, bone marrow aspiration, and biopsy, it is the prudent to get signed consent.

Procedure Room and Lighting

Separate procedure room is desirable. It should have good daylight and should be well illuminated and well equipped. All the equipment and drugs to perform the procedure as well as to manage any emergency if it arises should be made available.

Containers

It is very important to confirm that proper containers are available for collection and transferring the specimens.

Identification of the Patient

It should be a routine to identify the child before performing the procedure. It should be confirmed with hospital staff as well as the parents that you are dealing with the correct child.

Sedation

Children are afraid of procedures and their reactions in the form of crying and struggling, and frightened appearance increases the parental anxiety. It affects the performance of the person who is performing the procedure. It results in increased rate of failure and complications related to procedure. In this situation, sedation to the child may help.

Promethazine 1 mg/kg/dose or Triclofos sodium 20 mg/kg/dose by oral route will suffice in most of the cases. Diazepam, ketamine and general anesthesia are other options as per indications.

Restraint

Physical restraint of the frightened child may be essential for the successful outcome of any practical procedure. The child may be wrapped with a blanket taking care to prevent aspiration or airway obstruction. The help of the person who is assisting is very crucial in deciding the outcome of the procedure.

Anesthesia

Local anesthesia may be achieved by infiltrating tissues around the site with 0.5–2% lignocaine. The maximum dosage of 1% lignocaine that can be infiltrated is 0.3 mL/kg. An alternative is to apply lignocaine cream to small area of the skin 60 minutes prior to performing the procedure, protected by adhesive dressing. Sedation or general anesthesia may be needed in certain cases.

Asepsis

The physician should scrub hands and forearm using an effective cleaning agent like 4% chlorhexidine or hexachlorophane before undertaking any procedure. Wearing of sterile gloves by the doctor is very important both for his and the patient's safety. The site of the patient's skin is then cleaned with 70% isopropyl alcohol and the surface is allowed to dry, the surface is then again washed three times with 10% povidone-iodine or 0.5% chlorhexidine gluconate in 70% isopropyl alcohol. It should be cleaned in a circular fashion from the center outwards.

INTRAMUSCULAR INJECTION

Common Sites

Muscles commonly used for intramuscular (IM) injection are vastus lateralis, deltoid and gluteus medius. Children do not have well-developed gluteus medius and therefore it is not the site of preference for IM injections. It has been documented that some vaccines like hepatitis B and antirabies vaccines administered at gluteal region produce very poor antibody response.

The vastus lateralis (anterolateral aspect of thigh) is the preferred site in infants. The site in vastus lateralis is the middle-third of the area between the greater trochanter and lateral femoral condyle **(Fig. 1)**.

In case of deltoid, the site for injection is midway between acromion process and deltoid insertion; it comes to 3–5 cm below the acromion process. This site may be used in children above 5 years and adults. The quantity of drug should be less than 5 mL. Only watery injections with less viscosity should be injected at deltoid region.

Technique (WHO Technique)

- The site of injection should be exposed well
- For anterolateral aspect of thigh, the child may be laid supine or be held in mother's lap. For deltoid, child may be held in mother's lap or may sit
- The muscle selected for injection should be relaxed

Common Procedures in Pediatrics

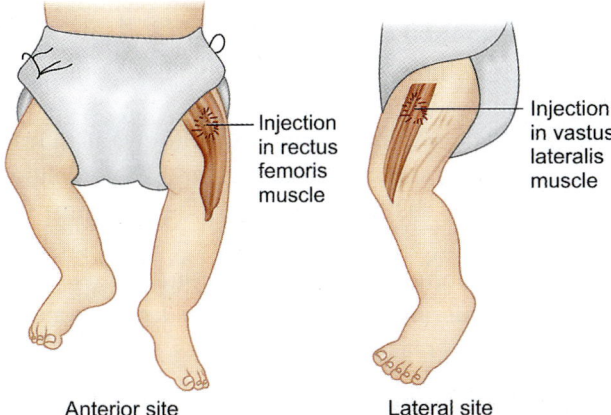

Fig. 1: Sites for intramuscular injections in an infant.
Source: Prajapati BS. Essential Procedures in Pediatrics, 1st edition. New Delhi: Jaypee Brothers Medical Publishers (P) Ltd.; 2003.

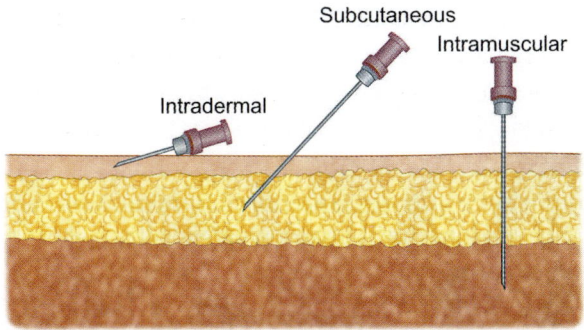

Fig. 2: The position of the needle during different ways of administering injections.
Source: Waechter EH, Philips J, Holaday B. Nursing Care of Children, 10th edition. Philadelphia: JB Lippincott Co.; 1985.

- The skin over injection site should be cleaned with spirit. A circular motion of swab is used proceeding from puncture site and extending outward for 5 cm. Let the spirit evaporate and skin become dry, otherwise spirit entering into tissues is painful
- The syringe is filled with the medicine
- In children, usually 23 G needle with 25 mm length is used for IM injections
- Stretch the skin flat and push the needle down at 90° **(Fig. 2)**

- Aspiration before injecting the vaccine is not required
- Inject the vaccine at the rate of 1 mL per 10 seconds
- The needle is withdrawn and injection site is pressed for few seconds. Do not rub the injection site
- Needle should be withdrawn smoothly with steady movement
- Discard the needle and syringe as per standard guidelines.

Alternative to WHO technique, Advisory Committee on Immunization Practices (ACIP) technique may be used. It is also called bunching technique. In this technique, bunch the muscle and direct needle inferiorly along long axis of leg at an angle of 45°. It stabilizes leg and increases the muscle mass.

SUBCUTANEOUS INJECTION

Drugs or vaccines are injected subcutaneously when slow absorption and long duration of action are desired. Another indication of subcutaneous (SC) injection route is a coagulopathy, which makes IM injection hazardous, for fear of development of IM hematoma. Insulin and heparin like drugs as well as measles, mumps, rubella (MMR), varicella, etc. Vaccines are given by SC route.

Technique

- Common sites are arm, anterior abdominal wall, and thighs. Atrophic and infected areas are avoided
- The skin is cleaned and disinfected with spirit
- 26 G needle with 13 mm length is commonly used for SC injection
- The skin is raised into a fold with thumb and index finger of the left hand
- The midpoint of the fold is pierced with the needle held at 45° with its surface. The tip of the needle is advanced into the SC tissue **(Fig. 2)**
- Aspiration is not required
- Drugs or vaccine is injected, needle is withdrawn, and site is pressed for few minutes.

INTRADERMAL INJECTION

Indications for intradermal (ID) injection are Bacillus Calmette-Guérin (BCG) vaccination, Mantoux test, skin tests for allergy, test for sensitization of certain drugs like penicillin. Antirabies vaccine also can be given by ID route.

Technique

- Ventral (volar) aspect of forearm is commonly used for ID injection
- Skin is cleaned with spirit or clean water
- A measured amount of antigen (usually 0.1 mL) is drawn into the syringe
- 26 or 27 G needle with ¼–½ inch (6.35–12.7 mm) length needle is used for ID injection
- The skin is held taut between thumb and index finger of the left hand. The syringe is held at an angle of 10–15° with the skin. Needle is inserted for about 2 mm, so that entire needle bevel penetrates the skin and the injected solution raises a small bleb of about 5 mm in diameter. The development of perifollicular puckering (Peau d'orange) indicates successful ID injection **(Fig. 2)**
- The needle is withdrawn
- The site is circled and it is recorded in patient's chart
- The reaction is observed in defined time.

RECTAL ADMINISTRATION OF DRUGS

It is a safe and easy way of administering drugs. The human rectum represents a body cavity in which drugs can be easily introduced and retained. The absorption of the drugs is well through this route. Rectal administration of drugs is indicated in patients who are not able to take orally due to nausea and vomiting, having convulsions, uncooperative children, before surgery, etc. If the child can understand, it should be explained to him. The child should be relaxed. He is kept in lateral position with knees flexed toward abdomen or in supine position with legs taken upward toward abdomen, and the drug is inserted into the rectum through anal orifice, and buttocks are held firmly to prevent expulsion of the drug. Paracetamol, diazepam, midazolam, paraldehyde, glycerine, bisacodyl, diclofenac sodium, steroids, neomycin, artesunate and many more drugs can be administered through rectal route. When rectal preparations are not available, some liquid preparations like injection Diazepam may be given per rectum. For this purpose, a lubricated tube is inserted into the rectum to a distance of about 5 cm and then the medication is administered through it using a syringe. The buttocks are held together for a couple of minutes. Local irritation and ulcerations in rectum may develop as complications of this procedure.

PERIPHERAL INTRAVENOUS ACCESS

Peripheral intravenous access is one of the mainstays of modern medicine. It allows blood sampling, administration of medicines, fluids, nutrients, blood and blood products. Intracaths and scalp vein needles are commonly used for this purpose. Various sites for venous access are as follows in order to preference **(Fig. 3)**:

- Veins on dorsum of hand
- Superficial radial vein on radial aspect of wrist
- Superficial veins over volar aspect of forearm
- Basilic vein and median cubital vein over antecubital fossa
- Superficial veins over dorsum of foot and long saphenous vein on medial aspect of leg above the ankle
- Veins of scalp in newborns and infants
- External jugular vein.

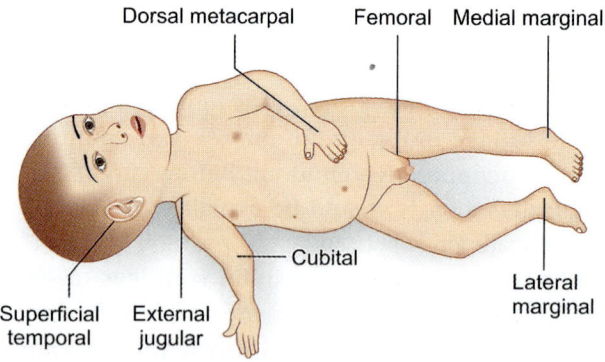

Fig. 3: Common sites for venipuncture.
Source: Prajapati BS. Essential Procedures in Pediatrics, 1st edition. New Delhi: Jaypee Brothers Medical Publishers (P) Ltd.; 2003.

Straight, large and easily accessible peripheral veins in healthy SC tissues are ideal for venous access. Veins of the upper extremities are preferred because there are many potential sites and more comfortable to the patient. The distal and superficial veins are preferred as complications are more following extravasation and thrombophlebitis in proximal and deep veins. When the veins are not visible, they can be palpated at common sites and can be accessed.

Scalp vein needle is a hollow needle with butterfly plastic handle and a plastic tube, at the other end of which, a syringe or infusion set can be attached. It is useful for venous sampling of blood and short-term use of intravenous (IV) route **(Fig. 4)**. Vein is counter punctured very easily on movement of the limb.

Intracaths are plastic catheters over a hollow metallic needle. The metallic needle just projects beyond the tip of plastic catheter. The metallic needle is to provide stiffness during insertion into the vein, after which it is withdrawn. The plastic catheter is then advanced further gently so that vein is not counter punctured. The plastic catheter is well tolerated. Intracaths and scalp vein needles are available in various sizes from 26 to 16 G. In children commonly, we use 26–21 G depending on age of the child and requirement.

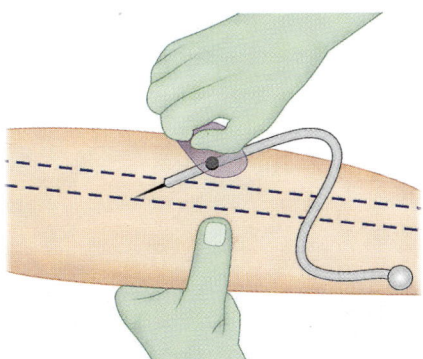

Fig. 4: Technique of venipuncture with scalp.
Source: Prajapati BS (Ed). Essential Procedures in Pediatrics, 1st edition. New Delhi: Jaypee Brothers Medical Publishers (P) Ltd.; 2003.

Technique

- A tourniquet is placed over the limb, 3–4 cm proximal to the site selected for venipuncture, taking care not to pinch the skin of the child. The pressure should be such that it occludes venous flow by continuous arterial blood flow
- Tapping sharply over the vein causes mechanical reflex dilatation of the vascular walls. It should be light otherwise pain will cause vasoconstriction
- Active or passive pumping of extremity enhances blood flow and distends veins
- A warm moist towel may be applied to the site for several minutes. It causes venous dilatation
- Aseptic precautions are mandatory
- The methylated spirit is applied over 4–5 cm area at planned site. Let it dry
- The skin is pulled taut distally to stabilize the vein with a nondominant hand. It is punctured by the needle bevel up at 15–30° angle parallel to the vein **(Fig. 5)**. After the entry into the SC tissue, the needle is aligned parallel to the skin surface and along the long axis of the vein. Its tip is depressed a little and is advanced until it penetrates the vein. Then, it is made parallel to the vein again and advanced until it is passed fully into the vein. Blood is collected if indicated and then the IV set is attached to it

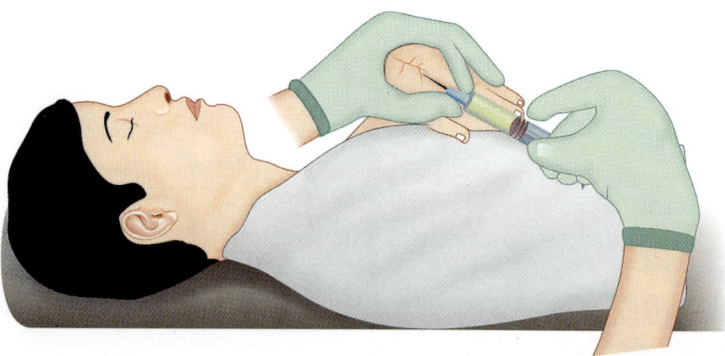

Fig. 5: For inserting the IV cannula on the dorsum of the hand. The hand may be held flexed at the wrist to occlude venous return and make the veins prominent.

- The tourniquet is removed and the infusion is started by releasing the clamp on the tubing. A hub of the cannula and IV set are secured to the skin with the adhesive plaster
- For flushing the cannula, normal saline should be used and not the distilled water. Distilled water causes pain at IV site and it also causes hemolysis
- If venipuncture is performed only for collection of blood, pull the needle gently after collecting the required sample and apply steady pressure at the site with a piece of spirit swab for few minutes.

INTRAOSSEOUS INFUSION

Peripheral percutaneous venous access is the fastest method of obtaining vascular access in children. However, during life-threatening emergencies, rapid access to venous compartment through peripheral or central venous route is occasionally difficult or an impossible procedure for a pediatrician to perform. Small peripheral vessels in children often collapse during shock and efforts at setting up an IV line in a peripheral vein may fail. When IV access cannot be established within three attempts or 90 seconds time, intraosseous route should be used as per the recommendations.

Common Sites

- Anteromedial surface of the proximal tibia, one or two finger breadths distal to tibial tuberosity to avoid damage to epiphyseal growth plate
- About 2–3 cm above the lateral condyle of the femur in the midline
- Medial surface of the distal tibia proximal to the medial malleolus.

Technique (Fig. 6)

- Especially designed needles, Jamshidi type available for intraosseous infusion should be used, if available. Hypodermic needle can also be used. 20–16 FG needle can be used for children below 18 months of age, and 16–12 FG for older children

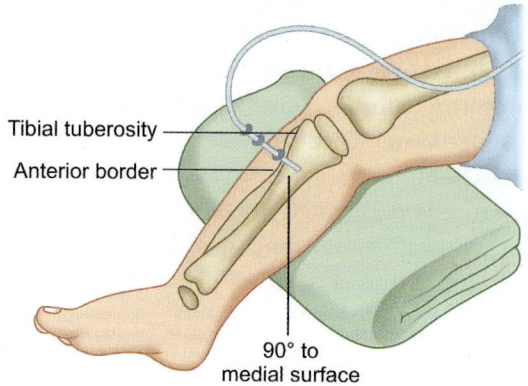

Fig. 6: Intraosseous cannulation technique.
Source: Chameides L. Textbook of Pediatrics Advanced Life Support. Texas: American Heart Association/American Academy of Pediatrics; 1988.

- Identify the site of placement
- Patient's leg should be restrained; a small sand bag is placed behind the knee
- The use of local anesthesia is optional, but usually recommended as it may be more painful once the child is resuscitated.
- Aseptic precautions are must
- Insert the needle perpendicular to the skin and advance to the periosteum and then with a screwing motion penetrate into the marrow. A distinct "give way" sensation indicates that your needle is in marrow. Confirm that the needle is firmly embedded in the bone
- Insertion of needle to a depth of 1 cm is usually adequate as the distance from skin through the cortex is rarely more than 1 cm in infants and children
- The needle should maintain erect posture without support
- Trocar is removed and correct position is verified by aspiration of marrow and easy flushing with 5–10 mL of normal saline without signs of extravasation
- The needle should be secured and apply sterile dressing over the site
- It should be watched for local complications like extravasation and infection

- As soon as the peripheral IV route is established, intraosseous needle should be removed
- Emergency drugs and fluids can be administered intraosseously essentially the same dosage and rates as given by IV route.

VENOUS CUTDOWN (VENESECTION)

Venous cutdown is now rarely resorted to in the present scenario of cannulas and intraosseous access. It is mainly useful when routine IV access has failed in conditions such as shock or when large amounts of fluids have to be given for a long time as in total parenteral nutrition.

Sites

- *Lower limb:* Most preferred site is saphenous vein near ankle
- *Upper limb:* Median cubital or basilic vein in front of elbow
- *Cephalic vein* at the wrist at anatomical snuff box
- *External jugular vein* in the neck.

Technique (Fig. 7)

- Get all the instruments ready
- Prepare the part aseptically. Then it is draped with sterile towels
- 0.5% Xylocaine is infiltrated subcutaneously at the site of incision. In emergency, local anesthesia can be skipped
- A 1–2 cm long transverse incision is made 1.5 cm above and in front of medial malleolus, over the saphenous vein
- The vein is exposed by blunt dissection, opening the blades of mosquito forceps parallel to the vein
- Pass the tip of mosquito artery forceps under beneath the vein and elevate atleast 1 cm above the vein
- Pass two silk ligatures under the vein
- Separate the proximal and distal ligatures for full length of exposed vein
- Tie the distal ligature and hold the ends with mosquito forceps
- With venesection scissors put "v" shaped cut on anterior wall of the vein at middle of the exposed part

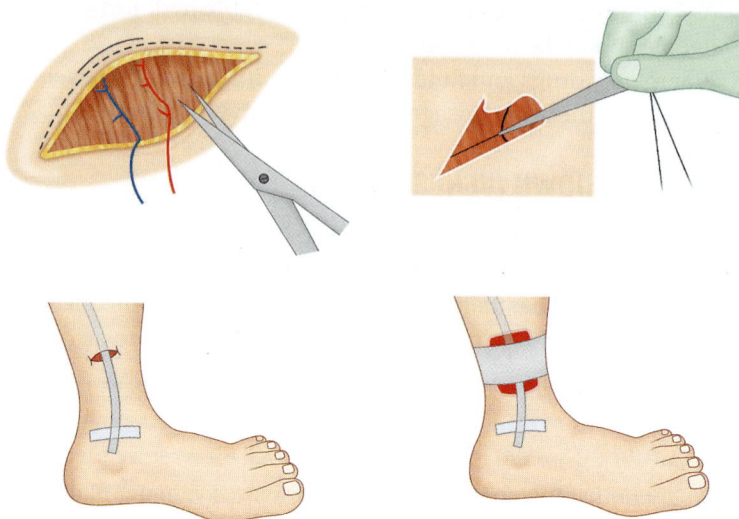

Fig. 7: Venous cutdown.
Source: Prajapati BS. Essential Procedures in Pediatrics, 1st edition. New Delhi: Jaypee Brothers Medical Publishers (P) Ltd.; 2003.

- Introduce polyethylene tube of suitable size proximally through the cut in the vein till the free flow of blood is obtained
- Cannula is fixed by tying proximal ligature on the vein with cannula in vein
- Ends of proximal and distal ligatures are trimmed
- Wound is sutured by silk sutures in a way so that cannula or tube does not get kinked or obstructed
- Dressing is applied and remaining part of the tube is properly fixed with dressing
- IV drip is connected to the venesection needle.

COMPLICATIONS
- Wound infections
- Thrombophlebitis
- Deep vein thrombosis
- Air embolism
- Injury to adjacent nerves and vessels.
  As alternate route is possible, earliest venesection tube should be removed.

EXTERNAL JUGULAR VEIN PUNCTURE

The external jugular vein is formed below the ear and behind the angle of mandible, passes downward and obliquely backward across the surface of sternocleidomastoid muscle, and ends in subclavian vein lateral to anterior scalene muscle.

Technique (Fig. 8)

- Place the patient in supine. Both the shoulders should touch the table and head is rotated fully to one side and extended partly over the end of the table so as to extend the vein. Making the child cry makes the vein prominent
- Restraining the child properly is very important
- Clean the overlying skin
- Use proper size of the cannula. Keep the cannula in the direction of the vein with the point aimed toward the same shoulder
- Make the venipuncture midway between the angle of mandible and midclavicular line
- Proceed as described for veins of extremities
- After removing the needle, apply constant pressure at puncture site for 5 minutes while the child is sitting.

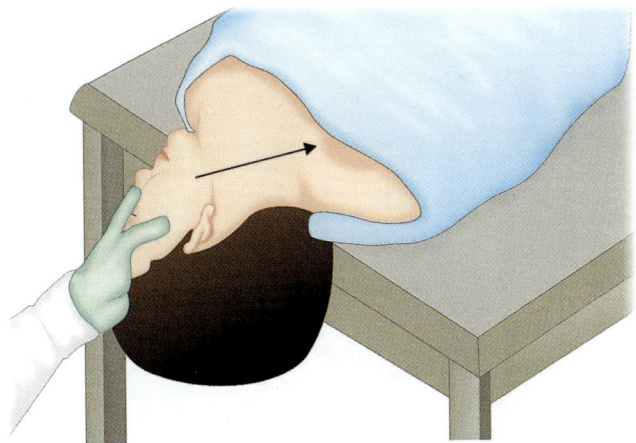

Fig. 8: Position for jugular vein (both internal and external) puncture. The arrow shows the direction of insertion of the needle for external jugular vein puncture.
Source: Silver HK, Kempe CH, Bruyn HB. Handbook of Pediatrics, 13th edition. Singapore: Lange-Maruzen Asia Publications; 1980.

FEMORAL VEIN PUNCTURE

In view of the risks of femoral venipuncture, it should be used as a last resort for collection of blood samples in neonates and infants.

Technique (Fig. 9)

- Restraining the infant in frog leg position
- Clean the inguinal area properly. The part is cleaned properly with spirit–iodine–spirit
- The femoral artery is located just below the midpoint of inguinal ligament
- The femoral vein lies medial to the artery
- Skin is pierced about 1–2 cm as below the inguinal ligament directly over the femoral vein and the needle is advanced at an angle of 30–45° with the skin while maintaining the gentle negative suction. As the vein is punctured, the blood is withdrawn in the syringe. If no blood is obtained while needle is inserted, suction should be maintained as the needle is slowly withdrawn. Sometimes needle passes through both the

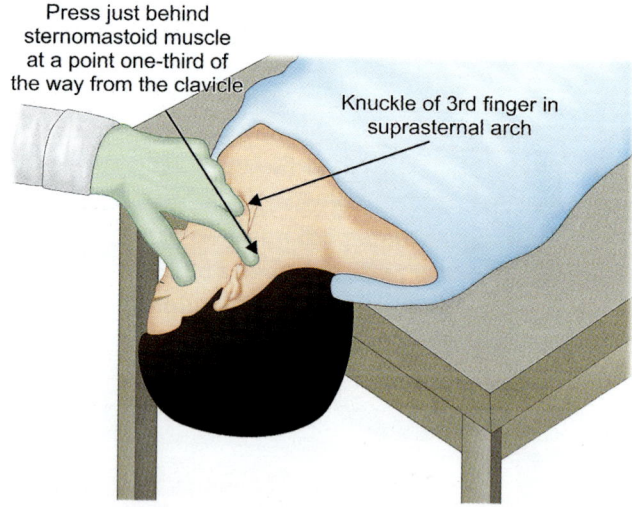

Fig. 9: Internal jugular vein puncture technique.
Source: Silver HK, Kempe CH, Bruyn HB. Handbook of Pediatrics, 13th edition. Singapore: Lange-Maruzen Asia Publications; 1980.

walls of the vein and blood is obtained only when the needle is being withdrawn
- On removal of needle, apply firm pressure over the site of puncture for atleast 3–5 minutes to avoid oozing and hematoma formation.

Precautions
- As far as possible avoid this procedure
- Strict asepsis is necessary as there is potential risk of septic arthritis and osteomyelitis
- Be careful regarding piercing the femoral artery, which can be identified by bright red color of blood as jet flow of it. If artery is pierced inadvertently, remove the needle and apply pressure for a long time and check the limb periodically for pulsations, color, and warmth.

UMBILICAL VEIN CATHETERIZATION

It is used for exchange transfusion. It may be used for rapid replacement of fluids and blood especially in extreme preterm neonates. Now-a-days, exchange transfusion is also preferred by peripheral route.

The umbilical vein spirals through the cord and is at 12 o'clock position at the level of the abdominal wall. Here it turns cephalad and runs slightly toward right to enter the porta hepatis. It continues with left portal vein, communicates with left hepatic vein and then with inferior vena cava. The umbilical vein is much wider than umbilical arteries.

Technique
- The child should be in supine position with gentle restraining. A padded crucifix splint is used to restrain the baby
- Sterilize and drape the skin around the umbilical stump
- The cord is then cut cleanly about 2 cm above the umbilicus and umbilical vein is located at 12 o'clock position. The blood clot in the vein is expressed or pulled out by fine forceps **(Figs. 10A and B)**

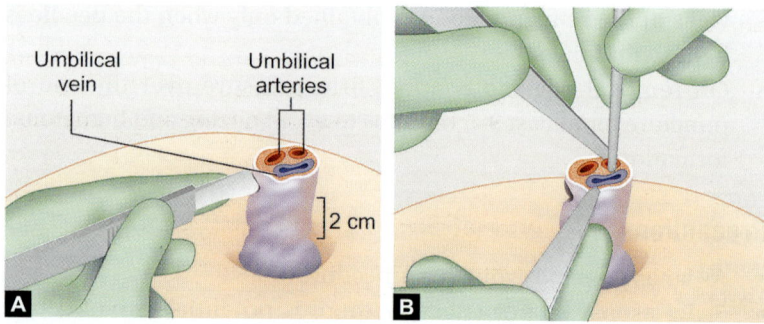

Figs. 10A and B: Cutting the umbilical cord for vessel catheterization insertion of umbilical catheter in umbilical vein.
Source: Prajapati BS. Essential Procedures in Pediatrics, 1st edition. New Delhi: Jaypee Brothers Medical Publishers (P) Ltd.; 2003.

- Mark the catheter for the correct distance to be inserted, which is about 20% of the crown heel length
- The catheter is passed into the vein slowly and gently, giving caudal traction on the cord stump till free flow of blood is obtained
- Flush the catheter with heparinized saline
- The free end of the catheter should be strapped to the abdominal wall.

Special Points

- If the cord is dried up, it can be excised flush with the umbilicus, which can expose the orifice of the umbilical vein at 12 o'clock position. This can be gently dilated with Hagar's dilator and then catheterized
- If both these methods fail, supraumbilical cutdown will become necessary
- Remove the umbilical vein catheter within 24–48 hours
- The catheter tip should be advanced up to thoracic portion of the inferior vena cava
- While passing the catheter, the resistance is felt at the ductus venosus. The catheter should be passed 1–2 cm beyond this point.

Complications
- Infection
- Vessel perforation
- Thrombosis of portal vein and portal hypertension in the future
- Liver infarction
- Liver abscess
- Necrotizing enterocolitis
- Cardiac arrhythmias.

UMBILICAL ARTERY CATHETERIZATION

It is used for periodic monitoring of arterial blood gases and for constant monitoring of blood pressure in a neonate. There are two umbilical arteries and the lumen appears patent.

Technique
- Prepare the umbilical stump as for venous catheterization
- Identify the artery and insert the catheter gently in the caudal direction, pulling the umbilical stump superiorly
- Position the tip of the catheter at either high (in the lower thoracic aorta above the diaphragm between T4 and T11 vertebrae) or low position (in the abdominal aorta opposite 14 vertebrae)
- Keep observing the color of the lower limbs during the procedure
- Fix the catheter in place using purse string sutures at the place
- Strap the free end of the catheter to the abdominal wall after filling it with heparinized saline and closing the end with a rubber stopper
- Every time before sampling, remove the heparinized saline in the syringe along with same blood, then collect the sample, and reinfuse the previously collected blood to the child

Complications
- Vessel perforation
- Thromboembolism
- Air embolism
- Hypertension
- Necrotizing enterocolitis
- Infarction of distal extremities
- Renal infarction.

RADIAL ARTERY CATHETERIZATION

It is very useful and frequently used for repeated sampling of arterial blood and for continuous arterial pressure monitoring. The radial artery is easily accessible at the wrist in the groove between the tendon of the flexor carpi radialis medially and the distal radius laterally.

Before puncturing the radial artery, carry out the Allen test to assess the ulnar collateral circulation.

Allen Test (Figs. 11A to D)

- Make the patient's hands warm to make pulsations easily demonstrable
- Have the patient open and close the hand held out in front and then clinch the fist tightly closed
- Occlude both radial and ulnar arteries for 30 seconds. Have the patient open the hand. Hand becomes pale due to occlusion of radial and ulnar arteries
- Release the pressure over the ulnar artery and observe the open hand for return of normal pink color. Return of normal color within 6 seconds indicates patency of the ulnar artery and an intact arch with good collateral circulation

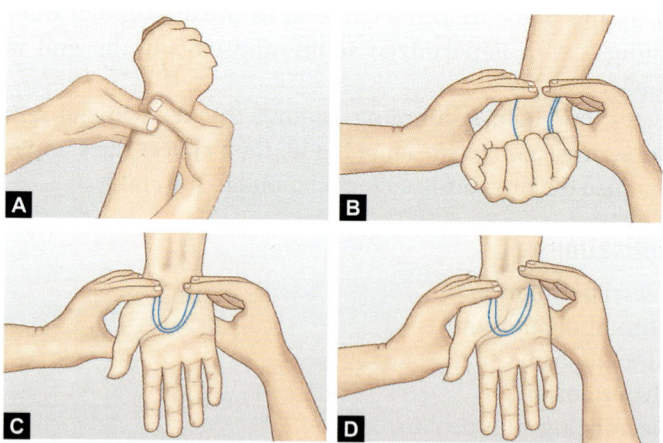

Figs. 11A to D: Allen test.
Source: Prajapati BS. Essential Procedures in Pediatrics, 1st edition. New Delhi: Jaypee Brothers Medical Publishers (P) Ltd.; 2003.

- Delay of appearance of normal color from 10 seconds to 15 seconds indicates slow filling of the ulnar artery and collaterals
- Persistent blanching for more than 15 seconds indicates an incomplete arch or poor collaterals
- Same test can be performed to check patency of radial artery
- If ulnar collateral circulation is good, radial artery puncture can be performed.

Technique (Figs. 12A and B)

Patient's hand should be supported and dorsiflexed at the wrist approximately 60° with both hands and lower forearm secured to a board. A roll of gauze behind the wrist will maintain dorsiflexion.
- Locate the radial artery just proximal to head of radius
- Clean the area and observe the absolutely aseptic precautions
- Infiltrate the skin with local anesthetic agent
- Insert the catheter needle at about 30° angle to the surface of the skin and advance the catheter and needle stylet into the artery until blood appears in hub of the needle
- Remove the needle and attach the hub of the catheter to the connecting tubing
- Secure the catheter at the place with silk sutures

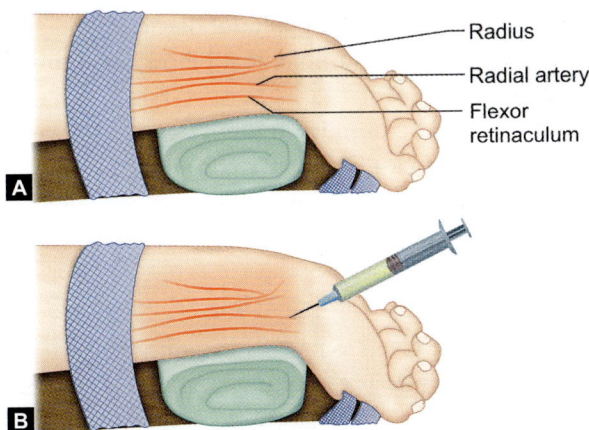

Figs. 12A and B: Radial artery—(A) Anatomy; and (B) Catheterization technique.

- Fix the wrist in a neutral position to the board. It is essential as flexion at wrist can disturb the arterial line
- Cover the insertion site with sterile dressing.

Special Points
- Do not perform the procedure if Allen test is delayed
- Observe the color of palm periodically after cannulation
- Before sampling blood, flush the line with 2% normal saline
- Do not infuse medications and blood products through the arterial line except flushing fluid.

BONE MARROW ASPIRATION

This is a very common ward procedure indicated in children with blood dyscrasias, malignancies, and undiagnosed fevers. Needle aspiration, trephine biopsy, and surgical biopsy are three methods available for bone marrow examination. Needle aspiration is commonly practiced in most of the cases in children. It should be done with caution when a defect in clotting mechanism is suspected.

Common Sites
- *Iliac crest:* This is the most preferred site in children. It is performed at 1 cm below the posterior iliac crest
- *Tibia:* At the upper end of tibia, just below tibial tuberosity on its medial aspect
- *Sternum:* It should be used in children beyond 7-8 years of age. Manubrium sterni can be used 1 cm above sternomanubrial angle, slightly to one side of the midline
- Rarely, lumbar spinous processes may be used.

Technique
- Atropine should be given as premedication
- Aseptic and antiseptic precautions are must during the whole procedure
- Local infiltration of 1% lignocaine from skin to periosteum. In some irritable children, general anesthesia is desirable for successful outcome of the procedure

- The needle for bone marrow aspiration should be stout and made of hard stainless steel. It is about 7–8 cm long with a well-fitting stylet and an adjustable guard **(Figs. 13A and B)**. The point of needle and edge of bevel should be sharp. The Sahan and Klima needles are most commonly used needles. Some people prefer to use stout hypodermic needles so that it can be disposed after use and complications of reuse of the needle can be avoided
- The needle with the guard adjusted 0.5–1 cm from the tip of the needle is introduced into the iliac crest or sternum with screwing or boring movements keeping the needle vertical. The force required varies but needs to be considerable. Sudden giving in of resistance indicates entry of the needle into the bone marrow. Leave the needle and if it remains steady, it indicates that the needle is in the bone marrow
- The stylet is withdrawn and marrow is aspirated with the syringe. About 0.2 mL of marrow is aspirated. This procedure is performed swiftly to obtain only bone marrow particles as slow sluggish aspiration causes dilution of marrow with blood
- To prevent dilution of marrow with blood, aspirate material only till it appears beyond nozzle of syringe. It is sufficient material for examination. Aspiration beyond it increases the chances of marrow dilution
- The needle is withdrawn and smear is prepared with marrow. With good material and well prepared smear marrow, particles can be seen by naked eyes

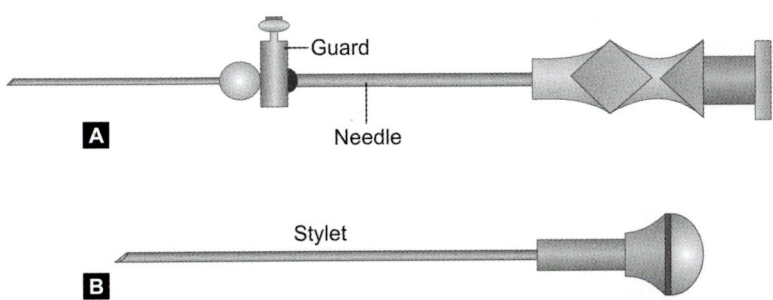

Figs. 13A and B: Bone marrow aspiration needles.
Source: Prajapati BS. Essential Procedures in Pediatrics, 1st edition. New Delhi: Jaypee Brothers Medical Publishers (P) Ltd.; 2003.

- Press the site for 5 minutes. Apply tincture of benzoin seal at puncture site
- Along with smears of bone marrow, smears from peripheral blood should be prepared and sent for examination.

Complications
- Local pain and hematoma
- Injury to mediastinal structures in case of aspiration at sternum
- Infection
- Dry tap.

LUMBAR PUNCTURE

This procedure is performed to obtain cerebrospinal fluid (CSF) sample for analysis in diagnosing infections and other disorders of central nervous system. It is also used for monitoring CSF pressure, intrathecal drug administration and removing CSF in some cases of hydrocephalus.

Contraindications
- Marked raised intracranial pressure with closed fontanel as shown by papilledema because of the risk of herniation of brain substance through foramen magnum
- Local infection
- Cardiovascular and respiratory instability.

Technique
- Informed written consent is must
- The patient is placed on his side at the edge of the table or bed with the knee drawn up toward abdomen and the head flexed to get maximum flexion of the spine **(Fig. 14)**. If the child is newborn or child has respiratory problem, child should be firmly fixed at shoulders and buttocks only without flexing neck and drawing up knees. In infants, sitting position allows easier identification of the midline. An experienced assistant has a vital role in positioning, restraining and comforting the patient
- Aseptic and antiseptic precautions are must

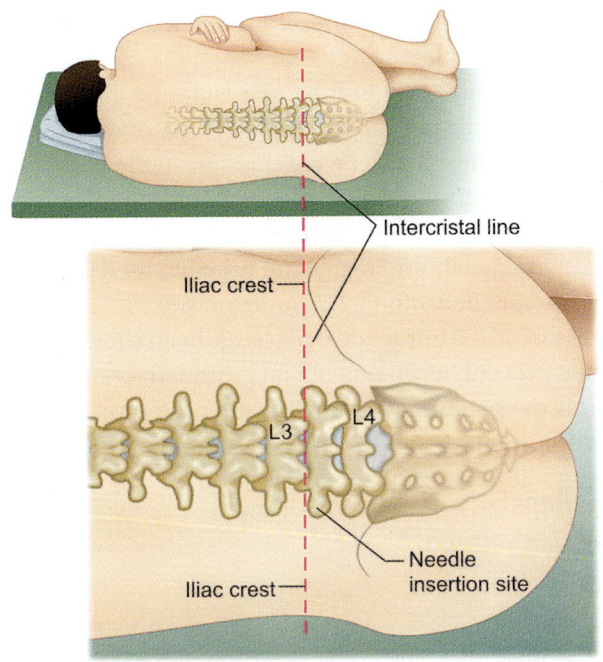

Fig. 14: Position for lumbar puncture.
Source: Prajapati BS. Essential Procedures in Pediatrics, 1st edition. New Delhi: Jaypee Brothers Medical Publishers (P) Ltd.; 2003.

- Routinely, local anesthesia is not used. But in older children those are irritable; local anesthesia may be useful for performing the procedure smoothly
- Site of puncture is defined by palpating the iliac crest, which corresponds to L3–L4. Hold the needle between index and middle fingers, the thumb acting as guard at open end
- In children instead of lumbar puncture needle with stylet, simple hypodermic needle is commonly used. 22–18 FG disposable needles are well suited for infants and children. Some people have good experience with the use of disposable scalp vein for lumbar puncture in neonates and children up to age of 2 years. Scalp vein set no. 23 with 2 cm length is suitable for neonates
- Gently introduce the needle in midline at abovementioned space, needle being directed toward umbilicus. Entry into the

subarachnoid space is indicated by giving the way sensation and free flow of CSF
- Collect the CSF 0.5 cc in Ethylene Diamine Tetra Acetic Acid (EDTA) bulb for cell count and 1 cc in plain bulb for biochemistry. It should also be collected in sterile bulb for culture. Cerebrospinal fluid for cell count should be examined at the earliest, usually within 30 minutes
- Remove the needle and apply firm pressure for few minutes
- Apply tincture benzoin seal at puncture site
- In a case of raised intracranial pressure, head should be kept little down to prevent herniation of brain through foramen magnum
- Monitor the patient for some time after the procedure for pulse and respiration.

Complications
- Infection
- Conning
- Headache
- Injury to local structures
- Epidermoid tumor.

SUBDURAL TAP

It is indicated for diagnosis of subdural hematoma, effusion, and empyema.

Technique
- Before subdural tapping, ultrasonography or CT scan study of cranium is desirable
- Informed written consent is must
- Scalp should be shared, atleast 5 cm posterior to the anterior fontanel and 5 cm lateral to midline and anteriorly up to forehead
- Sedation may be required in irritable infants
- Child should be in supine position with head at the edge of the table
- One person should hold the head at the middle position and another person hold the shoulders **(Fig. 15)**
- Strict aseptic and antiseptic precautions should be taken.

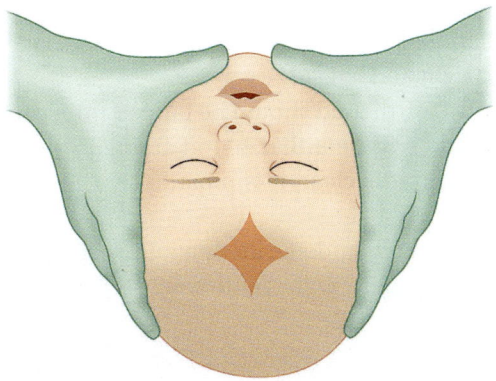

Fig. 15: Position of head for performing subdural tap.
Source: Prajapati BS. Essential Procedures in Pediatrics, 1st edition. New Delhi: Jaypee Brothers Medical Publishers (P) Ltd.; 2003.

- Sterilize the area
- Lateral margins of anterior fontanel are palpated along the coronal sutures and the site is chosen either for lateral as possible or at the area of maximum transillumination
- It should be atleast 2–3 cm from the midline to prevent injury to the underlying sagittal sinus
- A zig-zag puncture is used to prevent later leakage of subdural fluid
- A disposable no. 20 G needle is used. The skin is first pulled to one side and then needle is passed perpendicular to the scalp through the suture line and into the subdural space to a depth of approximately 0.3–0.6 cm. A definite pop giving the way is felt on entering the subdural space. The flow of fluid will be there on entering the subdural space. If flow of fluid is not there, slight adjustment or rotation of the needle may be necessary
- The subdural fluid is allowed to drain spontaneously. The fluid should not be aspirated for fear of drawing pial vessels into the point of needle
- The subdural fluid is collected in EDTA and plain bulbs for examination. Smear for Gram's stain should be prepared. It should also be collected for culture

- The subdural tap must be performed on both the sides. Samples from both the sides should be kept separate and labeled properly indicating right and left side
- Maximum 10 mL of fluid should be tapped from each side
- Subdural fluid will be either blood stained or xanthochromic but not clear. If it is clear, it is most likely CSF through ventricular tapping
- Remove the needle and sterile benzoin seal is done. Dressing should be done tightly with sterile gauze and adhesive tape.

Complications
- Trauma to blood vessels and hematoma formation
- Infection leading to subdural empyema.

VENTRICULAR TAP

This procedure is useful in newborns for diagnosis of ventriculitis and intraventricular hemorrhage. It is also performed to relieve the acute rise of intracranial pressure in non-communicating hydrocephalus. In some conditions, it may be done to administer intraventricular drugs.

Technique
- Before ventricular tapping, ultrasonography or CAT scan study of cranium should be done
- Informed written consent should be taken
- Shaving of scalp
- Sedation, if necessary
- Aseptic and antiseptic precautions
- Child should be in supine position with head at middle edge of the table
- One person should hold the head at middle position and another person should hold the shoulders
- The ventricle is entered by passing no. 23 FG needle in neonates and no. 22 FG in infants, 4–5 cm long disposable needle through lateral margin of anterior fontanel and keeping the direction of needle slightly inwards toward inner canthus of opposite eye or nasion **(Fig. 16)**

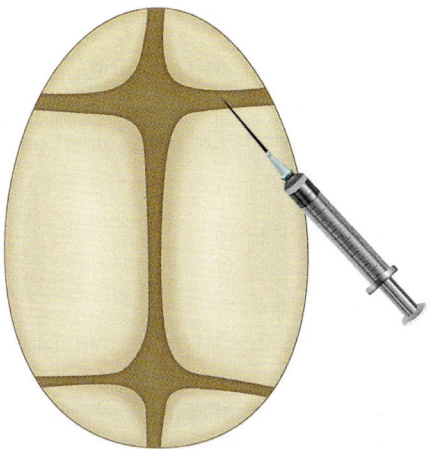

Fig. 16: Ventricular tapping. The needle should be directed forwards and inwards toward nasion.
Source: Prajapati BS. Essential Procedures in Pediatrics, 1st edition. New Delhi: Jaypee Brothers Medical Publishers (P) Ltd.; 2003.

- Depending on the degree of ventricular dilatation and size of the patient, the ventricle is reached at the depth of about 2.5 cm
- Entering the ventricle, gives the way
- No syringe suction should be applied
- CSF should be collected in EDTA and plain bulbs for examination. Smear should be prepared for Gram's stain
- After removing the needle, press at puncture site for some time
- Sterile benzoin seal is done. Dressing should be done with sterile gauze and adhesive tap
- In a case of hydrocephalus, CSF can be drained in large quantity
- For administering drugs in ventricles, drug should be taken in the syringe and after ventricular puncture it should be attached with the needle. Let the CSF come in syringe, get the medicine diluted in CSF, and then inject back into the ventricle. Drug should not be diluted in any solution.

Complications
- Ventriculitis
- Injury to brain tissues
- Intraventricular hemorrhage.

NASOGASTRIC TUBE INSERTION

Nasogastric tube is passed for either aspiration of gastric contents or administration of feeds or therapeutic substances. Nowadays, silastic and polyethylene tubes are being used because they have less tissue reactions.

Indications

Diagnostic

- Gastric aspirate test for diagnosis of neonatal septicemia
- Shake test for lung maturity in preterm babies
- Examination of gastric contents for *Mycobacterium tuberculosis*
- Assessment of upper gastrointestinal (GI) tract bleeding
- Measurement of gastric volume.

Therapeutic

- Paralytic ileus
- Intestinal obstruction
- Enteral feeding
- Administration of therapeutic substances.

Contraindications

- Esophageal stricture
- Ingestion of alkali may cause esophageal perforation
- Head and neck injury preventing passage of tube
- Nasal fracture.

Technique

- The head is raised in semiupright position
- The distance from nose to ear lobe and from ear lobe to xiphoid process is determined to measure the length of the tube to be passed. The point is marked on the tube **(Figs. 17A and B)**
- The more patent nostril is selected for passing the tube
- The terminal part of the tube is lubricated with a lubricant. It is avoided in newborns to prevent aspiration of an oily substance. In that case, it is wet with water

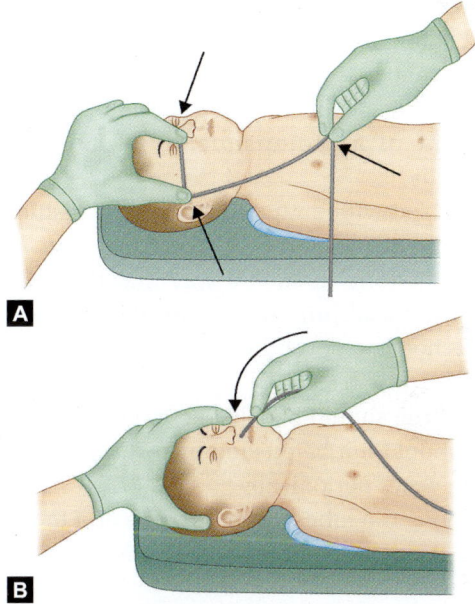

Figs. 17A and B: Method of inserting a nasogastric tube in a child.
Source: World Health Organization. Management of the Child with a serious Infection or Severe Malnutrition-Guidelines for care at the First-Referral level in Developing Countries Department of Child and Adolescent Health and Development. Geneva: World Health Organization; 2000.

- The tube is passed into the nostril, its curve directs downward. It is passing along the floor of the nose. In case of difficulty, it is tried in another nostril. Resistance is felt when it reaches the nasopharynx. Getting the patient to sip a little water helps to overcome it
- With swallowing of the saliva or water by the patients, the tube is advanced into the esophagus
- If the patient gags or the tube coils up in the mouth, the tube is withdrawn partly and again it is passed
- The tube is passed up to the mark which is decided as per size of the child
- Confirmation of proper placement is done by the following tests:
  • Aspiration of stomach contents on applying suction at the outer end of the tube with a syringe indicates that the tube lies in the stomach

- Air is injected into the tube while epigastric area is auscultated. A sound is heard if the tube is in the stomach
- Placing a tube in a glass of water and escape of air bubbles in the water indicate that the tube lies in the trachea
- Placement of a radiopaque tube can be assessed by radiography
- The tube is fixed with a tape in a butterfly fashion around the tube or with vertical tapping over the nose and the tube. The tapping is done in such a way that the tube rests in the middle of the nasal lumen and not directly in contact with mucosa. It is not taped over the forehead as it may cause pressure necrosis of the nose
- The feed or drug should be allowed to go in the tube by gravity method. It should not be pushed by piston. The tube should be flushed with water periodically
- While removing the tube, pinch the tube end to prevent spilling of the contents into the trachea.

Complications
- Pulmonary aspiration
- Esophageal perforation
- Gastric perforation
- Nasal necrosis
- Esophageal stricture.

Instead of nasogastric tubing, nowadays orogastric tubing is preferred to avoid certain complications.

GASTRIC LAVAGE

It is useful in poisoning to remove the substance from the stomach. In corrosives and hydrocarbons ingestion, gastric lavage is contraindicated. In corrosives, passing the tube may cause perforation. Since passing the gastric tube is likely to induce vomiting, it increases the risk of aspiration of hydrocarbons into the trachea and lungs, which causes pneumonia.

After passing the tube in the stomach as described in nasogastric tube insertion, lavage of the stomach using aliquots of normal saline is done in cases of poisoning. It is continued till the color of the lavage is normal.

ABDOMINAL PARACENTESIS

Abdominal paracentesis is performed for diagnostic purpose in case of ascites, peritonitis and hemorrhage. In huge ascites, it is also done to relieve discomfort and respiratory embarrassment. In some situations, drugs may be instilled in peritoneal cavity such as malignancies.

Technique

- The patient should be placed in supine position. If the patient is not comfortable in supine position, reclining or upright position may be used
- Site for paracentesis is selected in midline, midway between umbilicus and pubic symphysis or in an iliac fossa lateral to the rectus abdominis
- The needle should never be advanced through a surgical scar because it can penetrate bowel adherent to the under surface of the scar, or lacerate an omental or mesenteric vessel
- Informed written consent should be taken
- Aseptic and antiseptic measures must be taken
- Injection atropine as premedication
- 1% lignocaine is infiltrated under skin and into the deeper structures at the site selected for paracentesis. Wait for few minutes for full effect of anesthetic agent
- The hypodermic needle 20 FG is attached to 20 mL syringe. It is passed into the peritoneal cavity perpendicular to the skin. As the needle enters the peritoneal cavity, it gives the way and ascitic fluid starts to drain through the needle
- In a case of tense ascites, needle should be passed obliquely or skin should be retracted caudad before insertion of the needle to produce a Z track effect on withdrawing the needle so that needle tract after paracentesis gets sealed properly and persistent drainage can be prevented after removal of the needle
- After removal of fluid, 10–15 mL for diagnostic purpose, the needle is withdrawn and a seal of tincture benzoin is applied locally

- If the paracentesis is for therapeutic purpose, the needle should be connected with IV set and regulator of IV set is adjusted in such a way that ascitic fluid is drained slowly. One liter of fluid may be drained over a period of 2–3 hours
- The patient should be watched following the procedure.

Complications
- Intestinal perforation or laceration
- Peritonitis
- Postparacentesis shock
- Electrolyte imbalance
- Hypoproteinemia
- Perforation of urinary bladder
- Pneumoperitoneum.

LIVER BIOPSY
Nowadays, liver biopsy is done under the ultrasound guidance rather than blind biopsy.

Indications
- Chronic hepatitis
- Undiagnosed hepatomegaly
- Neonatal hepatitis
- Cirrhosis of liver
- Fever of unknown origin.

Contraindications
- Bleeding tendency
- Massive and tense ascites
- Severe portal hypertension.

Prerequisites
- Bleeding time, clotting time, platelets count and prothrombin time
- USG study of liver
- *Premedication:* Atropine 0.01 mg/kg IM 30 minutes before the procedure.

Technique

- Vim–Silverman needle, Menghini's needle, and Tru-Cut® needles are used for liver biopsy. Tru-Cut® needle is disposable, easy to operate and has more success rate, so it is common in use
- Informed written consent is must
- Patient is kept in supine position, near the edge of the bed or table with the right arm under the head and left arm by the side
- Preparation of the local area
- Aseptic and antiseptic precautions are must
- 1% lignocaine is infiltrated in the skin, intercostal muscles and Glisson's capsule. Wait for some time for good effect of the anesthetic agent. Some children may require sedation or general anesthesia
- The Tru-Cut® needle is introduced under ultrasound guidance into the liver substance with the inner needle retracted. The latter is then advanced, holding the outer cutting sheath steady. The outer sheath is then advanced to cut the liver in the biopsy notch. The whole apparatus is then withdrawn together quickly. The entire sequence should take only few seconds
- The Vim–Silverman needle has trocar and bifid needle to cut the liver tissue. In Menghini needle, the cut piece of liver is sucked into the syringe applied with negative pressure
- On removal of the needle, the puncture site is sealed with tincture of benzoin.

THORACOCENTESIS (INTERCOSTAL DRAINAGE)

Thoracocentesis refers to temporary insertion of a needle or a catheter into the pleural space for removal of fluid or air from the pleural cavity. The fluid is collected for diagnostic purpose and in some situations it is done for therapeutic purpose to remove fluid or air, which is in large quantity and causes respiratory embarrassment. Drugs can also be instilled in the pleural cavity by this procedure, if it is indicated, such as in a case of malignancy.

Technique

- Written consent is must
- Injection Atropine as premedication

- Site of insertion of needle can be decided by chest X-ray, dull note on percussion and ultrasound study of thorax. Best way to perform the procedure is under ultrasound guidance
- It should be performed in sitting position of the patient. Patient can lean forward on the teapoy (or chair) of suitable height with head resting on his forearms **(Fig. 18)**
- Strict aseptic and antiseptic measures should be taken
- 1% lignocaine is infiltrated at the upper border of the rib below the space chosen. Anesthetizing wide area and generous infiltration of local anesthetic agent for good anesthesia help to get good cooperation of the patient, performing the whole procedure comfortably leading to successful performance with minimal chances of complications. Wait for some time for good effect of anesthetic agent
- A wide bore needle is connected on one side of the three way stop cock and opposite to it a syringe is attached. Three-way stop cock is arranged in such a way that there is a single track between the needle, stop cock and syringe
- The needle is inserted into the chest in the same manner as for the anesthetic needle, finding the intercostal space and stepping

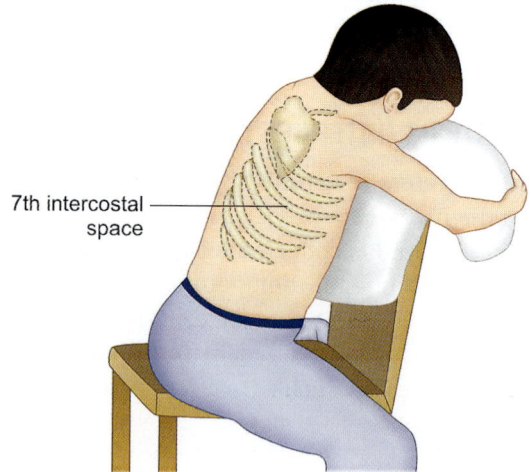

Fig. 18: Another position for doing thoracocentesis.
Source: Johnson KB. The Harriet Lane Handbook—A manual for Pediatric House Officers, 13th edition. New Delhi: Jaypee Brothers Medical Publishers (P) Ltd.; 1993.

over the lower rib with care, thereby preventing damage to underlying structures **(Fig. 19)**. Slight suction is applied to the syringe so that the fluid is aspirated in the syringe immediately as the needle enters the pleural space
- Fluid should be withdrawn slowly and steadily
- A forceps should be attached to the needle at the skin level, which helps to prevent excessively deep insertion of the needle into the thorax
- The fluid is aspirated in the syringe and then three-way stop cock is turned to connect the syringe with the outlet, which is attached to IV set
- Collect the fluid in EDTA and plain bulbs. It is also collected for culture. Smear should be prepared for Gram's stain and Ziehl–Neelsen stain.
- The three-way tap is now turned again to connect the syringe with the needle and the pleural space, a further aspiration is carried out. It is expelled into the drainage bag by turning the three-way tap. The drainage bag or bottle should be placed well below the level of the patient's chest
- As fluid is removed, the lung expands and this often makes the patient to cough

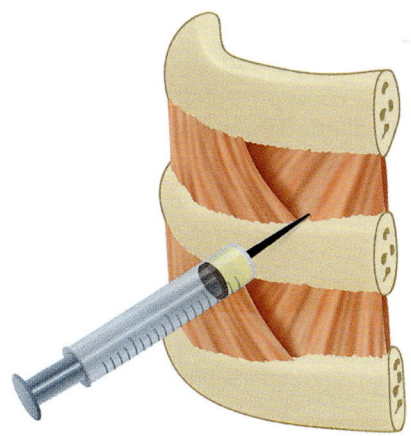

Fig. 19: Site of needle for pleural fluid aspiration.
Source: Prajapati BS. Essential Procedures in Pediatrics, 1st edition. New Delhi: Jaypee Brothers Medical Publishers (P) Ltd.; 2003.

- The needle is withdrawn and puncture site is covered with a benzoin seal. A sterile gauze is put over it and adhesive tape is applied.

Complications
- Pneumothorax
- Hemothorax
- Infection
- Unilateral pulmonary edema
- Hypoproteinemia.

ENDOTRACHEAL INTUBATION

Endotracheal intubation is a procedure, which every pediatrician and one working in intensive care units must be well conversant with. The critically ill patient often requires endotracheal intubation. It secures patent airway. It is a prerequisite for mechanical ventilation. Endotracheal suction can most efficiently be done through an endotracheal tube. It is indicated when bag and mask resuscitation fails in a case of an asphyxiated newborn.

Indications
- In neonatal asphyxia
  - Bag and mask resuscitation fails
  - Apparently still born baby after adequate suctioning of upper airways
  - Infants with diaphragmatic hernia
  - Meconium aspiration
- Cardiorespiratory arrest due to any cause
- Central nervous system depression in a case of head injury or comatose child
- Diseases of peripheral nervous system, poliomyelitis, Guillain-Barré syndrome, tetanus, organophosphorus poisoning, etc.
- Administration of general anesthesia.

Equipment
- Laryngoscope—with straight blade for neonates

- Endotracheal tubes (ETs) for various sizes with stylet:

Weight/age	ET size (ID in mm)
<1,000 g	2.5
1,000–2,000 g	3.0
2,000–3,000 g	3.5
>3,000 g	4.0
1–5 years	4–5
5–12 years	5–6.5

- Approximately size of ET, ID in mm = Age (years) + 16/4.

Technique
- The patient is placed in a supine position. The operator stands beyond the patient's head. Patient's neck is slightly extended with the head in midline
- Clear the oropharynx with gentle suctioning
- Empty the stomach
- Hold the handle of laryngoscope in left hand with thumb and first three fingers, stabilize the hand with fifth finger resting on patient's cheek. The blade should be pointing away from oneself
- Open the baby's mouth and push the tongue left with the back of right forefinger and steady the head with the rest of right hand
- While visualizing insert the blade midline until the tip is between base of tongue and epiglottis within the vallecula **(Figs. 20A and B)**
- If the infant is making respiratory effort, free flow of oxygen with an oxygen tubing held close to the infant's mouth and nose is to be provided during intubation
- Open the mouth further by pulling on laryngoscope handle, simultaneously tilt the blade tip upward slightly to elevate epiglottis and visualize the glottis. Use base of the tongue as pivot rather than maxilla
- Suction is needed
- Have the assistant to palpate suprasternal notch with index finger, applying gentle pressure if desired
- Hold the tube with concave curve anterior and pass it down to right side of the mouth, outside the blade, along with maintaining visualization

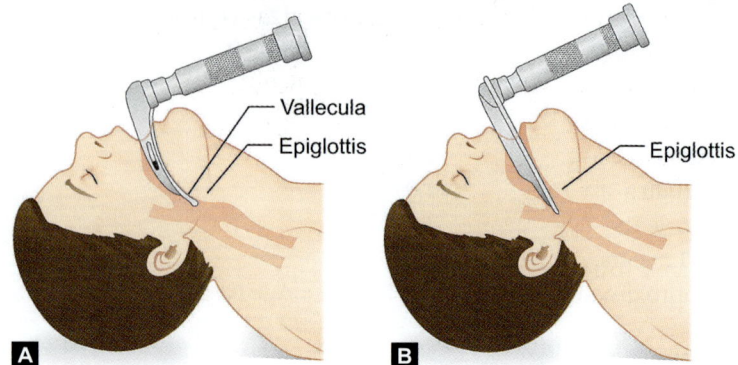

Figs. 20A and B: Position of laryngoscope blade when using—(A) Curved blade, it is in the vallecula; and (B) Straight blade, it is over the epiglottis.
Source: Prajapati BS. Essential Procedures in Pediatrics, 1st edition. New Delhi: Jaypee Brothers Medical Publishers (P) Ltd.; 2003.

- As the patient inspires, pass the tube through cords 2 cm into trachea or until immediately after tip passes under assistant's finger in suprasternal notch
- The tube is then held firmly at the lips with the right hand, and the laryngoscope and stylet are carefully removed
- Initially confirmation of the tube placement is accomplished by attaching a resuscitation bag with the connector and ventilating the infant. With correctly placed tube, the air entry is heard on both sides of the chest, breath sounds are of equal intensity, and air is not heard entering the stomach. While listening the breath sounds, the stethoscope is to be placed at approximately the nipple line
- Note the centimeter marks on the tube at the level of upper lips and then secure the tube to the infant's face
- Final confirmation of placement of the tube can be obtained by chest film, if it is needed
- Attempts to intubate should not exceed 30 seconds. If you are unable to intubate within 30 seconds, abort and continue with bag and mask and then try again after a few minutes. Repeated attempts may cause serious glottic edema and bleeding

- Intubation is not a matter of prestige. If you are unable to do so, please ask for help
- Endotracheal route is also used for administration of some drugs like epinephrine, atropine, naloxone, etc.

Complications
- Hypoxia
- Bradycardia
- Apnea
- Pneumothorax
- Injury and lacerations to tongue, gums, pharynx, epiglottis, trachea, vocal cords, etc.
- Infections
- Postextubation stridor can be managed by nebulized epinephrine or steroids.

Some physicians prefer nasotracheal intubation when long-term ventilation is required.

SUPRAPUBIC BLADDER ASPIRATION

This procedure is performed to collect non-contaminated urine sample in neonates and infants. It is a safe and reliable way of collecting urine samples. It is easy, especially in neonates, as bladder is an intra-abdominal organ in these patients unlike a pelvic organ in older children and adults.

Technique
- The infant is placed on a flat surface in supine position
- The assistant stands opposite the operator and immobilizes the infant by grasping the thorax with one hand and thighs and hips with the other
- Make sure that the bladder is full
- Local part is cleaned. Aseptic and antiseptic measures are must
- A 10 cc disposable syringe with 22 FG, 4–5 cm long needle is taken
- The symphysis is located with one finger and the needle is inserted 2 cm above the symphysis in the midline with syringe held at 10–20° angles from perpendicular **(Fig. 21)**

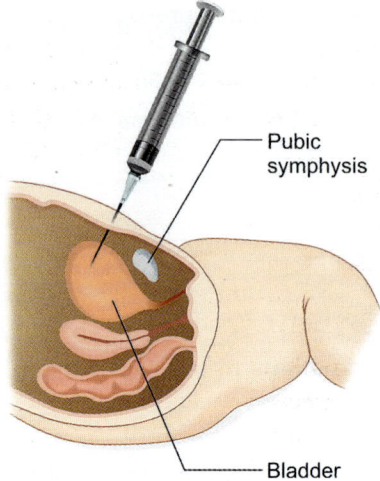

Fig. 21: Suprapubic bladder puncture technique.
Source: Prajapati BS. Essential Procedures in Pediatrics, 1st edition. New Delhi: Jaypee Brothers Medical Publishers (P) Ltd.; 2003.

- With a single steady motion the needle is inserted until a perceptive change in resistance is felt as the needle enters the bladder.
- Light aspiration is applied to aspirate the urine specimen.
- After removal of needle, a seal of tincture benzoin is applied at puncture site.

PERITONEAL DIALYSIS

Dialysis involves the use of semipermeable membranes that permit the simultaneous passage of smaller molecular weight solutes and water while retarding or inhibiting the movement of large sized particles. The basic principle controlling the transmembrane movement of solute and water are similar whether the membrane is artificial (hemodialysis) or natural (peritoneal dialysis).

Indications
- Blood urea more than 300 ms/dL
- Hyperkalemia, serum potassium more than 6.5 mEq/L not responding to medical line of treatment

- Severe acidosis
- Pulmonary edema
- Acute left ventricular failure
- Drug intoxications like barbiturates, salicylates, etc.
- Life-threatening electrolyte imbalance.

Contraindications
- Peritonitis
- Abdominal adhesions
- Laparotomy done
- Pleuroperitoneal communication.

Technique (Fig. 22)
- Informed written consent
- Aseptic and antiseptic precautions must be taken
- Injection atropine 0.01 mg/kg IM 30 minutes before the procedure as the premedication
- Sedation, if required
- Proper restraining
- Bladder is emptied by its own or catheterization, if it is necessary
- Abdominal wall is prepared, painting spirit–Betadine–spirit. Towel draping
- The catheter is usually placed in the midline few centimeters below the umbilicus. If midline insertion is not possible, the catheter can be inserted in the flank area, outside the line of inferior epigastric artery
- The site is anesthetized by injecting 1% lignocaine up to peritoneum
- If there is no ascites, distend the abdomen with 10 mL/kg dialysate solution using 17–20 FG angiocath or needle
- Needle is withdrawn and a knife blade is used to enlarge the puncture wound in the skin
- If ascites is present, a very small penetrating incision is made in the skin and the trocar with catheter is stabilized with the fingers of one hand on the skin while the other hand introduces the trocar through the abdominal wall with an alternating drilling motion

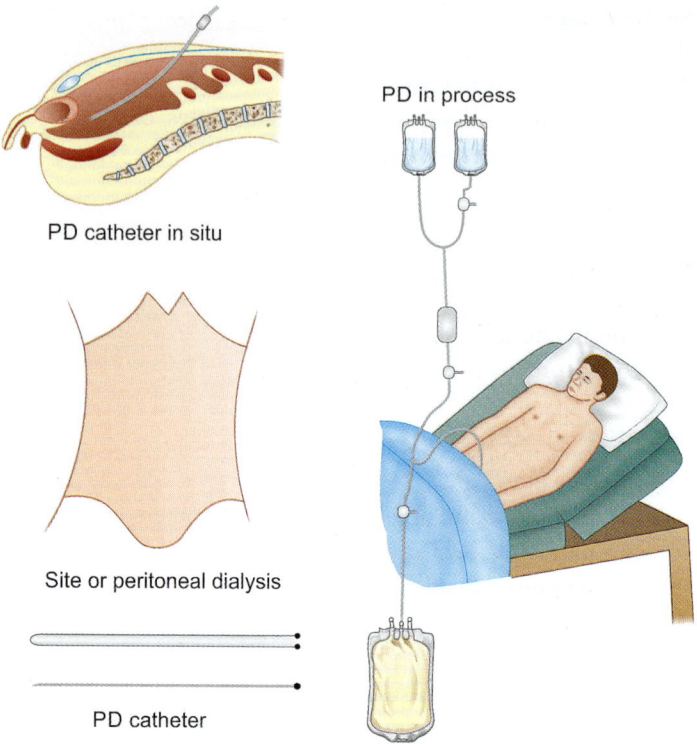

Fig. 22: Peritoneal dialysis (PD).
Source: Prajapati BS. Essential Procedures in Pediatrics, 1st edition. New Delhi: Jaypee Brothers Medical Publishers (P) Ltd.; 2003.

- Penetration up to peritoneum is detected by a definite sensation of giving the way and also by the appearance of fluid in the catheter when trocar is removed
- On reaching the peritoneal cavity and before removing the trocar, the catheter is gradually advanced in the peritoneal cavity in right or left paracolic gutter and trocar is gradually withdrawn
- When the catheter is sufficiently introduced in the peritoneal cavity, trocar is removed totally. All the fenestrations on the catheter must be within the peritoneal cavity to avoid subcutaneous fluid infiltration in the abdominal wall. In neonates and infants, IV catheters or simple feeding tube can be used

- The catheter should be stabilized with adhesive plaster
- The catheter is connected with the administration tubing through small connector, and dialysis fluid is flown
- Because hyperkalemia is often present, potassium free fluid is used for the first three–six cycles
- Time of input of dialysis fluid will be about 10–15 minutes. The fluid is kept in the peritoneal cavity for about 30 minutes. Time for output of dialysis fluid will be about 15–20 minutes. Each cycle will take about an hour. First few cycles should be of half an hour (rapid cycles)
- Record the weight of the patient prior to the procedure and every 12 hours
- Total duration of dialysis is about 40 hours depending on the clinical and biochemical parameters
- Warm the dialysate to body temperature
- Infuse it by gravity flow
- Each cycle should be of 30–50 mL/kg
- Blood sugar, blood urea, serum creatinine, serum electrolytes and serum proteins should be checked 12 hourly
- In the presence of fluid overload, use hypertonic dialysate
- Tip of the catheter should be sent for culture
- Close the site of dialysis by sterile bandage
- Peritoneal dialysis-related problems like, pain in abdomen, diarrhea, dyspnea, bleeding and fluid delivery should be sorted out appropriately.

Complications

- Pain may be due to over distention, peritonitis, etc.
- Bleeding
- Dialysate leak
- Outflow obstruction
- Peritonitis
- Metabolic complications
- Thrombosis
- Pulmonary complications.

RENAL BIOPSY

Indications
- Steroid resistant nephrotic syndrome
- Asymptomatic proteinuria
- Glomerulonephritis associated with conditions like systemic lupus erythematosus, Henoch-Schönlein purpura, etc.
- Rapidly progressive glomerulonephritis.

Contraindications
- Bleeding diathesis
- Solitary functioning kidney
- Ectopic/horseshoe shape kidney
- Severe uncontrolled hypertension.

Prerequisites
- Bleeding time, clotting time, partial thromboplastin time or activated partial thromboplastin time and platelets count
- Blood grouping and cross matching
- Hypertension and uremia should be controlled
- Informed written consent is must.

Technique
- Atropine 0.01 mg/kg IM before 30 minutes of the procedure
- The patient is placed in the prone position on a firm bed. A pillow is placed under patient's abdomen. This compresses and fixes the kidneys to the posterior abdominal wall, bringing the kidneys closer to the skin and limiting possible ballottement of the kidney by the biopsy needle
- Ultrasonography is commonly used to mark the location of kidneys and point of entry of the needle into the kidney perpendicular to the skin surface and to obtain depth of tissue from skin surface. Usually, lower pole of left kidney is selected for biopsy
- The area is prepared and local anesthesia is given. Irritable children may need general anesthesia
- A 23 G exploring lumbar puncture needle is passed downward and obliquely toward the lower pole of the kidney.

A needle can be felt going through different structures and renal capsule. On penetration of the renal capsule, an experienced person feels cessation of resistance.
- The patient is asked to take slow deep breathings. If the needle is in the kidney, a characteristic pendular movement is seen with respiration, the hub of needle swings through a wide arch, moving toward head during inspiration and toward buttock during expiration. If the needle is not in the kidney tissue, it is slightly advanced until it penetrates kidneys and moves characteristically on breathing. The depth of the kidney below the skin is measured on the stem of the needle
- A small nick is made over anesthetized area with a scalpel
- Franklin modified Vim–Silverman needle and Tru-cut® needle are commonly used in the practice. Tru-cut® needle is easy to use and having less failure rate. Therefore, Tru-cut® needle is preferred nowadays
- Tru-cut® needle is one piece apparatus with a length of 11.4 or 15 cm. The needle with cannula covering the obturator is advanced in the kidney to desired length in a direction perpendicular to skin surface
- The patient is asked to hold the breath in deep inspiration
- The obturator is advanced by firm tap on the handle. The specimen is cut by downward movement of cannula over obturator
- Entire assembly is removed
- The patient is asked to breathe normally
- Firm pressure is applied over biopsy site for few minutes and the site is sealed with tincture benzoin.
- Two good cores of tissue (8–10 mm long) are needed for adequate histological examination. One is immediately fixed in buffered formalin and other in saline (for immune fluorescence study).

Postprocedure Management
- The patient is asked to remain in prone position for 2 hours and in bed for 24 hours
- Monitoring temperature, pulse, RR and BP one hourly for 6 hours and then 4 hourly for 24 hours

- Urine should be collected in separate bottles during each voiding and should be checked for hematuria
- Patient is asked to take ample liquid orally
- Diuretics may be given in case of oliguria to flush any clot in the passage
- If no Frank hematuria and vitals are normal, patient can be discharged after 24 hours with instructions not to do exertion for a week.

Complications
- Hematuria
- Perinephric hematoma
- A-V fistula.

PERICARDIOCENTESIS

Pericardiocentesis is a procedure for removal of fluid from pericardial cavity for diagnostic purpose or to relieve cardiac tamponade. It is occasionally a life-saving procedure. It is a risky procedure. It should be performed only by skilled person under continuous cardiac monitoring. Echocardiographic diagnosis is must before performing the procedure. It gives idea regarding amount of fluid and also helps to determine the anatomical approach.

Prerequisites
- Echocardiographic diagnosis
- Coagulation profile
- Resuscitation kit including defibrillator
- Cardiac monitor
- IV line
- Premedication with injection atropine 0.01 mg/kg IM 30 minutes before the procedure.

Technique (Fig. 23)
- Informed written consent should be taken
- Sedation may be required in some patients. If possible, it should be avoided

- Child should be seated leaning backward at approximately 60° and carefully restrained
- The best site is xiphocostal angle. The other sites are fourth, fifth or sixth intercostal spaces 1–2 cm medial to the border of cardiac dullness on percussion **(Fig. 23)**
- Aseptic and antiseptic precautions are must
- 1% xylocaine is infiltrated in the skin at left xiphocostal angle, 3–4 cm below left costal margin.
  The needle is advanced initially perpendicular to the skin surface and after traversing the soft tissue under the rib cage, its tip is pointed to the left shoulder. While advancing the needle in the deeper structures if it reaches to pericardial cavity, the pericardial fluid is withdrawn in the syringe. Local anesthetic agent should not be injected in the pericardial cavity.
- The pericardiocentesis needle is passed along the same path until the fluid is obtained. The distance from skin to the pericardium is less than 5 cm in a child. A distinct "give" or "pop" is felt when the pericardium is punctured. Pericardial fluid can then be aspirated.
- Getting the fluid confirms the position of needle into the pericardial cavity. Normal saline can be injected under 2D echo monitoring, which shows bubbles of saline

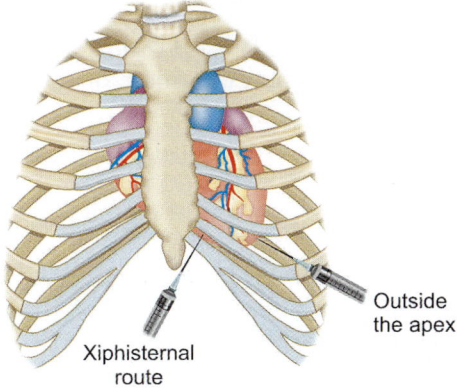

Fig. 23: Sites for pericardiocentesis.
Source: Prajapati BS. Essential Procedures in Pediatrics, 1st edition. New Delhi: Jaypee Brothers Medical Publishers (P) Ltd.; 2003.

- If the blood or bloody fluid is withdrawn, it is vital to determine if cardiac chamber or coronary artery has been punctured. Still uremia and malignant diseases can give rise to hemorrhagic pericardial effusion. Blood obtained from heart or coronary vessel clots immediately
- Fluid is sent for appropriate examinations
- The needle is withdrawn and benzoin seal is done at puncture site
- Postprocedure monitoring of heart rate, RR and BP should be done. 2D echo may be performed to study post-tapping condition.

Complications

- Hemopericardium
- Arrhythmias
- Vasovagal reactions
- Infection
- Pneumothorax
- Air embolism
- Perforation of an abdominal viscus, commonly stomach
- Cardiac arrest and death.

FINE-NEEDLE ASPIRATION BIOPSY

Fine-needle aspiration biopsy (FNAB) is very useful for cytological and bacteriological evaluation of a mass or a lymph node. It is minimally invasive and requires no sedation. It aids in tissue diagnosis and in determining the course of management.

Requirements

- 1–1.5" 20–25 FG needles. 22 FG 1" long is the most commonly used size of needle
- 10–20 mL plastic disposable syringes
- Clean glass slides
- About 70–90% ethanol for routine wet fixation
- Containers for culture media whenever needed.

TECHNIQUE
- Sterilize the area
- Anesthesia is usually not required; local anesthetic agent may be used in uncooperative and irritable children
- Immobilize the lump to be biopsied between your thumb and finger with one hand
- Hold the syringe in the other hand and insert needle into the assigned area, perpendicular to the skin surface and position the needle within the target tissue
- Pull the syringe plunger to apply negative pressure
- While maintaining suction, make several passes through the mass or node
- Release the negative pressure while needle remains in the target tissue
- Withdraw the needle
- Detach the needle, draw 2–3 mL air into the syringe, reattach the needle and blow the aspirates onto the slide
- Apply the pressure over the puncture site with cotton swab for 5 minutes
- Deep biopsies can be done with assistance of radiological imaging techniques like ultrasound.

The following situations can give unsatisfactory yield during FNAB:
- When needle misses the lesion tangentially
- When central area is cystic, necrotic or hemorrhagic and devoid of diagnostic material
- When there is a small malignant lesion close to a dominant benign mass
- When the target tissue is fibrosclerotic and poor in cells.

Index

Page numbers followed by *b* refer to box, *f* refer to figure, and *t* to table.

A

Abdomen 157, 351
    distention of 158, 165, 165*b*, 189*f*
    examination of 170, 172*f*
    inspection of 173*b*
    movements of 173
    palpation of 177*t*
    percussion of 188
    shape of 172, 173
Abdominal viscus, perforation of 498
Abducens nerve palsy 288
Abductor digiti minimi 310*f*
Abductor pollicis 310*f*
    brevis 310*f*
    card test 310*f*
Aberrant left coronary artery originating from pulmonary artery 224
Abscess 435
Acanthosis nigricans 68*f*
Acarus mite
    high power view of 392*f*
    low power of 392*f*
Achilles jerk 322
Acid-fast bacillus 25
Acidosis, severe 491
Acne 381
Acrocephaly 51
Acrocyanosis 348
Acrodermatitis enteropathica 381
Acromelia 72
Acute febrile encephalitic syndrome 19
Acute left ventricular failure 491
Acute respiratory failure 200*b*
    signs of 199
Addictive drugs 339
Adductor angle 146, 302, 303*f*
Adelaide coma scale 278
Adenoid
    enlarged 426*f*
    facies 426*f*
    hypertrophy 425
Adenoviruses 195
Adventitious sounds 44, 214, 217

Advisory Committee on Immunization Practices Technique 454
Age appropriate vision screening charts 408*t*
Age-specific normal respiratory rates 42*t*
Air embolism 462, 467, 498
Alae nasi, flaring of 199
Alimentary system 157
Alkali, ingestion of 478
Allen and tumbling E chart 410*f*
Allen cards 408
Allen test 468, 468*f*, 470
Allergic disorders 373
Allergy 454
Alopecia 386
    areata 381
Alport syndrome 419
Amaurotic cat's eye reflex 397
American Academy of Ophthalmology 395
American Academy of Pediatrics 395
American Association for Pediatric Ophthalmology and Strabismus 395
American Association of Certified Orthoptists 395
Amiel-Tison method 147*t*
Amino acids 98
Aminoglycosides 339
Amnionitis, history of 340
Anacrotic pulse 232
Anal fissure 167
Anal reflex 319
Ancillary testing 449
Anemia 259, 340
    hemolytic 182, 185
Anesthesia 313, 451
Angiofibroma, juvenile nasopharyngeal 428, 429
Angiotensin-converting enzyme 196
Aniridia 58
Ankle
    clonus, elicitation of 322*f*
    jerk 322

Anosmia 281
Anotia 419, 422
Antecubital fossa 456
Anterior horn cells 335
Anthropometric indices, interpretation of 122
Anthropometry 49, 111, 124, 344
Antinuclear antibody 366
Antithyroid drugs 339
Anxiety 15
Aorta 40
Aortic regurgitation 41, 229, 263
Aortic stenosis 222-224, 231, 264
Apert syndrome 55
Apex beat 243, 244, 259
    method of palpation of 243, 244f
    types of 245
Apgar scoring system 341, 344, 345t
Aplasia cutis congenital 381
Apnea 489
    test 446, 448
Apneic oxygenation method 448
Appetite 158, 169
Appropriate growth charts 344
Aqueous humor 396
Arachidonic acid 98
Arm span 121
Arm, midpoint of 117
Arnold Chiari malformation 329
Arrhythmias 224, 498
    cardiac 467
Arteriovenous fistula 229, 496
Arthralgia 369
Arthritis 259, 362, 366, 366t, 369, 370, 372
    acute 362, 370
    chronic 362, 370, 371
Articular cartilage 370
Articular diseases 363
Articulation, disorder of 280
Artificial CO_2 augmentation procedure 448
Ascites 165, 452
    signs of 189
Asthma
    acute severe bronchial 233
    bronchial 14, 163, 195
Asymmetric tonic neck reflex 151, 354
Ataxia 273, 326, 327
    telangiectasia 387
Atelectasis 218
Athetosis 312
Atopic dermatitis 368f, 381, 389

Atrial septal defect 222, 226, 253, 254, 261
Atrophy 379
Atropine 483
Auditory brainstem response 424
Auditory steady state response 424
Auricle, hematoma of 420f
Auscultation 212, 250, 350
    areas of 251
    cardiac 250, 251t
    method of 212
Autism 155
Autoinflammatory disorders 362
Autonomic nervous system 330
    manifestation of 331
Autonomic neuropathies 331
Autonomic system 331
AVPU pediatric response scale 278b
Axillary lymph nodes 80
    right anterior 81
    right apical 81
    right lateral 81
    right posterior 81
Axillary suspension 351, 352f
Axillary temperature 37

B

Baby friendly hospital initiative 91
Bacillus Calmette-Guérin 23
    vaccination 454
Back pain 273
Bacteremia 274
Bacterial endocarditis 286
    subacute 407
Bacterial infections 388, 391
Bacterial meningitis 266, 268, 269, 271, 295, 419
Ballismus 312
Barbiturates 491
Barlow tests 357
Barognosis 316
Basal ganglia diseases 301
Basal metabolic rate 229
Basilic vein 456
Beau's line 71, 387
Beckwith-Wiedemann syndrome 64
Behavioral audiometry 424
Bell's palsy 292
Bell's phenomenon 291
Benzodiazepine 329
Biceps jerk, elicitation of 320f
Bifid uvula 67f

Index

Bilious vomiting 161
Birth
    asphyxia 337, 342
    weight 222, 336, 425
Bisferiens pulse 231
Bladder 273
Bleeding 493
    causes of 167*b*
    diathesis 494
    manifestations 342
    per rectum 158, 168
    per vaginum, history of 340
    tendency 482
Blood
    flow, direction of 175, 176*f*
    group 338, 339
    in stool 161
    pressure 44, 47, 169, 346, 365
        arterial 233
        measurement of 45, 233, 234
Blue lips and nails 342
Blue sclera 58*f*, 347
Blueberry Muffin' spots 391
Body
    language 15
    mass index 122
    proportions 120
    temperature
        measurement of 37
        normal 37
Bone 70
    marrow aspiration 470
        needles 471*f*
Bordetella parapertussis 195
Botulism 297
Bounding pulse 41, 231
Bowel involvement 273
Bowel sounds 192
Brachioradialis 322
Brachycephaly 51, 331
Bradycardia 228, 228*t*, 489
    causes of 229*b*
Brain
    abscess 268
    death 443, 449
        assessment of 446
        diagnosis of 444, 448*b*
    function, cessation of 446
    injury, post-traumatic 271
    space occupying lesions of 155
    tissues 477
    tumors 268

Brainstem 334
    evoked response audiometry 424
    reflexes 446
    tumors 287, 296
Branchial cleft cyst 435
Breast
    abscess 102
    anatomy of 93, 95*f*
    engorgement of 101
    examination of 77
    milk 102
        composition of 97, 99*t*
        types of 97
Breastfeeding 5, 91, 93, 99, 103
    continuation of 104
    initiation of 93
    schedule of 102
Breath sounds 217
    mechanism of 212
Breathing
    difficulty in 195, 197*t*
    signs of 44*b*, 196, 199*b*
    types of 213, 213*f*
Broca's aphasia 280
Bronchial breathing 213
    types of 214
Bronchiolitis 18
Brucellosis 371
Bruckner's reflex 402
Bruckner's test 398, 402*f*
Brudzinski sign 325, 326*f*
    positive 324, 325
Buccal mucosa 63, 435
Budd-Chiari syndrome 84, 182
Bulbar palsy 296, 297
Bulla 375, 377*f*
Bullous disorders 391
Bullous impetigo 388
Buphthalmos 53

C

Café-au-lait spots 267
Candida infection 390
Capillary refill time 47, 348
Caput succedaneum 346
Cardiac arrest 498
Cardiac failure, congestive 77, 222
Cardiac murmur 255
    mechanisms of 256
Cardiff cards 408
Cardiovascular disorders 221
Cardiovascular malformations 222*b*

Cardiovascular system 221, 350, 372
    examination of 241
Carotid pulsations 252*f*
Cat scratch disease 435
Cataract 58, 143, 347, 359
    bilateral 413*f*
    congenital 397
Catford drum 408
Catheterization technique 469*f*
Celiac disease 164
Central cyanosis 79
Central nervous system 19, 130, 265,
        266*b*, 372, 402, 445
    infection 130, 268, 269
    malformations 266
Central venous pressure 237
Cephalic vein 461
Cephalohematoma 346
Cereal-pulse combinations 108
Cerebellar
    disorder 311*f*
    signs 277, 326, 327*b*, 329*b*
    tumors 329
Cerebellitis 275
Cerebral
    depression 339
    palsy 155*b*, 273, 274, 296, 333
Cerebrospinal fluid 472
Cervical lymph nodes 79, 80*b*, 80*f*
CHARGE syndrome 426
Chemoprophylaxis 103
Cherry red spot 286
Chest
    circumference 118, 119*f*
    examination of 203
    expansion 208, 209*f*
    indrawing 342, 350
    inspection of 205*f*
    movements of 207
    pain 198, 198*t*, 223, 224*f*
    percussion, method of 211*f*
    shape of 204
    unilateral retraction of 206*f*
Cheyne-stokes breathing 43
Child's physical growth 123
Chin 66
Chloroquine 339, 387
Choanal atresia 425
Cholesteatoma 419
Chorea 259, 312
Choreiform movements 224
Chromosomal disorders 331

Chronic sinusitis 202
    causes of 202
Circumduction gait 329
Clasp knife spasticity 301
Clavicle 357
Cleft lip 62, 62*f*
Cleft palate 202
Clinical digital thermometer 31
Clomiphene 339
Club fingers 69*f*
Clubbing 240, 241, 259
    causes of 202*b*
    grades of 202*b*
    mechanism of 201
Coagulation profile 496
Coarctation of aorta 222, 262, 345
Coffin-Siris syndrome 387
Coin test 216
Cold spatula test 431, 431*f*
Colonic polyp 167
Color vision 283, 285
Colostrum 97
Coma 278, 446
Comedo 380, 380*f*
Communication skills, nonverbal 4*b*
Concentration, lack of 281
Confrontation test 284, 285*f*
Congenital malformations 329, 339, 342
Congestive heart failure 77, 196, 235
    signs of 236*b*
    symptoms of 223, 236*b*
Conjunctiva 57, 396
Connective tissue
    diseases 17
    disorders 362
Consanguinity 425
    degree of 24*t*
Consciousness 277, 281
Constipation 158, 164
    causes of 165*b*
Contact dermatitis 381
Continuous murmur 257, 258
Convulsions 274, 342
Copper metabolic disorders 275
Cornea 57, 396
Corneal light reflex test 397, 399, 401*f*
Corneal reflex 288, 446, 449
    examination of 447
    method of elicitation of 289
Cornelia de Lange syndrome 56*f*, 387
Corona radiata 334
Corpus callosum, absence of 268

Corrigan's pulse 263
Corrigan's sign 263
Cortical sensations 315, 316*b*
Corticosteroids 339, 387
Coryza 194
Cough 194, 195, 196*t*, 446, 447
Cover test 399
Cow's milk
    composition of 98, 99*t*
    protein allergy 164
Coxsackie B virus 221
Cracked nipple 102
Cracked pot sign 52, 332
Cranial bruits 53
Cranial nerve 277, 282*b*, 283, 288, 290, 295, 297
    examination 282
Craniofacial abnormality 425
Craniofacial anomalies 295
Craniosynostosis 332
Craniotabes 52
Cremasteric reflex 319
Crepitations 215
Crepitus 430
Cretinism 339
Croup 433
Crust 378, 379*f*
Cryptotia 422
Cushing's syndrome 387
Cyanosis 78, 223, 236, 259, 349, 350
    causes of 79*b*
Cyst 377, 433
    epidermal 377
Cystine 98
Cytomegalovirus 221, 419
    infection, congenital 391

D

Danger signs 349, 350*b*
Deafness 339
Death
    cardiac 498
    diagnosis of 443
Decerebrate rigidity 301*f*
Decorticate rigidity 300*b*, 300*f*
Deep palpation 179
Deep tendon reflex 277, 318, 319, 321*t*, 323
    grades of 321*t*
Deep vein thrombosis 462
Degenerative diseases 273

Dehydration 332
    assessment of severity of 48*t*
    severe 44
    severity of 48
Dementia 281
Demyelinating disorders 419
Depressor angularis oris, congenital absence of 292*f*
Dermatitis artefacta 381
Dermatoglyphics 88
Dermatomyositis 387
    juvenile 366
Dermatophytes 393*f*
Dermatophytosis, diagnosis of 391
Dermoid 398
    cyst 435
Deviated nasal septum 427
Diabetes insipidus, features of 281
Diabetes mellitus 390
    gestational 221, 222
Diabetic ketoacidosis 44, 163, 271
Diaphragmatic paralysis 43
    unilateral 43
Diarrhea 158, 161, 162, 389
    acute 162, 163
    causes of 164*b*
    chronic 163
    drug induced 164
Diastolic blood pressure 46
Diastolic murmurs 257, 258
Diazepam 339
DiGeorge syndrome 60, 390
Digital clubbing 74*f*
Digital scale 343
Digital thermometer 32*f*, 38*f*
Digital trauma 429
Diphtheria 10, 297, 434
Diplopia 287
Direct ophthalmoscope 408*f*
Direct ophthalmoscopy, method of 404
Distal extremities, infarction of 467
Distance visual acuity 400
Docosahexaenoic acid 98
Dolichocephaly 51, 331
Doll's eye phenomenon 287
Doppler method 46, 233, 235
Dorsalis pedis, method of palpation of 230*f*
Dorsiflexion angle 302, 303, 304*f*
Double vision 272
Down syndrome 35*f*, 51, 54*f*, 58, 64, 88, 140, 222, 225, 276, 295, 323, 324, 332, 337
    anhidrotic ectodermal dysplasia 386

Drowsy 277
Drug 329
	allergy 14
	intoxications 491
	rectal administration of 455
	withdrawal syndrome 339
Dry tap 472
Duchenne muscular dystrophy 226, 309, 330, 333
Dugdale's index 122
Dull aching 161
Dysarthria 280, 327, 329
Dysdiadochokinesia 311, 327, 328
Dysentery 164, 167
Dysmetria 311*f*, 327, 328
Dysmorphism 86, 259
Dysphagia 198, 281, 431
Dysphonia 280, 433
Dysplasia 86, 87
Dyspnea 199, 223, 258
	grades of 223*b*
	inspiratory 199
Dystonia 313, 334
Dysuria 161

E

Ear 33
	examination 60, 417, 420
		method of 421*f*
	foreign body of 418
	hemangiomas 422
	itching of 418
	pain, causes of 418
	tag 422
Earache 269
Ectodermal dysplasia 56*f*
Ectopic kidney 494
Edema 83, 170, 259
	abdominal wall 178
	angioneurotic 62, 63*f*, 64
	causes of 85*b*
Edinger-Westphal nucleus 285
Edward syndrome 69*f*, 225
Elbow 117
Electrocardiogram 226
Electroencephalogram 449
Electrolyte imbalance 482
Ellis-van Creveld syndrome 226
Encephalitis 275, 296, 297
Encephalopathy 268, 274
Endocardial fibroelastosis 222
Endophthalmitis 397

Endothrix invasion 393*f*
Endotracheal intubation 486
Endotracheal tube 447, 487
Energy requirements 28*t*
Enophthalmos 53, 287
Enteral feeding 478
Enthesitis-related arthritis 366
Epidermoid tumor 474
Epigastric pulsations 246
	palpation for 246*f*
Epigastrium 159
Epiglottitis 434
Epilepsy 155, 268, 271
	abdominal 158
Epileptic encephalopathies 271
Epiphora 59, 429
Episode, duration of 267
Epistaxis 428
	causes of 429*b*
Epstein pearls 349
Epstein-Barr virus 397
Erosion 378
Erythema marginatum 259
Erythema multiforme 70, 381, 390
Erythema toxicum 349
Erythematous skin rash 347
Esophageal perforation 478, 480
Esophageal stricture 478, 480
Esophagus, foreign body in 432*f*
Estrogen 222
Ethylene diamine tetra acetic acid 474
Eustachian tube dysfunction 418
Evoked otoacoustic emissions 424
Excessive sneezing 429
Excoriation 378
Exophthalmos 287
Extensor pollicis
	brevis 310*f*
	longus 310*f*
External auditory canal 422
	atresia of 419
External ear anomalies 60
External genitalia 175
External jugular vein 456, 461
	puncture 463
Extracardiac murmurs 260
Extremely low birth weight 337
Eye 33, 53, 143, 169
	anatomy of 396, 396*f*
	discharge 396
	examination of 347, 357, 395
	external evaluation of 401*f*

itching of 397
screening 397
  age appropriate methods of 399*t*
  methods of 397
slanting of 54
Eyeballs, size of 53
Eyebrows 55, 56*f*
Eyelashes 55, 56*f*
Eyelids 55, 415
  drooping of 55
  vicinity of 397

F

Face 53
Facial dysmorphism 34
Facial nerve 290
  motor function 291*f*
  palsy 292*f*
Failure to thrive 158
Fallot's tetrad 257
Febrile seizures 18, 268
Fecoliths 187
Feeding twins 95*f*
Femoral vein puncture 464
Fetal scalp 339
Fetor hepaticus 171
Fever 194, 241, 270, 340
  acute rheumatic 363
  history of 417
  of unknown origin 482
Fibrosis, cystic 202
Filariasis 83
Fine motor
  development 135
  milestones 137*t*
Fine-needle aspiration biopsy 498
Finger
  abductors 310*f*
  adductors 310*f*
Finger-finger and finger-nose
    test 309, 311*f*
Fingertip patterns 88
Fix and follow test 399
Flat chest 206*f*
Flexion creases 89
Flexor digitorum
  profundus 310*f*
  sublimus 310*f*
Flexor pollicis
  brevis 410*f*
  longus 310*f*
Floating spots 272

Fluid
  overload 238
  thrill 191
    demonstration of 192*f*
Flush method 46, 233, 234
Follicular hyperkeratosis 73*f*
Fontanels 50
Food poisoning 164
Foot 68
  dorsiflexion angle of 146, 303
Football holding method 95*f*
Fossa tumor, posterior 297
Frankfort's horizontal plane 115, 121
Friedreich ataxia 333
Frontal lobe dysfunction 281
Fundoscopy 59
Fundus
  evaluation 407, 408*f*
  examination 240, 283, 286, 286*f*
    normal 406*f*
Fungal infection 417
Funnel chest 206*f*, 207*f*

G

Gag reflex 296
Gait 277
  ataxia 327
  broad based 330
  disturbances 266
  examination 329
  hemiplegic 329
Galactosemia 103
Galeazzi's sign 356, 356*f*
Gallop rhythm 350
Gangliosidosis 59*f*, 286
Gastric
  aspirate test 478
  lavage 480
  perforation 480
  volume, measurement of 478
Gastroesophageal reflux disease 21,
    195, 196
Gastrointestinal bleeding 166
Gastrointestinal system 157
Gastrointestinal tract 167*b*
Gaucher disease 182, 296
Genetic syndromes 155
Genitalia 74, 348
Genitourinary system 157
Genodermatoses 373
Geographic tongue 65*f*, 381

Gestational age
  adequate for 337
  large for 337
  small for 337, 348
Gianotti-Crosti syndrome 381
Giardiasis 164
Giddiness 266, 420
Glabellar tap 354
Glasgow coma scale 277, 278, 278*t*
Glaucoma 272
Glossopharyngeal nerve 295
Glucose 6 phosphate dehydrogenase deficiency 18
Glycogen storage disease 226
Gower sign 309
Gram's stain 485
Granuloma annulare 381, 384*f*
Graphesthesia 316
Grasp reflex 130
Great arteries, transposition of 222
Great vessels, transposition of 261
Gross motor milestones 131, 132*t*
Growth 33, 259
  assessment of 111, 226
  based on
    height 115
    weight 112
  charts 123
  pubertal acceleration of 112
Guarded prognosis 440
Guillain-Barré syndrome 275, 287, 292, 297, 301, 329, 331, 486
Gums 64, 435
Gynecomastia 171

H

Hackett's grading 184, 185*f*
Haemophilia
  A 429
  B 429
  influenzae 10, 275
Hair 386
  color of 387
Hairpins 116
Hairy pinna 347
Haloperidol 339
Hand 68
  and feet, cyanosis of 348
  dorsum of 458*f*
  muscles 310*f*
Hand-foot-and-mouth disease 377*f*
Hand-to-mouth reflex 137
Hansen's disease 381, 383

Harrison's sulcus 205, 207*f*
Head 346
  and neck injury 478
  circumference 115
  examination of 49
  injury 296
    history of 272
  shape of 331
  size of 332
Headache 224, 266, 268, 269, 269*b*, 270, 273, 274, 416, 474
  causes of 269*b*
  cluster 269
  during fever 269
  in migraine 270
Hearing 131, 143
  assessment 293, 424
  deficit 295*b*, 360
  loss 143, 155, 345, 418
    causes of 419*t*
    conductive 419
    family history of 425
Heart
  block, congenital 222
  defect, congenital 222, 224
  disease
    congenital 221, 224
    cyanotic 348
  rate 40, 169, 226, 345
  sound
    abnormal 253*t*
    first 251
    fourth 254
    second 252
    third 252
Hemangioma 64, 386*f*, 398, 434
  capillary 347
Hematemesis 158, 161, 167
Hematochezia 168
Hematoma 427, 472
Hematuria 158, 161, 168, 169, 496
Hemiballismus 334
Hemiparesis 273
Hemiplegia 273
Hemoglobin level 22
Hemoglobinuria 169
Hemopericardium 498
Hemophilia 365
Hemophilic arthropathy 364
Hemoptysis 198
Hemorrhage 268
  intracranial 266, 271
  intraventricular 342, 477

Hemorrhoids 167
Hemothorax 486
Henoch-Schönlein purpura 71*f*, 365, 366, 372
Hepatic encephalopathy 171, 271
Hepatitis
    B 10, 22, 23, 342
        vaccines 342
    C virus 22
    chronic 482
Hepatobiliary system 157
Hepatoblastoma 182
Hepatocellular failure, signs of 171*b*
Hepatojugular reflux 238
Hepatomegaly 237
    causes of 182*b*
Hepatosplenomegaly 241
Hernia, inguinal 348
Herpes simplex 62
    virus 221
Herpes zoster 381, 382*f*
High stepping gait 330
Hind milk 98
Hip 357
    circumference 119
    congenital dislocation of 358*f*
    developmental dysplasia of 356
    examination of 357*f*
Hirschsprung's disease 341
Hissing sound ceases 46
Hodgkins tumor 435
Hoffman sign 323
Holt-Oram syndrome 226
Homocystinuria 58
Homonymous hemianopia 281
Hormonal therapy 339
HOTV matching cards 411*f*
Human immunodeficiency virus 22
Human milk
    components of 99
    composition of 98
    immunological components of 100*t*
Hurler's syndrome 202, 226
Hyaline membrane disease 342
Hydration, assessment of 47, 352*f*
Hydrocele 348
Hydrocephalus 51*f*, 155, 268-271, 329
Hydroxychloroquine 416
Hygroma, cystic 435
Hyperbilirubinemia 425
Hyperesthesia 313
Hypernatremia 268, 271

Hypertelorism 347
Hypertension 229, 269, 365, 467
    pregnancy-induced 340
    severe uncontrolled 494
Hypertensive encephalopathy 271
Hyperthermia 350
Hyperthyroidism 312, 387
Hypertonia 301
    types of 301
Hypertrichosis 386, 387*b*
Hypertrophic obstructive cardiomyopathy 222, 231
Hypocalcemia 140, 266, 268
Hypoglossal nerve 297
Hypoglycemia 130, 266, 268, 271
Hypokalemia 165
Hypokinetic pulse 42, 232
Hypomagnesemia 266, 268
Hyponatremia 268, 271
Hypoproteinemia 482, 486
Hypothalamic dysfunction 281
Hypothermia 342, 350, 445
Hypothyroidism 36*f*, 165, 332
Hypotonia 301, 323, 327, 339
Hypotonic cerebral palsy 323
Hypoxia 489
Hypoxic ischemic encephalopathy 130, 266

I

Ichthyosis, congenital 347
Icterus 78, 348
Iliac crest 470
Immaturity 143
Immotile cilia syndrome 202
Immune thrombocytopenic purpura 428
Immunization 14
    history 16, 27, 342
Impetigo 379*f*, 388
In utero infection 419, 425
Indian Academy of Pediatrics classification 128
Infantile tremor syndrome 18
Infantometer 113*f*, 343
Infection 271, 429, 467, 472, 486, 489, 498
Infective endocarditis 372
    signs of 241*b*
    symptoms of 241*b*
Inflammatory articular diseases 363
Inflammatory bowel disease 164, 365, 366
Infrared thermometer 38*f*
Injury 434, 489

Innocent murmurs 257
Intellectual disability 273
Intelligence quotient 277
Intensive care units 449
Intention tremor 312, 327
Internal jugular vein puncture
        technique 464*f*
Intertrigo 381
Intestinal laceration 482
Intestinal obstruction 165, 478
Intestinal perforation 482
Intra-articular ligaments 370
Intradermal injection 454
Intramuscular injection 452
  sites for 453*f*
Intraosseous cannulation technique 460*f*
Intraosseous infusion 459
Intrauterine growth retardation 338, 339
Intrauterine infections 391
Inverted syringe technique 100, 101*f*
Iris 58, 396
Iron deficiency anemia 75*f*, 275
Irritable bowel syndrome 164

J

Janeway lesions 241
Jaundice 57, 78, 158, 161, 166, 259, 339,
        342, 349
  acute 166
Jaw
  abnormalities 434
  jerk 290
Joint 70, 240
    capsules 370
    examination 370
    involvement, distribution of 372
    pain 223, 366, 370
    position, sense of 315
    swelling 161
Jugular vein puncture, position for 463*f*
Jugular venous pressure 237, 238*f*
Juvenile idiopathic arthritis 362, 366
    systemic onset 364, 366
Juxta-articular bones 370

K

Kanawati index 122
Kangaroo mother care 94*f*
Kartagener syndrome 202
Kawasaki disease 18, 63, 74, 223, 224, 292,
        364, 355, 366, 379, 387

Kayser-Fleischer ring 58*f*
Keratosis pilaris 381
Kernicterus 130
Kernig sign 324, 325, 326*f*
Kidney
  bimanual palpation for 186*f*
  horseshoe shape 494
  palpation of 184
Kiesselbach's plexus 428
Knee
  asymmetry of 356*f*
  extensors, testing power of 308*f*
  flexion 308*f*
  flexors, testing power of 308*f*
  jerk 319, 322
    elicitation of 320*f*
  joint 365
Koilonychia 74, 75*f*, 387
Koplik spots 63
Korotkoff sound 45, 46
Kuppuswamy scale 29
  modified 29*t*
Kyphoscoliotic chest 206*f*

L

Labyrinthine function 293
Lacrimal glands 59
Lacrimal sac, distention of 398
Lactation, physiology of 95
Lactiferous ducts 93
Lactose intolerance 164
  congenital 103
Landau reflex 355
Language
  development 138, 139*t*
  loss of 280
Laparotomy 491
Laryngeal edema 434
Laryngeal examination 436
Laryngeal web 434
Laryngitis, acute 434
Laryngomalacia 434
Laryngoscope 433, 486
    blade, position of 488*f*
Laryngotracheobronchitis 195, 433, 434
Lea symbols 410*f*
Lead
  encephalopathy 329
  poisoning 271
Left axillary BCG adenitis 82*f*
Left bundle branch block 253, 254
Left hypochondrium 159

Index

Left iliac fossa 160
Left kidney 186
Leishman's staining 392
Lens 58, 396
Lenticular opacity 58
Leprosy 381
Lethargy 342
Leukemia 77, 182, 429, 435
Leukocoria 143, 397
Lichen planus 381
Lichenification 378
Limb 68
    length 72
Lipomas 435
Lips 62, 435
    swelling of 63f
Little's area 428
Liver
    abscess 467
    biopsy 482
    cirrhosis of 482
    failure 429
    infarction 467
    lower border of 179
    palpation of 179, 180f
    upper border of 180
Lobar pneumonia 210, 216
Lobe functions 280
Local pain 472
Logmar chart 408
Loud murmurs 258
Low Apgar score 425
Low birth weight 295, 337
Low pulse volume 77
Lower limb 461
    hypertonia of 299
    scissoring of 305f
Lower motor nerve palsy 292
Lower motor neuron 333
    disease 333t
    facial palsy 291
    lesion 291
        localization of 335t
Lower respiratory tract infections, recurrent 222
Ludwig's angle 204
Lumbar puncture 472
    position for 473f
Lumbar regions 160
Lumbosacral meningomyelocele 358f
Lumbricals 310f
Lump, abdominal 187
Lurching gait 330
Lyme disease 419
Lymphadenitis
    acute 435
    inguinal 82f
Lymphadenopathy 79, 170, 259
    significant 81
Lymphangiectasis 83
Lymphangioma 64

M

MacEwen sign 52, 332
Macrocephaly 332
    causes of 51b
Macroglossia 64
Macula lutea 407
Macular means spot 374
Macule 374
    over face 375f
Magnesium sulfate 339
Magnetic resonance imaging 265
Malformation syndromes 87
Malignant tumors 435
Malnutrition 27, 124
    grades of 128
    moderate 128
    severe 128
Mandible 66
Mantoux test 454
Marasmus 34f
Marfan syndrome 58, 225, 276
Mass
    abdominal 187b
    lesions 397
        around eyelids 398t
Massive ascites 192f
Massive edema over face 84f
Mastitis 102
Mastoid abscess 419f
Maternal endocrine disorders, history of 338
Maternal rubella 419
McCune-Albright syndrome 77
Measles 419
    mumps, rubella 454
    rubella vaccine 9
    vaccine 275
Measuring digital clubbing 200, 201f
Mechanical ventilation 425
Meckel's diverticulum 167
Median cubital vein 456
Mediastinal structures 472

Megaloblastic anemia 77
Melena 158, 167
Membrane's temperature 39
Memory 277, 279
Meningeal irritation, signs of 277, 324
Meningism 324
Meningitis 287, 292, 324
    acute bacterial 19
Meningococcal meningitis 275
Meningococcal vaccine 275
Meningococcemia 71*f*
Meningoencephalitis 269, 271
Menke's syndrome 275
Mercury clinical thermometer 38*f*
Mesomelia 72
Metabolic acidosis 44
Metabolic disorder 155, 360
Metabolism, inborn error of 44, 140, 163, 266, 268, 271
Metastasis 435
Microcephaly 332
Micromelia 72
Micronutrient deficiency
    clinical signs of 85
    diagnostic signs of 85*b*
Microphthalmos 53
Microtia 419, 421*f*
Micturition disturbances 281
Middle ear infection 292
Midline neck swelling 68*f*
Mid-upper arm circumference 117, 118
Migraine 269
    abdominal 158
Migratory arthritis 362
Milia 347, 349, 381
Miliaria rubra 376*f*
Milk ejection reflex 96, 97*f*
Milk production reflex 96*f*
Mitochondrial disorders 331
Mitral regurgitation 41, 229, 263
Mitral stenosis 263
Mitral valve prolapse 223, 224
Mongolian spots 349
Monocular vision assessment 411*f*
Monoparesis 273
Moro reflex 152*f*, 352, 353, 355*f*
    asymmetric 353
    exaggerated 353
    incomplete 352
    reverse 353
Morphine 339
Motor deficits 273

Motor system 277
    examination 298
        components of 298*b*
Mouth 62
Movement disorders 273
Mucopolysaccharidosis 36*f*, 54*f*, 165
Mucosa 431
Multinucleate giant cells 392
Mumps 222, 419
Murmurs 255*b*
    conduction of 256*b*
    radiation of 256*b*
Muscle 335
    bulk 298, 304
    nutrition 304
    power 277, 298, 306
        grades of 306*t*
    tone 277, 298, 299, 301, 345
    wasting 304
    weakness 273
Muscular disorders 155
Muscular dystrophy 329
Musculoskeletal pain 198
Musculoskeletal system 356, 362
    examination 363
    pediatric regional examination of 369
Myasthenia gravis 55*f*, 292
Mycobacterial lymphadenitis 435
Mycobacterium tuberculosis 478
Myocarditis 264
Myoclonus 313
Myoepithelium 96
Myoglobinuria 169
Myopathy 273, 329

N

Nail 70, 74, 241, 387
    clubbing of 387
    pitting 387
Narcotic withdrawal syndrome 339
Nasal
    blocks 270
    cavity 61, 430
    discharge 270
    fractures 429, 478
    intubation 429
    itching 429
    necrosis 480
    obstruction 425, 429
    patency 431
    polyps 427
    regurgitation 296
    septum 430

Nasogastric tube 429, 478, 479f
Nasolacrimal system 415
Nasopharyngeal carcinoma 435
Nasopharynx 426f
Nausea 270
Neck 67
    masses, causes of 435t
    rigidity 324
    stiffness 324
    swellings 435
    vessels 259
Necrotizing enterocolitis 342, 467
Neonatal
    death 337
    disorder 339, 339t
    hepatitis 482
    hyperbilirubinemia 295
    intensive care unit 2, 341, 425
    jaundice, history of 341
    reflexes 150t, 352, 353t, 355f
    septicemia, diagnosis of 478
Nephrotic syndrome 14, 18, 77
Nerve roots 335
    involvement 273
Nervous system 265
Neuroblastoma 329, 331
Neurocutaneous syndromes 268
Neurodegenerative disorders 155, 296, 419
Neurofibroma 435
Neurofibromatosis 268
Neurologic system 351
Neurological deficits 241
Neurological lesion, localization of 333
Neutral thermal environment 344
Nevus
    achromicus 383
    sebaceous 381
        over scalp 384f
Niacin 86
Niemann-Pick disease 182, 286
Nikolsky sign 391
Nipples, inverted 99
Nitrofurantoin 339
Nodular rash 365
Nodules 70, 374, 433
    over scalp 376f
Nonaccidental injuries 416
Nonarticular pain 370
Non-Hodgkins tumor 435
Nonpitting edema 35f
Noonan syndrome 35f, 55, 225

Nose 33
    examination of 61, 417, 429
    foreign body in 427f
    method of examination of 430f
Nuchal rigidity 324, 325f
Nutrient gap 108
Nutrition 33, 109
    assessment of 118
Nutritional status 123t
    assessment of 124
Nystagmus 327, 328

O

Obesity 27, 281
Obstruction 434f
Obstructive lung diseases 199
Occipital lobe dysfunction 281
Ocular media opacities 415
Ocular movements 402
Oculocephalic reflex 287
Oculocephalic response 445, 448
Oculomotor nerve
    Edinger-Westphal nucleus 285
    palsy, manifestations of 287b
Oculovestibular response 445, 448
Oilgoarticular juvenile arthritis 371
Olfactory nerve 282
Oligoarticular idiopathic arthritis 372
Ophthalmoplegia 272
Ophthalmoscope 32f, 286f, 344
Opisthotonus 299f
Opponens pollicis 310
Optic nerve 283
    atrophy 286
    examination of 283b
    head 405
    pathway of 283
Optic neuritis 272
Optimum nutrition 90
Oral cavity 169
    examination of 62, 435
Oral mucosa 381
Oral poliovirus vaccines 9, 23
Orchidometer 75f
Organophosphorus poisoning 486
Oropharynx, examination of 435
Ortolani's tests 357
Oscillometer method 46, 233, 235
Osler nodes 241, 259
Ossicular disruption 419
Ossicular malformations 419
Otitis externa 418

Otitis media 418, 419
   acute 418
      acute suppurative 417, 423, 423f
      chronic suppurative 417, 423, 424f
Otoscope 32f
Otoscopic examination 61
Ototoxic drug 295, 425
Oxycephaly 51, 331
Oxygen saturation 48
Oxytocin 96, 339
   reflex 97f

P

Pain 364, 417, 493
   abdominal 157, 158, 161t
   character of 160
   esophagitic 198
   nature of 160
   radiation of 160
   site of 158
   types of 160
Palate 64, 435
Pallor 77, 241, 348, 349
Palmar erythema 171, 241
Palmar grasp 150, 353, 354, 355f
Palpable heart sounds 243
Palpable lymph nodes 79
Palpatory method 45, 234
Pansystolic murmur 257, 258
Papilledema 286, 406f
Papillitis 407
Papillomatosis 433, 434
Papular urticaria 70, 389
Papule 374
Paracentesis, abdominal 481
Parachute reflex 356
Paralytic ileus 478
Paraparesis 273
Paraphimosis 76f
Paraplegia 273
Parasternal heave, palpation for 245f
Parental diarrhea 164
Paresthesia 273
Paronychia 387
Parotid gland 292
Parotid swelling 171
Paroxysmal hypertension 331
Patau syndrome 225
Patch 374
Patellar clonus, elicitation of 323f
Patellar jerk 322

Patent ductus arteriosus 41, 221, 222, 260, 342
Pathologic signs 349
Pectus carinatum 206f
Pectus excavatum 207f
Pedal edema 236f
   demonstration of 179f
Pediatric
   intensive care unit 2
   ophthalmologist 415t
Pedigree chart 26f
   typical 25f
Pellagra 381
Pendred syndrome 419
Pendular knee jerk 327, 328
Pentavalent vaccine, doses of 9
Perforated tympanic membrane 424f
Periarticular pain 370
Pericardial friction rub 255
Pericardial knock 255
Pericardial pain 198
Pericardial rub 260
Pericardiocentesis 496
   sites for 497f
Pericarditis 223, 224
   constrictive 233
Perinatal asphyxia 295
Perinatal birth asphyxia 23
Perinatal mortality rate 337
Perinatal period 221, 337
Perinephric hematoma 496
Periodic breathing 43
Perioral dermatitis 381
Peripheral cyanosis 79
Peripheral intravenous access 456
Peripheral nerves 335
Peripheral nervous system 372
   diseases of 486
Peripheral pulsations 40, 227, 230
Peripheral pulses 365
Peritoneal dialysis 490, 492f
Peritonitis 482, 491, 493
Peritonsillar abscess 431
Pernicious anemia 387
Persistent diarrhea 163
Persistent neonatal jaundice 36f
Pertussis 10, 163
Petechial spots 16, 71f
Pethidine 339
Pharyngeal reflex 446, 447
Pharynx 66
Phenobarbitone 339, 339f
Phenytoin 222, 329, 339, 387

Index

Pheochromocytoma 331
Philtrum 63
Photophobia 270
Phrynoderma 73, 73*f*, 381, 383*f*
Pigeon chest 206*f*
Pinna 420
   congenital deformities of 422*b*
Pityriasis alba 381, 383, 389
   over face 385*f*
Pityriasis rosea 379*f*, 381
Pityriasis rubra pilaris 381
Pityriasis versicolor 375*f*, 381, 383, 391
Plantar grasp 353, 354, 355*f*
Plantar reflex 319
   elicitation of 318*f*
Plaque 374
Platynychia 74, 75*f*
Plethora 349
Pleural effusion 208, 210, 218
Pleural rub 216
Pleuritic pain 198
Pleuroperitoneal communication 491
Pneumococcal meningitis 275
Pneumococcal vaccine 275
Pneumonia 164
Pneumoperitoneum 482
Pneumothorax 208, 210, 211, 219, 486, 489, 498
Poliomyelitis 275, 297, 301, 486
Polycystic ovarian disease 77, 68*f*
Polycythemia 348
Polydactyly 69*f*
Polymorphous light eruption 381
Pompe disease 64, 226
Ponderal index 122
Popliteal angle 302, 303
Porphyria 169
   cutanea tarda 387
Portal hypertension, severe 482
Portal vein, thrombosis of 467
Positron emission tomography 449
Postextubation stridor 489
Postinflammatory hypopigmentation 383
Postlumbar puncture 269
Postnasal drip 195
Postparacentesis shock 482
Postpartum psychosis 103
Poststernotomy, post-thoracotomy of 242
Post-tussive vomiting 163
Postural hypotension 331
Post-viral cerebellitis 329
Potassium hydroxide 391, 393*f*
Preauricular sinus 422*f*

Preauricular skin tags 60*f*
Precordial pulsations 243, 259
Precordium 242, 259
Preferential looking test 408
Premature birth 419
Prepregnancy health status 338
Primaquine 339
Primary microcephaly, causes of 50*t*
Primitive reflexes, evaluate for 147
Progesterone 222
Prolactin reflex 95, 96*f*
Prone position 132
Propranolol 339
Protection of Children from Sexual Offences Act 438
Protein
   energy malnutrition 165, 275
   requirements 28*t*
Proximal finger 41
Pruritis 390
Pseudobulbar palsy 296
Pseudostrabismus 401*f*
Psoriasis 381
   vulgaris 376*f*, 381, 383*f*
Ptosis 55*f*
Puddle sign 189, 189*f*
Puffy face 84*f*
Pulmonary artery 223
   hypertension, severe 237
Pulmonary aspiration 480
Pulmonary edema 491
   unilateral 486
Pulmonary stenosis 222, 254, 262
Pulmonary valve obstruction 223, 224
Pulse 40, 227
   abnormal 231
   apex deficit 229
   examination of 40
   oximetry, advantages of 49
   rate 40, 226, 228
   volume 365
Pulsus
   alternans 231
   bigeminus 231
   paradoxus 42, 233
      causes of 233*b*
   tardus 232
   trigeminy 231
Punctuate erythematous spots 331
Pupil 58
   examination of 446
   white reflex in 397
Pupillary examination 399, 402

Pupillary light reflex 449
Pupillary reaction 283, 285
Pure tone audiogram 425
Purpuric spots 16
Pustule 375
Pyloric stenosis, congenital hypertrophic 162
Pyoderma 347
Pyridoxine 86

Q

Q-T syndrome, prolonged 224
Quinine 339

R

Radial artery 469*f*
    catheterization 468
    method of palpation of 230*f*
Radiofemoral delay 41, 229
Radioradial delay 41, 229
Raised intracranial pressure 19, 52, 163, 268, 269, 273-275
Raised jugular venous pressure, causes of 238*b*
Rao's index 122
Rattling sounds 214
Reactive arthritis 362, 365, 366
Rectal temperature 39
Red eye 397
Red flag signs 34*b*
Red reflex 359*f*
    examination 399, 403*f*
    test 359*t*, 398
Red-colored urine, causes of 169*b*
Reflex 277, 319, 321, 322
    abdominal 317*f*, 319
    examination of 316
    response 345
    superficial 277, 317, 319*t*
Refractive errors 269, 359
Regional lymphadenopathy 388
Renal biopsy 494
Renal bruit 192
Renal failure, acute 44
Renal infarction 467
Renal lump 186, 187*b*
Renal tenderness 186
Respiration 42, 200, 345
    depth of 44
    muscle of 44
    rate 42, 169
    types of 43

Respiratory diseases 216
Respiratory distress syndrome 16, 342
Respiratory signs 197*t*
Respiratory sounds 44*t*
Respiratory system 194, 350, 372
Responsive feeding 109
Retina 402, 407
Retinal detachment 272, 397
Retinal hemorrhage 286
Retinal infarcts 286
Retinal vessels 405
Retinoblastoma 359
Retinopathy of prematurity 342, 416, 416
Retractions 197, 199
Retropharyngeal abscess 433*f*, 434
Rheumatic activity, signs of 259
Rheumatic chorea 224, 273, 301
Rheumatic fever 18, 241*f*
Rheumatoid arthritis, juvenile 365
Rheumatologic disorder 369
Rhinitis 429
    allergic 202
Rhinorrhea 429
Rhizomelia 72
Rhonchus 214
Rhythm 40, 228
Rickets 86, 165, 332
Rifampicin 339
Right bundle branch block 253
Right cardiac border 248
Right heart failure 238
Right hypochondrium 158
Right iliac fossa 160
Right kidney 184
Rigid direct laryngoscopy 436
Rinne's test 294, 294*f*
Risus sardonicus 54*f*
Rocker-bottom feet 69*f*
Romberg sign 327, 328*f*
    positive 327
Root pain 273
Rooting reflex 150, 353, 354
Roth's spots 241, 407
Rubella 58, 222, 419
    congenital 295
    syndrome 226

S

Salbutamol 312
Salicylates 339, 491
Salivary gland disorders 435
Salmon patches 347

Index

Sarcoidosis 372
Scabies 70, 381, 388
Scale 378, 379f
Scalp 381
    hairs, loss of 389
    veins of 456
Scaphocephaly 51, 331
Scaphoid abdomen 173
Scar 378
Scarf sign 146, 302, 304
Schönlein purpura 158
Schwabach test 294
Scissoring gait 330
Sclera 57
Sclerosis 379
Scrotal swelling 158, 168
Scurvy 86, 364
Seborrheic dermatitis 381, 389
Secondary microcephaly, causes of 50t
Sedation 451
Seizures 265, 266, 268b, 339, 350
    causes of 266b, 268b
    history of 341
    types of 267
Select appropriate growth chart 124
Sensorimotor system 415
Sensorineural hearing loss 419
Sensory
    extinction 316
    loss 314t
    system 277, 313
Sepsis 425
Septate hyphae 393f
Septic arthritis 362, 365, 372
Septicemia 342
Shakir tape 118
Shock 77
Sickle cell disease 185, 365
Simian crease 72f, 89
Single photon emission computed tomography 449
Sinus
    bradycardia 40
    tachycardia 40
Sinusitis 269, 270
Sjögren's syndrome 59
Skeletal deformities 259
Skeletal system, examination of 367b
Skin 16, 34, 240, 347
    appendages of 386
    elasticity 47
    examination of 373, 386
    lesions 73b
    pain 198
    scars 174
    striae 173
    tests 454
    turgor 47, 73
Skinfold thickness 120
Skull 277
    abnormal shapes of 51b, 331b
    examination of 331
    frontal bossing of 52
Sleep disturbances 266, 281
Slipped upper femoral epiphyses 18
Smell, loss of 281
Snake bite 271
Snellen chart 408, 412f
Soft palate 436
Sore nipple 102
Sore throat 194, 223
Spasmodic cough 195
Spastic gait 330
Spatula 344
Speech 131, 277, 280
    functional disorder of 280
Spherocytosis 185
Sphygmomanometer method 45, 233
Spider angioma 171
Spinal accessory nerve 297
Spinal cord 273
    involvement 273
Spinal nerve roots 321, 322
Spinal shock, features of 335
Spine 277, 357
    examination of 333
Spinomuscular atrophy 298, 330
Spleen 187b
    bimanual palpation of 183f
    differentiation of 183
    palpation of 181
    size of 184
Splenomegaly 240
    causes of 185b
Splinter hemorrhage 241
Spondyloarthropathy, juvenile 362
Stahl's ear 422
Staphylococcal scalded skin syndrome 70f, 381
Staphylococcus aureus 388
Status epilepticus 271
Stepping reflex 151, 353, 355f
Stereognosis 315, 316
Sternomastoid tumor 347, 435
Sternum 470
Steroid toxicity 84f

Stethoscope 32f, 250, 343
Stevens-Johnson syndrome 381, 391
Stool, consistency and color of 163
Strawberry tongues, white and red 64f
Streptomycin 339
Stress 15
Stridor 197, 296, 433
    causes of 434t
    types of 434f
Stroke, cerebrovascular 224, 271
Stupor 278
Sturge-Weber syndrome 268
Subconjunctival hemorrhage 57f, 347f
Subcutaneous nodules 241f, 259
Subglottic stenosis 434
Subhyaloid hemorrhage 407
Sublingual temperature 39
Subscapular skinfold 120
Sucking reflex 150, 353-355
Sun-setting sign 51f
Superficial veins, abdominal 189f
Suprapubic bladder
    aspiration 489
    puncture technique 490f
Suprapubic region 160
Suprasternal pulsations 247
    palpation of 247f
Swollen breast 102
Sydenham chorea 312
Sydney crease 89
Symmetrical edema 128
Symmetrical tonic neck reflex 354
Syncope 223, 224
Syndactyly 69f
Synovial fluid 370
Syphilis, congenital 70, 347, 391
Systemic lupus erythematosus 17, 18, 222, 362, 365, 366, 387, 397
Systolic murmur 256
    grading of 256t

T

Tache cerebrale 331
Tachycardia 77, 228, 228t, 350
Tachypnea 44, 196, 197, 199, 345, 350
    cut-off for 43t
Tactile vocal fremitus 217
Takayasu arteritis 228
Tandem walking 327
Taurine 98
Tay-Sachs disease 59f, 286
Tears 59

Telangiectasia 380
Telemedicine, concept of 439
Teller acuity chart 408, 409f
Temporal artery thermometer 39
Temporal lobe dysfunctions 281
Tenderness 177, 430
    abdominal 340
Tenesmus 164
Tense
    abdomen 177
    ascites 482
Tension 41, 229
    headache 269
Teratoma 77, 435
Tetanus 10, 54f, 299f, 486
    toxoid vaccination 338
    maternal status of 342
Tetralogy of Fallot 254, 261
Thalassemia 182, 185, 339
Therapeutic hypothermia, use of 445
Therapeutic substances,
    administration of 478
Thermometers 38f
Thoracocentesis 483, 484f
Thrills 243, 247
Throat
    examination of 417
    pain 431
Thrombocytopenia 339, 391, 429
Thromboembolism 467
Thrombophlebitis 462
Thrombosis 493
Thyroglossal duct cyst 435
Thyroid
    disorders 331
    tumors vascular malformations 435
Tibia 470
Tics 312
Tinea
    capitis 381, 390
    corporis 381, 390
    cruris 381
    versicolor 390
Tinnitus 420
Toe walking 330
Tongue 64, 434, 436
    fasciculation of 298
    spatula 31, 32f
Tonic neck reflex 353, 355f
Tonsillitis, acute 432f
Tonsils 66, 436
Tooth 56f, 66, 435
Topognosis 316

TORCH infection 339, 391
Toxic epidermal necrolysis 391
Toxic look 16
Toxins 271
Tracheal position 208
Tracheal reflex 446, 447
Tracheoesophageal fistula 21
Trachoma 57
Traction response 351, 352*f*
Transient pustular melanosis 347
Transient tone abnormalities 155
Transillumination test 332
Trauma 269, 297, 365, 419
Traumatic cataract 397
Traumatic ulcer 65*f*
Treacher Collins syndrome 55, 387
Tremors 312, 328
Triceps
    muscles 307*f*
    skinfold 120
Trichotillomania 387
Tricuspid
    atresia 262
    stenosis 238
Trigeminal nerve 288
Trigonocephaly 331
Trisomy 13 225
Trisomy 18 225
Trisomy 21 88, 222, 225, 337
Trivandrum development screening
    chart 140*f*
Trochlear nerve palsy 288
Truncal ataxia 326
Trunk 381
Tuberculoma 268
Tuberculosis 342, 371
Tuberculous arthritis 362
Tuberculous meningitis 268, 269, 271,
    273, 297, 299*f*
Tuberous sclerosis 268, 387
Tumors 428
    benign 435
Tuning fork test 424
Turner syndrome 55, 83, 225, 276
Turricephaly 51
Tympanic membrane 423
    appearance of 423*t*
    malformations 419
    perforation 419
Tympanic thermometer 39
Tympanometry 425
Tzanck cells 393
Tzanck smear 391

U

Ulcer 378
Umbilical artery catheterization 467
Umbilical catheter 466*f*
Umbilical cord 466*f*
Umbilical hernia 36*f*, 174, 175*f*
Umbilical vein 466*f*
    catheterization 465
Umbilicus 173, 174
Unconsciousness 274, 278
Undescended testes 76*f*
Unilateral facial palsy, causes of 292
Upper gastrointestinal tract bleeding,
    assessment of 478
Upper limb 461
Upper motor neuron 291, 333, 333*t*
    facial palsy
        bilateral 292
        unilateral 292
    lesion 291
Upper respiratory tract infection 196, 270
    history of 417
Uremia 163
Uremic encephalopathy 271
Urinary bladder 187
    perforation of 482
Urinary tract infection 163
Urticaria 377, 378*f*
Usher syndrome 419
Uvula 436

V

Vague psychiatric disorders 281
Vagus nerve 295, 296
Valproic acid 339
Varicella 454
    vaccine 275
Vascular thrombosis 268
Vasculitis 362
Vasovagal reactions 498
Veins, superficial 173, 456
Vena cava obstruction, superior 238
Ventricular septal defect 222, 226, 260
Ventricular tap 476
Ventricular tapping 477*f*
Ventriculitis 477
Vertigo, benign paroxysmal
    positional 420
Very low birth weight 337
Vesicle 374
Vesicular breathing 213

Vessel
    perforation 467
    wall, condition of 230
Vestibular function 293
Vestibulocochlear nerve 293
Vestibulo-ocular reflex 446
Vibration sensation 315
Viral arthritis 362
Viral infection 163, 195, 221, 372, 391
Viral meningoencephalitis 268
Vision 59, 155
    assessment 409*f*
    disturbances 266, 272
    field of 283
    screening method 407, 408
Visual acuity 283, 415
Visual aura 270
Visual behavior 415
Visual field defects 272
Visual hallucination 281
Visual milestones 413
Vitamin
    A 105
        deficiency 57, 59, 73*f*, 85, 86*b*
    B
        complex 105
        deficiency 85
    B_1 85, 105
    B_{11} 105
    B_{12} 86, 105
    B_2 85, 105
    B_3 105
    B_6 105
    C 105
        deficiency 86
    D 105
        deficiency 86
            signs of 62
    E 105
        deficiency 86
    K 339
        dependent bleeding
            manifestations 339

Vitiligo 375*f*, 381, 382*f*, 384
Vocal cord
    disorder of 280
    paralysis 434
Vocal resonance 215
Voice
    hoarseness of 296, 433
    nasal quality of 296
Vomiting 158, 161, 162, 266, 270, 273, 274, 342
    causes of 163*t*
    contents of 162
    types of 162
von Willebrand disease 429

W

Waddling gait 330
Waist-hip ratio 122
Water hammer pulse 42, 231, 232*f*
Watering eye 59
Weber test 294, 295*f*
Weighing machine 31, 32*f*
Weight loss 342
Weight-for-age 122, 126*f*
Weight-for-height 128
Wernicke's aphasia 280
Wheeze 197, 214
William syndrome 87, 226
Wilms tumor 168
Wilson disease 18, 58*f*, 275
Wood's lamp 383
World Breastfeeding Week 91
World Health Organization 395, 443
Wound infections 462

Y

Yellow sclera 57
Yellow white papules 347

Z

Ziehl-Neelsen stain 485
Zinc deficiency 389